'QUICK REVIEW OF OPHTHALMOLOGY'

{Jiffy Ophthalmology Revision in Detail by Exclusive Notes}

VINAY VIJAY BURADKAR

Contains standard, systematic answers for the most important and frequently asked topics in various Undergraduate Professional Exams.

"The only thing worse than being blind is having sight but no vision".

First Edition : 2018

ISBN : 978-93-83794-03-4

Published by :

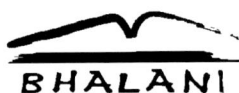

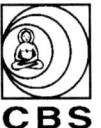

Rajesh Bhalani for
Bhalani Publishers
1201, Avanti-Neelkanth Kingdom,
Vidyavihar (West), Mumbai - 400 0086.
Mobile : 098672 14519
E-mail : bhalanipublishers@gmail.com

Satish Kumar Jain for
CBS PUBLISHERS & DISTRIBUTORS PVT. LTD.
4819/XI Prahlad Street,
24 Ansari Road, Daryaganj,
New Delhi - 110002, India.
Ph.: 011-23289259, 23266861/67 Fax: 23243014
Email : delhi@cbspd.com/cbspubs@airtelmail.in
Website: www.cbspd.com

Corporate Office: 204 FIE, Industrial Area,
Patparganj, Delhi - 110092
Ph.: 49344934, Fax: 49344935
Email : publishing@cbspd.com

Dedicated to :

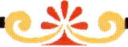 My parents Mr. Vijay & Mrs. Vidhya Buradkar, My brother Vineet for their love and affection.

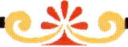 My late grandfathers Ghularamji, Bhagawanji, Nilkanthrao Buradkar & late grandmothers Indirabai, Subhadrabai and Shevantabai Buradkar.

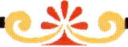 Department of Ophthalmology, SMBT IMSRC Nashik for their guidance, insights and for teaching the core of Ophthalmology.

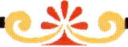 Dr. Ashok Balaji Bhukte, Consulting General Surgeon, Sushrut Hospital Chandrapur for his guidance and support right from childhood.

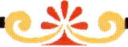 Dr. Nitin Baste, Associate Professor of Surgery, SMBT IMSRC, Nashik for his unstinted support.

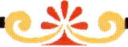 SMBT Trust, SMBT Family, My batchmates, Juniors for their constant love and encouragement.

Preface

Present book has been written with primary objective of undergraduate learning, to provide them state of the art information but in a concise and simplified format which will help UG students to refresh their knowledge, speed up their revision of the important topics before the exam and attempt the paper in systematic format. This is not a text book of Ophthalmology but is based on the most important and frequently asked topics in Undergraduate Professional Exams. This book covers almost all the important topics of Ophthalmology in notes format that an Undergraduate Student must know at IIIrd Minor level.

Although many excellent textbooks on Ophthalmology have been published during past few decades, most of them concentrate on the training at post graduate level and are often considered too advanced for Undergraduates. In this book, I have tried to include all those most important topics asked in Undergraduate Professional Exams after going through past 28 years question papers thoroughly. This has helped me to restrict the size of the book to a manageable level so that the Undergraduate medical students may find it handy and useful.

There is no better way to learn Ophthalmology than working sincerely in the wards and attending the clinics. There is no shortcut to this approach. The principal object of this book is to help an Undergraduate Medical Student in his/her hard work and is not intended to be a substitute to ward-work.

This book should not be considered as an alternative to the best standard text books available out there in the market, but should be used as an adjuvant to speed up the learning process and to revise the subject speedily without missing the important points.

I hope the book will be received well by the Ophthalmology fraternity. Despite the best efforts, some mistakes might have crept in, which I request all the readers to kindly bring to my notice. Your suggestions, appreciation and criticism regarding the book will help in improving its quality and are most welcome.

Vinay Vijay Buradkar
(vinayburadkar007@gmail.com)

Acknowledgement

The foundation of a career is laid down in the school days and hence I would like to begin with thanking all my teachers in MCCHS, Chandrapur and Allen Career Institute, Kota. A special thanks to my father Mr. Vijay G. Buradkar for shaping my Mathematics, Science, Handwriting in my initial days of school and junior college.

I would like to thank and extend fathomless gratitude to Dr. Shubhangi Sathe (HOD, Department of Ophthalmology, SMBT IMSRC, Nashik), Dr. Shubhangi Pimprikar, Dr. Rucha Gulhane, Dr. Gopal Sir and other faculty members of Ophthalmology at SMBT IMSRC, Nashik for their guidance, immense support and their beautiful teaching methodology while in MBBS IIIrd year. I would also like to thank our Dean at SMBT IMSRC, Nashik Dr. Vidya Paranjape Mam, Dr. Anil Mane (HOD, Department of Medicine), Dr. Meenal Mohgaonkar (HOD, Department of Radiology), all the members of SMBT Family and Trust for playing a substantial role in framing the career of the students at SMBT IMSRC, Nashik. Special thanks to Dr. Nitin Baste, Associate Professor, Department of Surgery, SMBT IMSRC Nashik not only for his constant support but also for the art he taught me, to remain grounded always in life.

I am deeply indebted to all my teachers, professors from all other departments at SMBT IMSRC, Nashik for the help and support that I have received during the first three years of M.B.B.S. I take the opportunity to extend my heartfelt reverence to Dr. Ranjan Kumar Patel, the author of Conceptual Review of Pharmacology and Dr. Deepak Marwah, the author of Complete Review of Medicine for their guidance and encouragement while preparing this book. I am grateful to Miss. Pruthvi Joshi who diligently kept me motivated while preparing the manuscript of this book.

I would like to thank Miss. Asmita Suryavanshi (SMBT IMSRC Nashik), Mr. Saket Mundhada (Grant Medical College and Sir JJ group of Hospitals, Mumbai) for helping me while preparing the general format and image section of this book. Special thanks to Dr. Piyush Gadegone (Senior Resident, Department of Orthopaedics, LTMC & Sion Hospital Mumbai), Dr. Sushrut Bhukte (General Surgeon, Sushrut Hospital Chandrapur), Mr. Vishwanath Jatkar (GMC Nagpur), Mr. Shubham Bodhe (GMC Nagpur), Mr. Abhishek Pethe (MIMER Pune), Miss. Shubhali Salunkhe (MIMER Pune), Mr. Nirzar Burande (VSPM Lata Mangeshkar Hospital, Nagpur) for their constant support and encouragement throughout. I would also like to thank all my relatives for their unconditional love.

I would like to thank all my batchmates (SMBTians 2014 batch), Juniors for their immense love and support ; Kalpak Garmade, Shadman Shaikh, Shaibaz Sawant, Shivam Chaturvedi, Imtiyaz Ansari, Suyash Gunjal, Yash Jakhotia, Shreay Gaikwad, Ajeet Gupta, Digvijay Mote, Dinesh Pawar, Umang Yagyi, Pratik Gajbe, Prathamesh Patil, Rohit Gupta, Kapil Honrao Patil, Shrikant Pulkantwar, Vaibhav Gange, Saurabh Patil, Sohail Shaikh, Madhav Khandare, Henil Ahir, Chirag Godara, Siddharth Sanap, Abhishek Raut, Sachin Sanap, Ashish Totawar, Arif Qureshi, Arshad Dukka, Nazar, Saquib, Suwaid, Talib, Sejol Kashyap, Sakshi Gawande, Sayali Darunde, Gargi Ambade, Kadambari Ubarhande, Tejaswini Chavan, Mary Ajayan, Sharyu Gaoture, Utsavi Modi.

Finally I wish to place on record my appreciation for **Mr. Rajesh Bhalani** and **CBS Publishers** and **Sunita Tikare** for speedy publication of the book and for the prompt, skilled publication work. In conclusion, I would like to admit that only few names appear in this acknowledgement, many too much unsung, have also contributed in one way or the other.

Vinay Vijay Buradkar
Final Year M.B.B.S. Student,
SMBT IMSRC,
Nashik.

Contents

Dedication iii

Preface v

Acknowledgement vii

Contents ix

Annexure .... x-xiv

SECTION – I

1.   Conjunctiva 1-15

2.   Cornea 16-31

3.   Lens 32-51

4.   Glaucoma 52-64

5.   Uveal Tract 65-71

6.   Lacrimal Apparatus 72-77

7.   Retina 78-93

8.   Neuro-Ophthalmology 94-102

9.   Ocular Motility 103-108

10. Sclera 109-113

11. Eyelids 114-124

12. Ocular Injuries 125-131

13. Errors of Refraction & Accommodation 132-141

14. Ocular Pharmacology 142-149

15. Darkroom Procedures 150-155

16. Community Ophthalmology 156-159

17. Systemic Ophthalmology 160-164

SECTION – II — INSTRUMENTS & LENS

18. Ophthalmic Instruments 165-180

19. Ophthalmic Lens 181-185

Annexure

□ DIFFERENTIAL DIAGNOSIS OF RED EYE :

I) Conjunctiva :
1) Conjunctivitis.
2) Subconjunctival hemorrhage
3) Trauma
4) Dry eye

II) Cornea :
1) Corneal ulcer
2) Keratitis
3) Foreign body
4) Laceration
5) Abrasion
6) Contact lens wear

III) Sclera :
1) Episcleritis
2) Scleritis

IV) Iris & ciliary body :
1) Iridocyclitis
2) Iritis

V) Anterior chamber :
1) Acute angle closure glaucoma
2) Hyphaema

VI) Eyelid :
1) Entropion
2) Ectropion
3) Trichiasis

VII) Orbit :
1) Orbital cellulitis

VIII) Lacrimal apparatus :
1) Acute dacryocystitis

◨ LOSS OF VISION (LOV) :

☞ It may be sudden or gradual loss of vision.

A) Sudden LOV causes :

i) Painful

1) Acute congestive (angle closure) Glaucoma
2) Acute Iridocyclitis (Uveitis)
3) Endophthalmitis
4) Optic neuritis

ii) Painless

1) Central Retinal Artery occlusion (CRAO)
2) Central Retinal Vein Occlusion (CRVO)
3) Macular edema
4) Retinal Detachment
5) 'Exudative' Age related macular degeneration (ARMD)
6) Vitreous & Retinal hemorrhage
7) Subluxation/Dislocation of lens.
8) Methyl alcohol amblyopia

B) Gradual LOV Causes :

i) Painful

1) Corneal ulcer
2) Chronic simple Glaucoma
3) Chronic Iridocyclitis

ii) Painless

1) Cataract (Senile & developmental)
2) 'Dry type' age related macular degeneration (ARMD)
3) Diabetic Retinopathy (Uveitis)
4) Refractive errors
5) Progressive pterygium
6) Corneal dystrophy
7) Corneal degeneration
8) Chorioretinal degeneration
9) Presbyopia

❑ EPIPHORA CAUSES :

Mechanical obstruction	Lacrimal Pump failure
1) Congenital absence or occlusion of puncta	1) Lower lid laxity
2) Congenital dacryocystitis	2) Bell's palsy (weakness of orbicularis oculi)
3) Chronic/Acute dacryocystitis	3) Ectropion
4) Canaliculitis	
5) Canaliculi obstruction	
6) Neoplasms of lacrimal sac	

◘ DIFFERENTIAL DIAGNOSIS OF WHITE PUPILLARY REFLEX : (LEUKOCORIA)

I) Hereditary :
1) Norrie's disease.
2) Congenital Retinoschisis.
3) Dominant exudative vitreoretinopathy.

II) Developmental :
1) PHPV (Persistent hyperplastic primary vitreous).
2) Congenital Cataract.
3) Coloboma.
4) Congenital corneal opacity.
5) Myelinated nerve fibres.
6) Morning glory syndrome.
7) Congenital Retinal fold.

III) Inflammatory :
1) Congenital CMV Retinitis.
2) HSV Retinitis.
3) Toxoplasmosis.
4) Toxocariasis
5) Uveoretinitis
6) Endophthalmitis
7) Orbital cellulitis

IV) Tumors :
1) Retinal Astrocytic Hamartoma.
2) Glioneuroma.
3) Lymphoma, Leukemia, Hemangioma.

V) Miscellaneous :
1) Coat's Disease.
2) Retinopathy of Prematurity. (Retrolental fibroplasia).

◘ DIFFERENTIAL DIAGNOSIS OF NODULE AT LIMBUS :

I) Congenital :
1) Dermoid
2) Dermolipoma
3) Naevi

II) Inflammatory :
1) Episcleritis
2) Scleritis

III) Allergy :
1) Phlycten
2) Vernal Catarrh
3) Ophthalmia nodosa

IV) Vascular :
1) Hemangioma

V) Traumatic :
1) Granuloma
2) Implantation cyst
3) Iris prolapse covered by conjunctiva

VI) Degenerative :
1) Pinguecula
2) Cystic pterygium

VII) Nutritional :
1) Bitot's spot

VIII) Neoplastic :
1) Papilloma
2) Squamous cell carcinoma
3) Primary melanoma
4) Intraepithelial epithelioma

IX) Miscellaneous :
1) Intercalary or ciliary staphyloma
2) Retention cyst
3) Parasitic cyst
4) Filtering bleb

SECTION

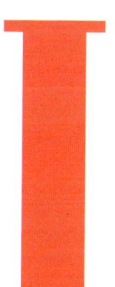

Chapter

1

Conjunctiva

Most Important (Must Read Topics)	Elective Topics
1) Ophthalmia Neonatorum	1) Conjunctivitis Classification
2) Trachoma	2) Phlyctenular keratoconjunctivitis
3) Vernal keratoconjunctivitis	3) Epidemic keratoconjunctivitis
4) Pterygium	4) Follicular conjunctivitis
5) Differential diagnosis of nodule at limbus	
6) Pterygium vs Pseudopterygium	

◘ CONJUNCTIVITIS & CLASSIFICATION :

✍ Conjunctivitis is inflammation of conjunctiva associated with watery, mucoid, mucopurulent or purulent discharge.

✍ Also called as "Pink Eye" or "Madras Eye".

A) Infective conjunctivitis :

1) Bacterial :
- ➢ Acute bacterial conjunctivitis.
- ➢ Hyperacute bacterial conjunctivitis.
- ➢ Chronic bacterial conjunctivitis.
- ➢ Angular bacterial conjunctivitis.

2) Chlamydial :
- ➢ Trachoma.
- ➢ Neonatal chlamydial conjunctivitis.
- ➢ Adult inclusion conjunctivitis.

3) Viral :
- ➢ Adenovirus conjunctivitis.
- ➢ Enterovirus conjunctivitis.
- ➢ Herpes simplex conjunctivitis.
- ➢ Molluscum contagiosum conjunctivitis.

4) Ophthalmia neonatorum.

5) Granulomatous conjunctivitis :
- ➢ Parinaud oculoglandular syndrome.

B) Allergic conjunctivitis :

1) Simplex allergic conjunctivitis :
- ➢ Hay fever conjunctivitis
- ➢ Seasonal allergic conjunctivitis
- ➢ Perennial allergic conjunctivitis

2) Vernal keratoconjunctivitis (VKC)

3) Phlyctenular conjunctivitis (PKC)

4) Giant papillary conjunctivitis (GPC)

5) Atopic keratoconjunctivitis

6) Contact (drop) dermoconjunctivitis.

C) Cicatrical conjunctivitis :

- Ocular mucous membrane pemphigoid
- Stevens Johnson Syndrome
- Toxic epidermal necrolysis
- Secondary cicatrical conjunctivitis

D) Toxic conjunctivitis.

❏ OPHTHALMIA NEONATORUM : (Fig. 1.1)

Also called as neonatal conjunctivitis, is the conjunctivitis in the first month of life.

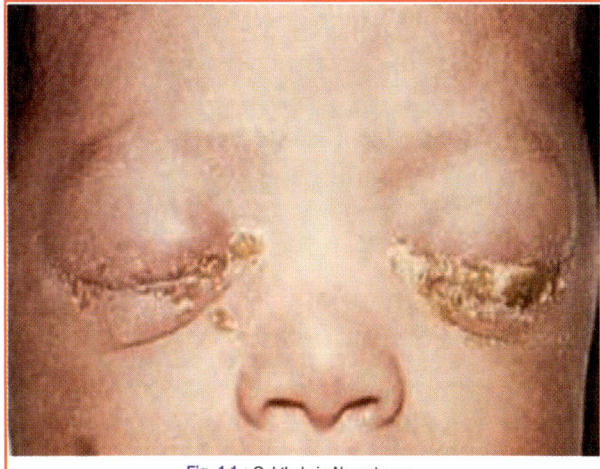

Fig. 1.1 : Ophthalmia Neonatorum.

Etiology :

- Infection acquired during the birth from infected birth canal (most common) or
- After the birth.
- Common organisms :

  1) C. trachomatis, C. oculogenitalis

  2) Gonococcus

  3) HSV

  4) Staphylococcus, Streptococcus, Pneumococcus.

  5) Pseudomonas, Serratia, Kleibsiella.

- Chemical conjunctivitis is caused by use of silver nitrate or antibiotic prophylaxis.

Clinical features :

Depends upon the type of Ophthalmia neonatorum:

i) *Infective :*

- Pain, tenderness.
- Purulent/mucopurulent discharge
- Swollen lids
- Chemosis
- Conjunctival hyperaemia.

ii) *Chemical :*

- 'Watery discharge'.
- 'Minimal or no edema or chemosis'.
- Self limited (1-2 days post partum)

Treatment :

i) *Curative :*

depends upon the causative organism.

a) *C. trachomatis D-K (inclusion conjunctivitis)*

  ➢ Erythromycin/chlortetracyclin eye ointment.

  ➢ Oral erythromycin.

b) *Gonococcus :*

  ➢ Topical penicillin drops/bacitracin ointment.

  ➢ Systemic (for 7 days) :

  Ceftriaxone, cefotaxime, ciprofloxacin, penicillin G.

c) *HSV :*

  Acyclovir ointment, systemic acyclovir.

d) *Other bacteria :*

  Bacitracin-neomycin eye ointment, Gentamycin/Tobramycin drops.

ii) *Prophylaxis :*

- 0.5% Erythromycin & 1% Tetracycline ointment have replaced 1% silver nitrate (Crede's method) for prophylactic use.
- Single injection of ceftriaxone should be given to infant born to mothers with untreated gonococcal infection.

🔲 TRACHOMA :

- ✒ Also called as 'Egyptian Ophthalmia'.

- ✒ Trachoma is chronic keratoconjunctivitis primarily affecting superficial epithelium of conjunctiva and cornea simultaneously.

- ✒ Characterised by mixed follicular & papillary conjunctivitis. **(Fig. 1.2)**

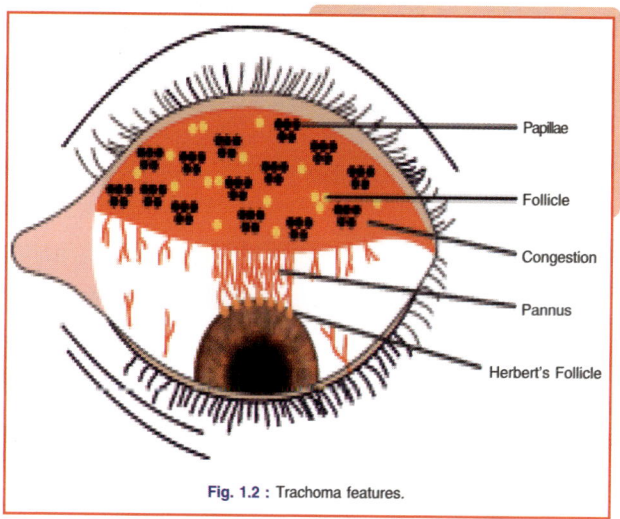

Fig. 1.2 : Trachoma features.

Etiology :

1) C. trachomatis A, B, Ba & C.

   Organism is epitheliotropic & produces intracytoplasmic inclusion bodies called Halberstaedler Prowazeke (HP) bodies.

2) Eye seeking flies.

3) Use of kajal/surma by same family members from same container.

4) Poor, unhygienic conditions.

5) Close person to person contact.

Clinical features :

- ✒ Determined by presence or absence of secondary infection.

- ✒ In absence of such infection, a pure trachoma is so mild and symptomless that disease is usually neglected and symptoms include mild foreign body sensation & occasionally lacrimation.

- ✒ Picture is complicated by secondary infection and starts with typical symptoms of acute mucopurulent conjunctivitis.

- ✒ On examination : conjunctiva, cornea both are involved.

A) Conjunctival signs :

1) Congestion of upper tarsal & forniceal conjunctiva.

2) Conjunctiva follicles :

   ➢ 'Boiled sago grain like follicles' on upper tarsal & forniceal conjunctiva (Fig. 1.3).

   ➢ 'Presence of follicles on bulbar conjunctiva' is pathognomic of trachoma.

   ➢ Characteristic feature of trachoma follicle is presence of necrosis & leber cells (large multinucleated cells) which differentiate it from follicular conjunctivitis.

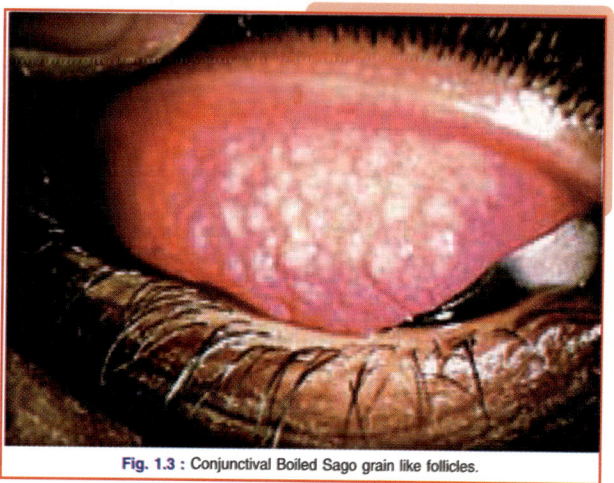

Fig. 1.3 : Conjunctival Boiled Sago grain like follicles.

3) Papillary hyperplasia :

   Reddish, flat topped raised areas which give red & velvety appearance to tarsal conjunctiva **(Fig. 1.4)**.

4) Conjunctival scarring :

   Linear scar in sulcus subtarsalis called as 'Arlt's line'. **(Fig. 1.5)**

5) Concretion :

   due to accumulation of dead epithelial cells and inspissated mucus in depressions called glands of Henle.

B) Corneal signs :

1) Superficial keratitis.

2) Herbert follicles : in limbal area.

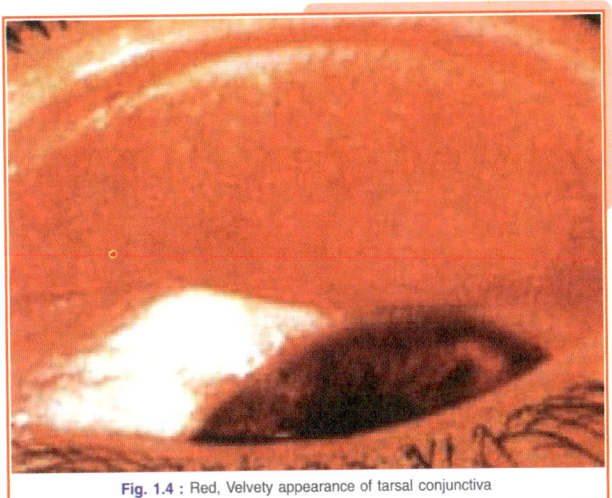

Fig. 1.4 : Red, Velvety appearance of tarsal conjunctiva

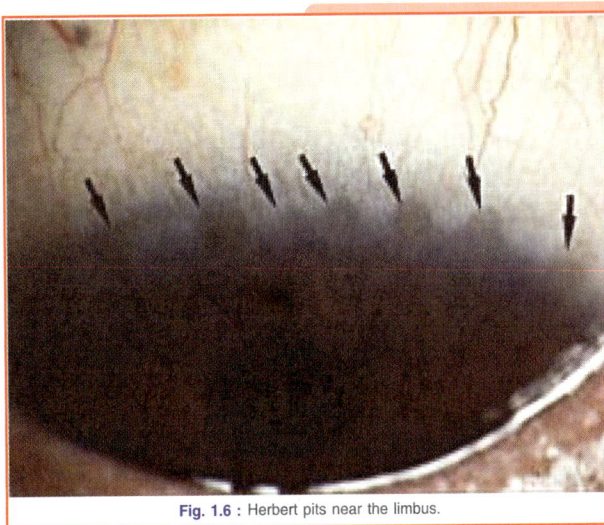

Fig. 1.6 : Herbert pits near the limbus.

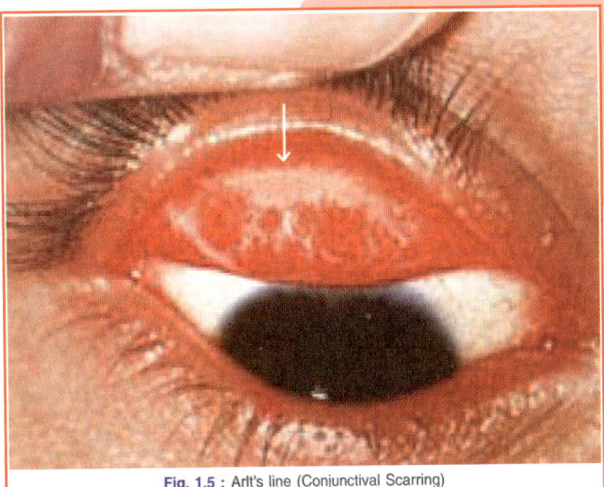

Fig. 1.5 : Arlt's line (Conjunctival Scarring)

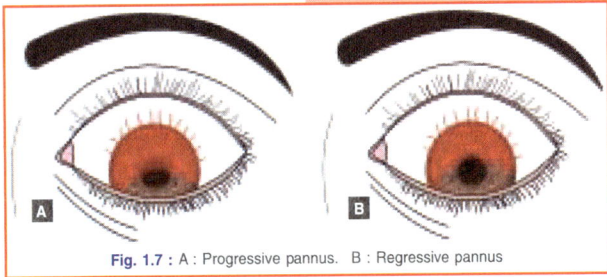

Fig. 1.7 : A : Progressive pannus. B : Regressive pannus

3) *Herbert pits :* left after healing of Herbert follicles in limbal area. **(Fig. 1.6)**

4) *Pannus :* Infiltration of cornea with vascularization. **(Fig. 1.7)**

   2 types : ➢ Regressive pannus
   ➢ Progressive pannus

5) Corneal ulcer.

6) Corneal Opacity.

Sequelae & Complications of Trachoma :

1) *Conjunctiva :*
   ➢ Xerosis (dryness)
   ➢ Concretions
   ➢ Pseudocyst
   ➢ Symblepharon

2) *Cornea :*
   ➢ Xerosis
   ➢ Corneal opacity
   ➢ Corneal ulcer
   ➢ Total corneal pannus
   ➢ Ectasia

3) *Lids :*
   ➢ Entropion
   ➢ Trichiasis
   ➢ Ptosis
   ➢ Tylosis
   ➢ Madarosis
   ➢ Ankyloblepharon

4) *Others :*
   ➢ Chronic dacryocystitis, dacryoadenitis.

5) Blindness.

WHO Classification of Trachoma : ☺ *FISTO* (Fig. 1.8)

Replaced all the previous classifications *i.e.* McCallan's & Jone's classification.

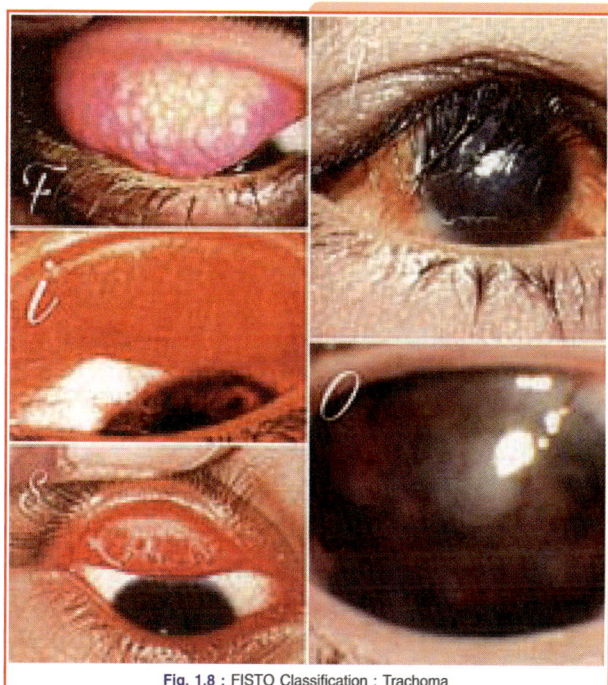

Fig. 1.8 : FISTO Classification : Trachoma

1) *Trachomatous Inflammation Follicular (TF) :*
   ➢ at least 5 or > 5 follicles of atleast 0.5 mm in diameter on upper tarsal conjunctiva.

2) *Trachomatous Inflammation Intense (TI) :*
   ➢ Follicles & Papillae are so numerous & inflammed that > 50% of palpebral conjunctival blood vessels cannot be seen.

3) *Trachomatous Scarring (TS) : (Cicatrising)*
   ➢ presence of scar in tarsal conjunctiva

4) *Trachomatous Trichiasis (TT) :*
   ➢ atleast one eyelash rubs the eye ball.

5) *Trachomatous Opacity (TO) :*
   ➢ easily visible corneal opacity.

Management :

Investigations :
1) Clinical diagnosis.
2) Conjunctival cytology by Giemsa stain.
3) Detection of Inclusion bodies.
4) ELISA.
5) PCR.

6) Isolation of Chlamydia by tissue culture, yolk sac inoculation.
7) Serotyping of TRIC agents.
8) Monoclonal fluoroscent antibody microscopy.

Treatment :

A) *Therapeutic :* ☺ **REST**

Chlamydiae are sensitive to Rifampicin, Erythromycin, Sulfonamides, Tetracycline.

Local :
☙ Sulphacetamide (20% or 30% drops)
   4 times daily for 6 weeks continuously.
☙ Tetracycline ointment (1%) twice daily for 6 weeks continuously.
☙ Followed by intermittent treatment with Tetracycline eye ointment.

in each month for 6 months { BD for 5 consecutive days OR OD for 10 consecutive days

Systemic :
☙ Oral Sulphonamides in full therapeutic dose for 3 weeks.
                    OR
☙ Tetracycline 4 times daily for 3-4 weeks.
                    OR
☙ Oral Doxycycline OD for 3-4 weeks.
☙ Oral Azithromycin, Erythromycin.

B) *Prophylactic :*
1) Improvement of personal hygiene & environmental sanitation.
2) Avoid kajal, surma.
3) Avoid person to person close contact.
4) Periodic treatment with Sulphacetamide (20%) or Tetracycline (1%) as intermittent therapy.

C) *Treatment of Complications :*
1) Excision of fornix.
2) Tarsectomy.
3) Surgery for trichiasis, entropion.
4) Pannus treatment by cryoapplication or peritomy.

5) Mechanical expression of follicles by Roller (Knaopp's forceps), AgNO$_3$ painting, Diathermy.

SAFE strategy for Trachoma in Vision 2020 :

S : Surgery for trichiasis / entropion

A : Antibiotics

F : Facial cleanliness

E : Environmental sanitation

◻ VERNAL KERATOCONJUNCTIVITIS (Spring Catarrh) (VKC) : (Fig. 1.9)

⚘ Allergic inflammation of conjunctiva which is characterised by Recurrent, bilateral, interstitial, self limiting conjunctivitis that becomes aggravated during spring and summer period.

⚘ Considered to be Type I Hypersensitivity Reaction (immediate type) to exogenous allergenes such as grass, pollens.

⚘ More common in boys, 4-20 years of age.

⚘ More common in summer, hence the name spring catarrh looks a misnomer.

⚘ Recently it is labelled as "Warm weather conjunctivitis".

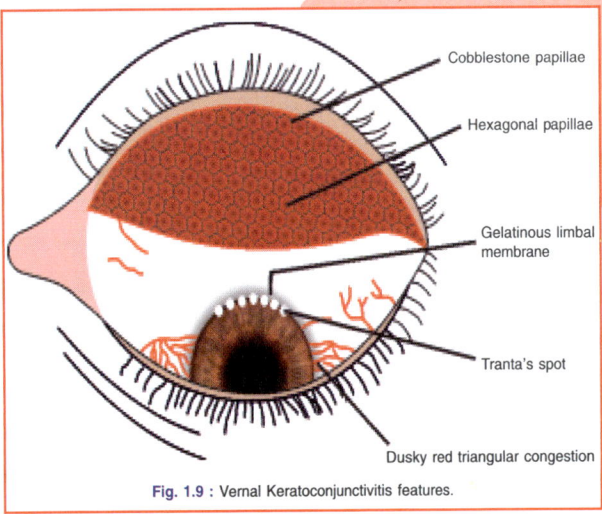

Cobblestone papillae

Hexagonal papillae

Gelatinous limbal membrane

Tranta's spot

Dusky red triangular congestion

Fig. 1.9 : Vernal Keratoconjunctivitis features.

Clinical features :

⚘ Characterised by marked itching & burning.

⚘ Stringy (ropy) discharge.

⚘ Lacrimation.

⚘ Photophobia.

⚘ heaviness of lids.

Clinically, divided into 3 types :

1) Palpebral form :

⧖ most common.

⧖ upper palpebral conjunctiva shows papillary hypertrophy.

⧖ large & flat topped papillae.

⧖ Cobble stone (pavement) appearance. (Fig. 1.10)

⧖ papillae heal without scarring.

2) Bulbar form :

⧖ dusky red triangular congestion of bulbar conjunctiva in palpebral area.

⧖ gelatinous thickened accumulation of tissue around the limbus.

⧖ presence of discrete whitish raised dots along the limbus (Horner Tranta's spot). (Fig. 1.11)

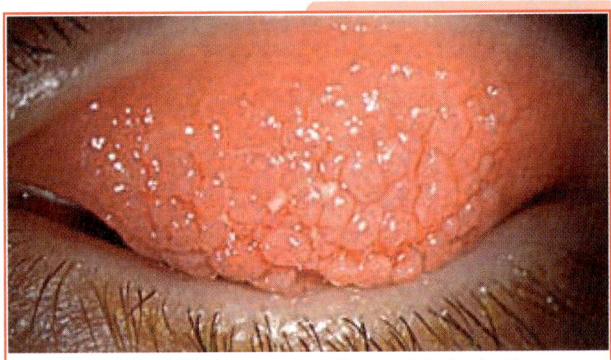

Fig. 1.10 : Cobblestone appearance of upper palpebral conjunctiva

Fig. 1.11 : Horner Tranta's spot (dots) along the limbus.

3) Mixed form :

both bulbar & palpebral manifestations occur together.

Corneal signs (Vernal keratopathy) :

- Punctate epithelial keratitis.
- Ulcerative vernal keratitis. (shallow transverse ulcer/shield ulcer). **(Fig. 1.12)**
- Vernal corneal plaques.
- Subepithelial scarring.
- Pseudogerontoxon : **(Fig. 1.13)**

  arc like 'whitish peripheral corneal deposition 'Cupid's bow' outline in inflammed segment of the limbus.

Treatment :

1) Anti inflammatory agents :

a) Topical steroids (Dexamethasone).

b) Mast cell stabilizers (Olapatadine, di sodium chromoglycate, idoxamide tromethamine)

c) Topical antihistaminics (Azelastine).

d) NSAID eyedrops (Ketotifen)

e) Topical cyclosporine.

f) Tacrolimus.

2) Lubricants/Mucolytics :

- Acetyl cysteine, artificial tears.

3) Systemic :

- Oral Steroids.
- Oral Antihistaminics.

4) Large papillae :

- Supratarsal steroid injection.
- Cryoapplication.
- Surgical excision.

5) General measures :

- Use dark goggles.
- Cold compress / ice packs.

☐ PHLYCTENULAR KERATOCONJUNCTIVITIS : (Fascicular ulcer) (Fig. 1.14)

- Allergic response of conjunctival and corneal epithelium to some endogenous allergens and is characterized by formation of Phlyctens (grey, yellow, pinkish, white nodules) slightly raised above the surface, seen on bulbar conjunctiva near the limbus.
- Common in girls, 3-15 years of age.

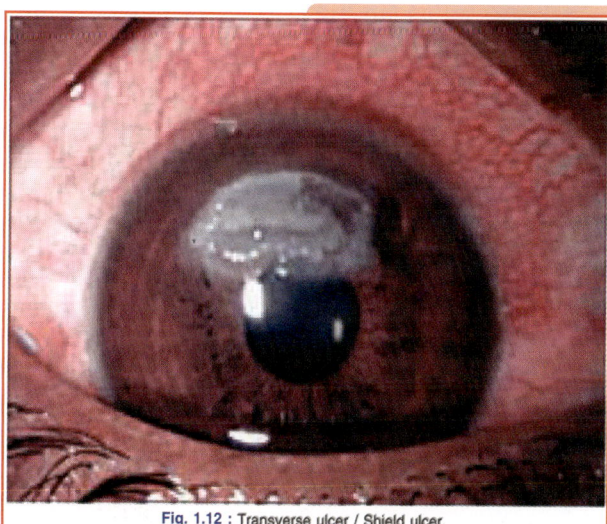

Fig. 1.12 : Transverse ulcer / Shield ulcer.

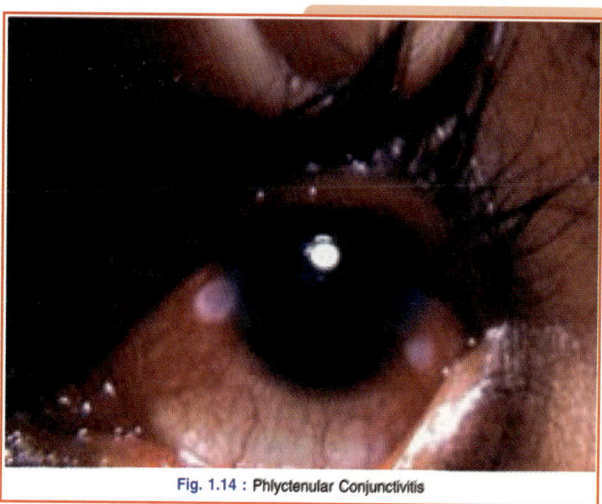

Fig. 1.13 : Pseudogerontoxon (Cupid's bow outline along the limbus)

Fig. 1.14 : Phlyctenular Conjunctivitis

Etiology :

Delayed Hypersensitivity (type IV) response to endogenous microbial proteins.

Causative allergens :

i) Staphylococcus protein (most common).

ii) Tuberculous protein.

iii) Proteins of Moraxella axenfield bacillus and certain parasites.

Symptoms :

⚬ Unilateral (vernal is bilateral) mild irritation, discomfort, lacrimation.

⚬ Itching is not prominent as seen in vernal.

⚬ Pain, photophobia if cornea is involved.

Signs :

⚬ Phlyctens are pinkish, white nodules at limbus.

⚬ Surrounded by hyperaemia (congestion) and is limited to the area around phlyctens.

⚬ Phlyctens ulcerate at the apex (Ring ulcer).

⚬ Corneal involvement shows :

    Miliary ulcer, Ring ulcer.

    Sacrofulous ulcer, Fascicular ulcer (Fig. 1.15) diffuse infiltrative phlyctenular keratitis.

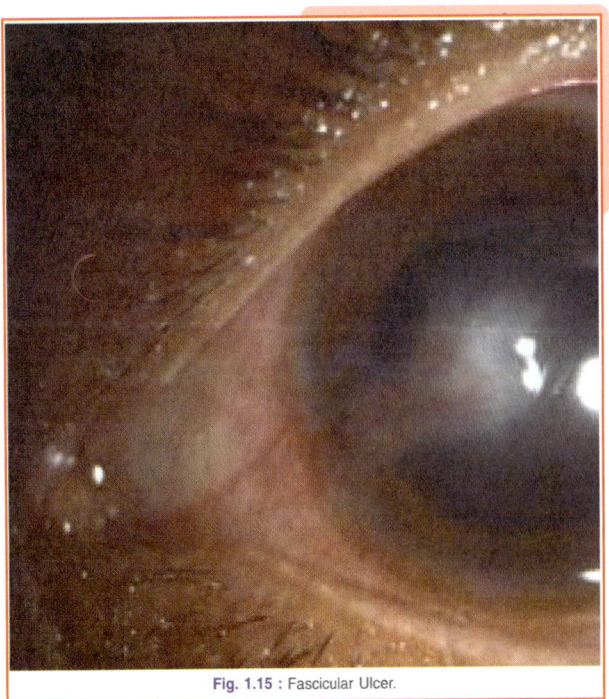

Fig. 1.15 : Fascicular Ulcer.

Treatment :

⚬ Topical steroids (Dexamethasone) → DOC.

⚬ Antibiotic drops.

⚬ Atropine.

⚬ Attempts must be made to rule out :

    a) TB   : if present → start ATT.

    b) septic forms : if there   → systemic
                                   antibiotics

⚬ General measures :

    High protein diet, supplementation of vit. A, C, D.

◘ PTERYGIUM (Pterygion = wing)

⚬ Pterygium is non-cancerous growth (non neoplastic) of conjunctiva, characterized by wing shaped fold of conjunctiva encroaching upon the cornea from either side within interpalpebral fissure. (Fig. 1.16)

⚬ Pterygium is always situated in the palpebral aperture.

⚬ Pathologically, it is degenerative & hyperplastic condition of conjunctiva, subconjunctival tissue undergoes elastotic degeneration and proliferates as vascularised granulation tissue under the epithelium, which ultimately encroaches the cornea.

⚬ Corneal epithelium, Bowman's layer, stroma are destroyed.

Etiology :

Not precisely known, but it is common in :

1) People with excessive outdoor exposure to

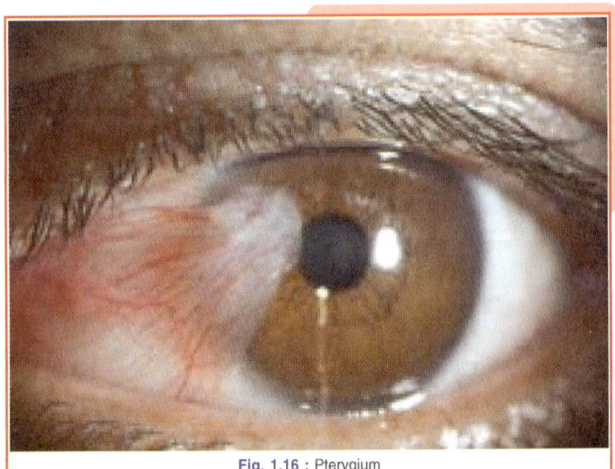

Fig. 1.16 : Pterygium

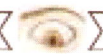

sunlight (UV rays), dry heat, high wind, abundance of dust.

2) Those who work outdoors.

3) Pinguecula may act as a precursor.

Stages : (Fig. 1.17)

<u>2 stages</u> : 1) Progressive stage
    2) Atrophic stage

1) Progressive stage :

- ⤳ It is thick, fleshy with prominent vascularity.
- ⤳ Gradually increases in size and starts encroaching the centre of cornea.
- ⤳ Opaque infiltrative spot (cap) is seen in front of the apex of pterygium also known as Fuch's spots or Islets of Vogt.

2) Atrophic / Stationary / Regressive Stage :

- ⤳ It is thin, attenuated with poor vascularity.
- ⤳ No cap is seen.
- ⤳ Deposition of iron as a line known as Stocker's line is seen in corneal epithelium infront of the apex.

Parts : (Fig. 1.18)

1) *Apex or Head :*
- ⤳ Apex of triangular mass.

2) *Neck :*
- ⤳ Constricted portion at the limbus.

3) *Body :*
- ⤳ Bulky part

4) *Cap :*
- ⤳ Semilunar infiltrative opaque spot just infront of the apex.

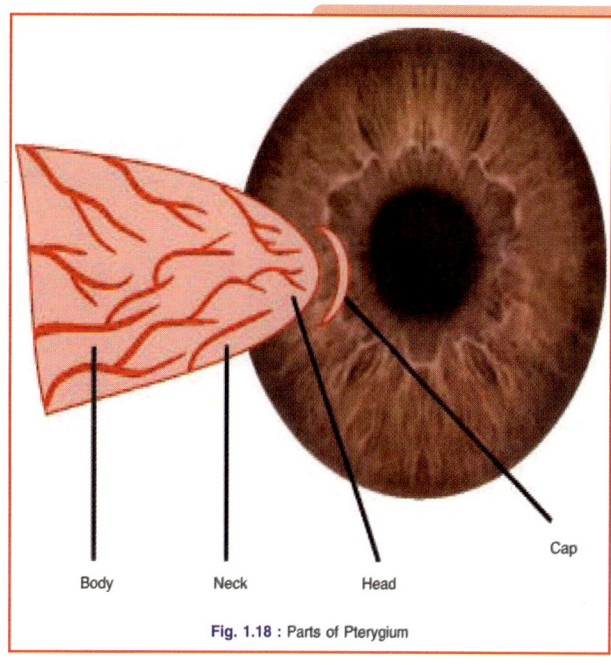

Fig. 1.18 : Parts of Pterygium

Clinical features :

Symptoms :

1) Cosmetic intolerance, or is asymptomatic in early stages.

2) Foreign body sensation, irritation.

3) Appearance of a mass on nasal, or rarely on temporal side of the cornea. Sometimes both nasal and temporal sides are involved (double headed pterygium).

4) Defective vision when it encroaches pupillary area or is due to corneal astigmatism.

5) Rarely diplopia may occur, due to the limitation of ocular movements, especially when associated with symblepharon.

Signs :

1) Triangular fold of conjunctiva encroaching upon the cornea in palpebral aperture, usually on nasal side.

2) Decreased visual acuity.

3) Folds at upper and lower borders of the mass.

4) Stocker's line may be seen. **(Fig. 1.19)**

Complications :

1) Cystic degeneration, infection.

2) Neoplastic change.

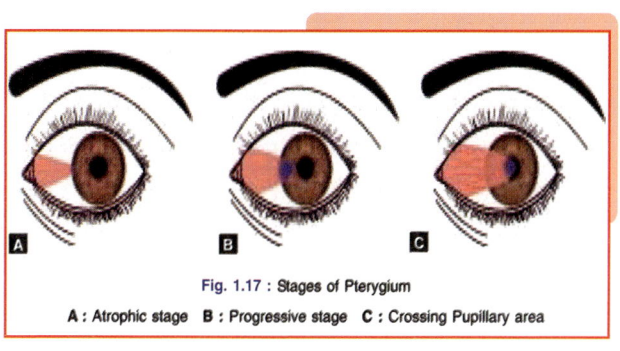

Fig. 1.17 : Stages of Pterygium

A : Atrophic stage B : Progressive stage C : Crossing Pupillary area

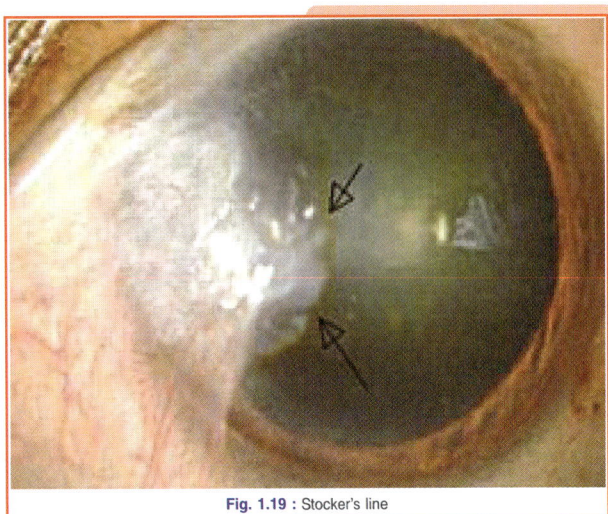
Fig. 1.19 : Stocker's line

Treatment :

Depends upon the type of pterygium :

1) Atrophic pterygium and if if is just on the cornea:

Best left alone with periodic follow up.

2) Progressive pterygium :

a) Bare-sclera technique : excision of pterygium with conjunctiva, keeping limbus and adjacent sclera bare. But associated with high recurrence (80%).

b) Subconjunctival pterygium dissection and then excision with bare sclera.

c) Transposition operation (Mc Reynolds operation)

➤ Older method not done nowadays.

3) Recurrent pterygium : (and also to prevent recurrence)

✎ After excision, bare sclera is treated with mitomycin C, Beta irradiation, thio TEPA.

✎ CLAU (Conjunctival Limbal Autograft) technique is most preferred technique. Recurrence rate is lowest here.

✎ Lamellar keratoplasty of affected part, along with excision of pterygium.

4) Pterygium involving pupillary area :

Resection of pterygium with anterior lamellar keratoplasty is treatment of choice.

◻ DIFFERENTIAL DIAGNOSIS OF NODULE AT LIMBUS :

☞ 'A limbal nodule is any nodular lesion at the limbus *i.e.* junction of the cornea and sclera of the eye'.

☞ It can be divided into following groups :

I) Congenital.

II) Inflammatory.

III) Allergic.

IV) Vascular

V) Traumatic.

VI) Degenerative.

VII) Nutritional.

VIII) Neoplastic.

IX) Miscellaneous.

I) Congenital :

1) Dermoid :

⇨ Yellowish white mass.

⇨ Consists of epithelium, sebaceous glands, hair.

⇨ *Rx* : Excision.

2) Dermolipoma :

⇨ soft, yellow and movable.

⇨ subconjunctival mass.

⇨ consists of adipose tissue and dermis around.

⇨ associated with Goldenhar's syndrome.

⇨ *Rx* : Excision.

3) Naevi :

⇨ Flat or raised, grey gelatinous, brown/black.

⇨ Tendency to grow during puberty and pregnancy.

⇨ may undergo malignant change.

⇨ *Rx* : Excision if it grows.

II) Inflammatory :

1) Episcleritis :

⇨ Inflammation of deep conjunctival tissue.

⇨ Pinkish elevated tender nodule, which is diffuse.

⇨ Occurs in Gout, Rheumatism, endogenous allergy to bacteria.

⇨ *Rx* : Topical steroids or NSAIDs.

Systemic Indomethacin.

<u>Recurrence</u> : Systemic therapy.

2) *Scleritis :*

⇨ nodular / diffuse form.

⇨ nodular form is fixed to the sclera.

⇨ due to collagen disorders, endogenous infections.

⇨ *Rx* : Steroids.

III) Allergy :

1) *Phlycten :*

⇨ pinkish, whitish nodules surrounded by congestion.

⇨ due to endogenous reaction to tuberculous protein.

⇨ *Rx* : Topical steroids.

Treatment of the cause.

2) *Vernal Catarrh :*

⇨ multiple nodules in upper limbus, which are white superficial spots.

⇨ associated with stringy white ropy discharge.

⇨ due to hypersensitivity to exogenous allergen - pollen and dust.

⇨ recurrence in summer.

⇨ *Rx* : Steroids, Mast cell stabilizers, NSAIDs.

3) *Ophthalmia nodosa :*

⇨ due to granulomatous inflammation to caterpillar hair.

⇨ *Rx* : Steroids or Excision.

IV) Vascular :

1) *Hemangioma :*

⇨ benign red lesion which blanches on pressure.

⇨ bleeds on trivial trauma.

⇨ may be associated with hemangioma of lid and orbit.

V) Traumatic :

1) *Granuloma :*

⇨ after surgical wound (squint or pterygium surgery)

⇨ at the site of foreign body.

⇨ *Rx* : Surgical excision.

2) *Implantation cyst.*

3) *Iris prolapse covered by conjunctiva.*

VI) Degenerative :

1) *Pinguecula :*

⇨ Triangular yellowish patch on bulbar conjunctiva near the limbus.

⇨ in elderly.

⇨ hyaline infiltration & elastotic degeneration of subconjunctival tissue.

⇨ precursor of pterygium.

⇨ *Rx* : Excision for cosmetic purpose.

2) *Cystic pterygium :*

⇨ Triangular sheet of fibrovascular tissue invading the cornea.

⇨ Occurs after recurrence.

⇨ *Rx* : Excision and conjunctival limbal autograft.

VII) Nutritional :

1) *Bitot's spot :*

⇨ Silvery white, foamy or cheesy patch.

⇨ Seen in vit. A deficiency.

VIII) Neoplastic :

1) *Papilloma :*

⇨ benign polypoid tumor.

⇨ sessile/pedunculated.

⇨ can become malignant.

⇨ *Rx* : Surgical excision.

2) *Squamous cell carcinoma :*

⇨ flat granular growth.

⇨ invades underlying structures.

⇨ *Rx* : Early excision.

3) *Primary melanoma :*

⇨ nodular form, may be pigmented or non pigmented.

⇨ *Rx* : Excision.

4) *Intraepithelial epithelioma.*

IX) Miscellaneous :

1) *Intercalary or ciliary staphyloma :*

⇨ bulge in the limbal area.

⇨ lined by the root of iris due to ectasia of weak scar tissue.

⇨ occurs following healed perforation injuries or corneal ulcer.

2) *Retention cyst :*

⇨ thin walled cyst with clear fluid.

⇨ *Rx* : Excision for irritation,

foreign body sensation, or

cosmetic reasons.

3) *Parasitic cyst –* due to cysticercosis.

4) *Filtering bleb :*

⇨ occurs following trabeculectomy.

◻ XEROSIS :

⚘ Xerosis of conjunctiva is a condition in which conjunctiva becomes dry and lustreless.

⚘ 2 types :

1) Parenchymatous xerosis.

2) Epithelial xerosis.

1) *Parenchymatous Xerosis : (Fig. 1.20)*

➢ due to cicatrical disorganization of the conjunctiva caused by :

a) Trachoma.

b) Steven-Johnsons Syndrome.

c) Pemphigus.

d) Thermal, Chemical, Radiational burns of conjunctiva.

➢ due to exposure of conjunctiva to air as seen in :

a) Proptosis.

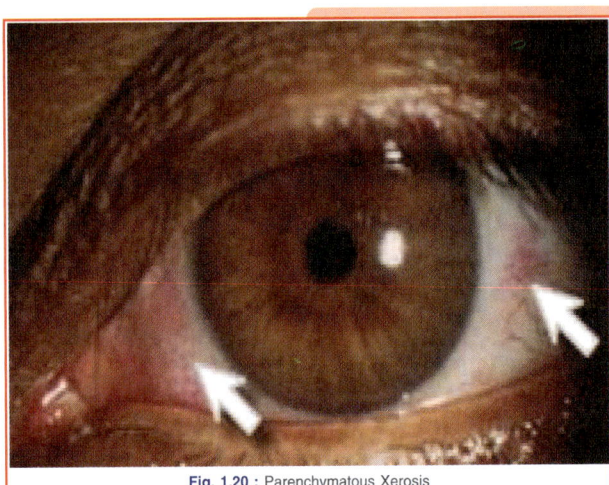

Fig. 1.20 : Parenchymatous Xerosis

b) Facial Palsy.

c) Ectropion.

d) Lack of blinking (as in coma).

e) Lagophthalmos due to symblepharon.

2) *Epithelial xerosis :* (Fig. 1.21)

➢ due to hypovitaminosis A.

Clinical features :

1) Conjunctival dryness.

2) Conjunctival thickening.

3) Wrinkling of conjunctiva.

4) Conjunctival pigmentation.

Treatment :

1) Treatment of the cause.

2) Symptomatic local treatment with Artificial tears (methyl cellulose), to be instilled frequently.

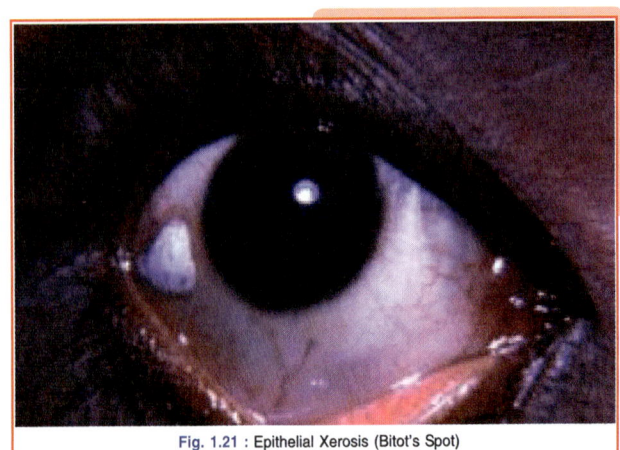

Fig. 1.21 : Epithelial Xerosis (Bitot's Spot)

☐ PTERYGIUM vs PSEUDOPTERYGIUM :

Character	Pterygium	Pseudopterygium
1) Age	Usually in elderly	At any age
2) Etiology	Degenerative process	Inflammatory process
3) Site	In interpalpebral fissure	At any site
4) Stages	Progressive, Regressive or Stationary	Always stationary
5) Probe test	Probe cannot be passed underneath	Probe can be passed under the neck

☐ EPIDEMIC KERATOCONJUNCTIVITIS (EKC):

- ✒ An acute follicular conjunctivitis mostly associated with superficial punctate keratitis.

- ✒ Usually occurs in epidemics, hence the name EKC.

Etiology :

1) Adenovirus type 8 and 19 (most common).

2) Spreads through the contact with contaminated fingers, solutions and tonometers, and is contagious.

Clinical features :

A) Symptoms :

1) Redness of sudden onset.

2) Profuse watering with mild mucoid discharge.

3) Foreign body sensation, discomfort.

4) Photophobia and is marked when cornea is involved.

B) Signs :

- ✎ *Conjunctival signs :*

  1) Hyperaemia, Chemosis. **(Fig. 1.22)**

  2) Characteristic small to moderate size follicles involving lower fornix and palpebral conjunctiva.

  3) Papillae in some cases.

  4) Petechial subconjunctival hemorrhage.

  5) Pseudomembrane lining the lower fornix and palpebral conjunctiva. **(Fig. 1.23)**

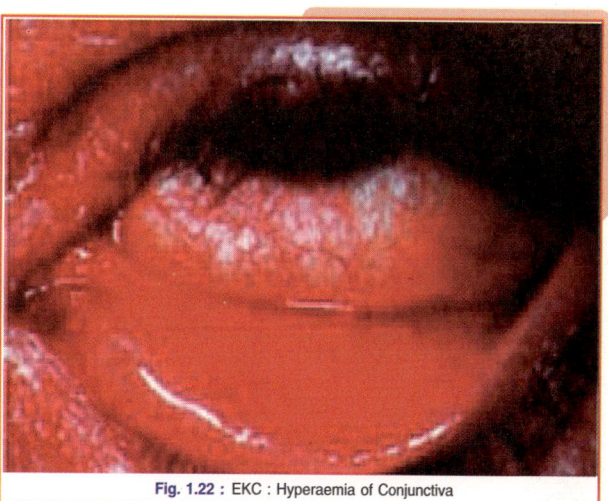

Fig. 1.22 : EKC : Hyperaemia of Conjunctiva

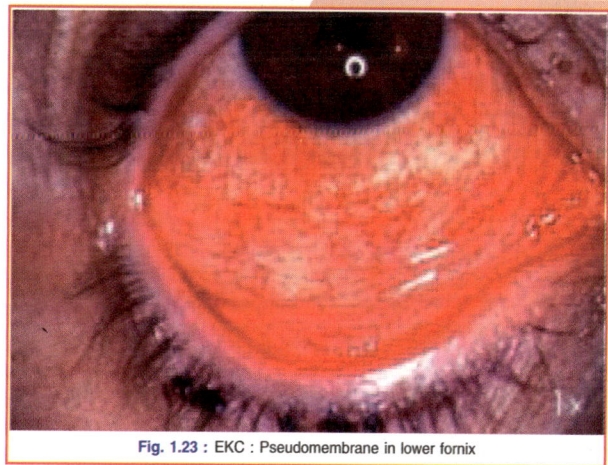

Fig. 1.23 : EKC : Pseudomembrane in lower fornix

- ✎ *Corneal signs :*

  1) Characteristic superficial punctate keratitis. **(Fig. 1.24)**

  2) Epithelial microcystic diffuse fine non staining lesions in early stages.

  3) Subepithelial infiltrates.

- ✎ **'Pre auricular lymphadenopathy'** in almost all cases of EKC.

Management :

A) Investigations :

1) *Conjunctival cytology with Giema stain :*

   - ➤ 'Mononuclear cells' are seen.

   - ➤ multinucleated cells are seen in herpetic conjunctivitis.

2) *Polymerase Chain Reaction :*

   - ➤ sensitive & specific.

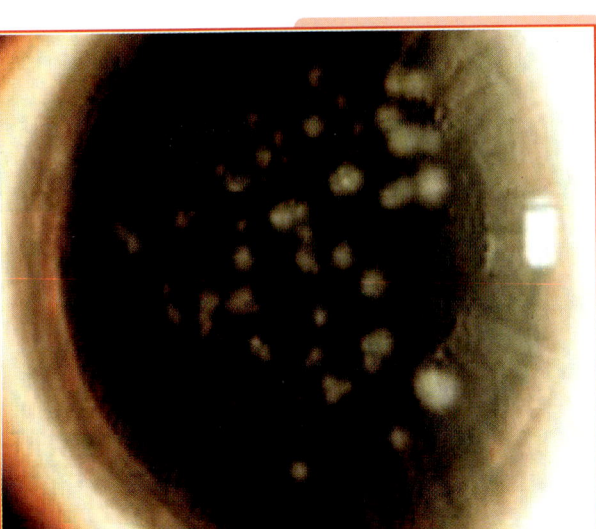

Fig. 1.24 : EKC : Superficial Punctate Keratitis

3) Immunochromatography.

4) Viral Cultures.

B) *Treatment :*

1) *Supportive treatment :*
   - ➢ Cold compresses, sunglasses.
   - ➢ Decongestant, lubricant tear drops.

2) *Topical antibiotics :*
   - ➢ to prevent superadded bacterial infection.

3) *Topical antivirals :*
   - ➢ Adenine arabinosides (Ara-A)
   - ➢ Cidofovir.

4) *Topical steroids :*
   - ➢ not to be used in active stage.
   - ➢ if membrane formation, subepithelial infiltrates exists : weak steroids are used

     such as : Fluorometholone or

     Loteprednol.

C) *As it is contagious, preventive measures to be used are :*

1) Frequent handwashing.

2) Isolation of infected individual.

3) Avoid eye rubbing and common use of towel, handkerchief sharing.

4) Disinfection of ophthalmic instruments and clinical surfaces after examination of the patient.

❑ FOLLICULAR CONJUNCTIVITIS :

✍ Conjunctivitis associated with hypertrophic lymphoid tissue is seen as pinkish round bodies in the conjunctiva.

Types :

A) *Acute follicular Conjunctivitis :*

1) Inclusion conjunctivitis.

2) *Adenovirus conjunctivitis :*
   a) Epidemic keratoconjunctivitis (EKC)
   b) Pharyngoconjunctival fever.

3) Acute herpetic conjunctivitis.

4) Allergic conjunctivitis.

5) Newcastle conjunctivitis.

6) Trachoma (acute) in foreigners.

B) *Chronic follicular conjunctivitis :*

1) Trachoma.

C) *Toxic follicular conjunctivitis :*

1) Molluscum contagiosum.

D) *Folliculosis.*

I) **Adult inclusion conjunctivitis :**

➢ acute follicular conjunctivitis.

➢ usually affects sexually active young adults.

Etiology :

1) Chlamydia trachomatis D to K.

2) Due to : urethritis in males,

   cervicitis in females.

3) Transmission to eye occurs commonly through contaminated water in swimming pools, 'Swimming Pool Conjunctivitis' and also by contaminated fingers.

Clinical features :

Symptoms :

1) Mucopurulent discharge.

2) Photophobia.

3) Ocular discomfort, foreign body sensation.

Signs :

1) Hyperaemia.
2) Acute follicular hypertrophy in lower palpebral conjunctiva. **(Fig. 1.25)**
3) Superficial keratitis (punctate).
4) Pre auricular lymphadenopathy.

Management :

Investigations :

1) Clinical diagnosis.
2) Conjunctival cytology by Giemsa stain.
3) Detection of Inclusion bodies.
4) ELISA.
5) PCR.
6) Isolation of Chlamydia by tissue culture, yolk sac inoculation.
7) Serotyping of TRIC agents.
8) Monoclonal fluoroscent antibody microscopy.

Treatment :

1) Topical Tetracycline ointment 4 times a day for 6 weeks.

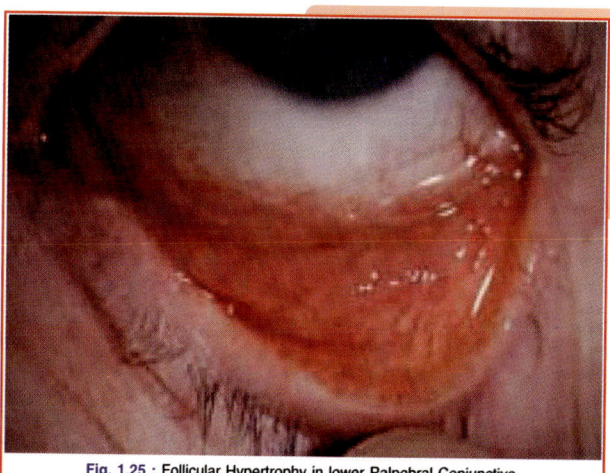

Fig. 1.25 : Follicular Hypertrophy in lower Palpebral Conjunctiva

2) Systemic Therapy ☺ DATE.

Doxycycline, Azithromycin, Tetracycline, Erythromycin.

3) Referral to Genitourinary specialist is mandatory.

II) Adenovirus Conjunctivitis (EKC) :

✍ discussed above.

III) Acute Herpetic Conjunctivitis :

✍ always accompanied by primary herpetic infection in children, adolescents.

Etiology :

1) HSV-1 – by kissing, personal contacts.
2) HSV-2 – by genital infections.

Clinical features :

1) *Typical form :*
   ➢ vesicular lesions of face and lids.

2) *Atypical form :*
   ➢ resembles EKC.
   ➢ hyperaemia, follicular hyperplasia, pseudomembrane formation.

3) *Corneal involvement is rare :*
   ➢ epithelial, dendritic keratitis.

4) Preauricular lymphadenopathy.

Treatment :

1) Topical antivirals.
2) Supportive measures like EKC.

IV) Trachoma :

discussed above.

Chapter

2

Cornea

Most Important (Must Read Topics)	Elective Topics
1) Bacterial corneal ulcer	1) Anatomy of cornea
2) Hypopyon corneal ulcer	2) Histology of cornea
3) Fungal corneal ulcer	3) Corneal Transparency
4) Herpes simplex (viral) keratitis	4) Interstitial keratitis
5) Corneal opacities	5) Keratoconus
6) Keratoplasty	
7) Differential diagnosis of Red eye	

❏ ANATOMY OF CORNEA :

⚵ Cornea is transparent, avascular, watch glass like structure.

  a) Surfaces : 2 surfaces → Anterior & Posterior

   ➢ Anterior is elliptical; posterior is circular

   ➢ Horizontal diameter of both surfaces   : 11.7 mm

   ➢ Vertical diameter of posterior surface   : 11.7 mm

   ➢ Vertical diameter of anterior surface   : 10.6 mm

   ➢ Radius of curvature of anterior surface   : 7.8 mm

   ➢ Radius of curvature of : 6.5 mm posterior surface

➢ Vertical meridian of cornea is 0.05 D steeper than horizontal meridian, resulting in astigmatism with the rule.

  b) Refractive power : 43-44D (3/4th of total diopteric power of eye).

   ➢ Most of the refraction in eye occur at the anterior surface of cornea (air tear interface).

   ➢ Cornea has Refractive Index : 1.376

   ➢ Refractive power of anterior surface is about + 48D but overall corneal power is less. *i.e.* +43 to 44 D as a result of negative power (-5.80 D) of posterior corneal surface.

  c) Change in size :

   ➢ Horizontal diameter of : 10 mm cornea at birth

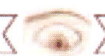

➤ Horizontal diameter of : 11.7 mm
cornea at adult size
(by age of 2 years)

Megalocornea :

☞ Horizontal diameter is of adult size at birth OR ≥ 13 mm after 2 years of age.

☞ Due to : Marfan syndrome

Ehler Danlos Syndrome

Apert syndrome

Down syndrome

Microcornea :

☞ Corneal diameter is < 10 mm.

◘ HISTOLOGY OF CORNEA : (Fig. 2.1)

5 layers (Superficial to Deep)

1) *Epithelium :*

   ☙ Stratified squamous non-keratinized

2) *Bowman's membrane :*

   ☙ Once destroyed, doesn't regenerate.

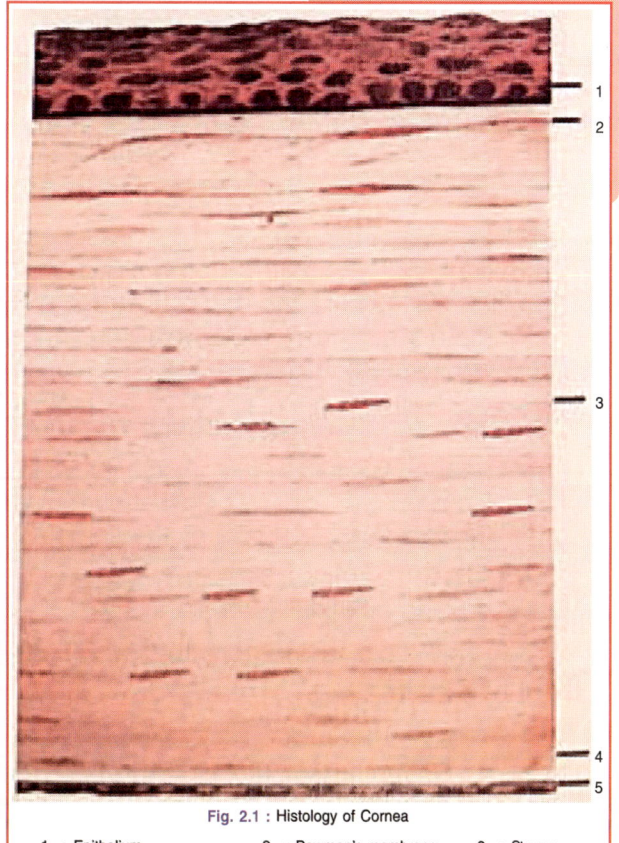

Fig. 2.1 : Histology of Cornea

1 → Epithelium	2 → Bowman's membrane	3 → Stroma
4 → Descemet's membrane	5 → Endothelium	

3) *Stroma :*

   ☙ Constitutes 90% thickness of the cornea, more in periphery than in centre.

   ☙ Collagen fibrils are present.

4) *Pre Descemet's (Dua's layer) :*

   ☙ Newly discovered

5) *Descemet's membrane :*

   ☙ Schwable's ring is present.

6) *Endothelium :*

   ☙ Most important layer maintaining the transparency of cornea.

   ☙ Cell density : 3000 cells/mm² in adults.

   ☙ Have active pump mechanism.

   ☙ Regenerates rapidly after injury.

◘ CORNEAL TRANSPARENCY :

Maintained by :

A) Anatomical factors :

i) Corneal epithelium & tear film :

   Homogenity of R.I. (Refractive index) throughout the epithelium.

ii) Absence of blood vessels.

iii) Presence of unmyelinated nerves.

iv) Regular lattice arrangement of collagen.

B) Physiological factors :

i) Stromal swelling & imbibition pressure

ii) Barrier function of epithelium & endothelium

iii) Endothelial Na⁺/K⁺ ATPase pump, Na⁺/H⁺ pump

iv) Evaporation from corneal surface.

v) Normal IOP.

These 5 factors helps to maintain corneal hydration in a state of relative dehydration.

◘ BACTERIAL CORNEAL ULCER :

☞ Corneal ulcer refers to discontinuation of normal epithelial surface of cornea associated with necrosis of surrounding corneal tissue.

☞ also called as suppurative keratitis.

Etiology :

1) *Damage to corneal epithelium :*

   by injury, foreign body, entropion, contact lens wear.

2) *Infection of eroded area :*

   by infected foreign body, lacrimal sac, conjunctival sac.

3) *Causative organisms :*

   Gram positive cocci – S. aureus, epidermidis (most common)

   Gram negative cocci – N. gonorrhoea, meningitidis

   Gram positive bacilli – C. diphtheria.

   Gram negative bacilli – Enterobacteriaceae

   Gram positive filamentous – Nocardia.

   Mycobacteria – M. tuberculosis.

☞ As long as cornea is healthy, majority of bacteria are unable to cross or adhere to corneal epithelium.

   Organisms which penetrate the intact epithelium are :

   a) N. gonorrhoea   d) N. meningitidis

   b) H. influenza   e) Listeria

   c) C. diphtheria.   f) H. aegyptus

Pathogenesis : (Fig. 2.2)

1) *Stage of progressive Infiltration :*

   ➢ by polymorphonuclear lymphocytes into the epithelium from peripheral circulation.

   ➢ Subsequently tissue oedema, necrosis occur.

2) *Stage of Active ulceration :*

   ➢ due to the necrosis and sloughing off the epithelium, basement membrane and stroma.

   ➢ Hyperaemia of circumcorneal vessels, congestion of iris and ciliary body occurs.

   ➢ Ulceration progresses further.

3) *Stage of Regression :*

   ➢ 'Line of demarcation' develops around the ulcer consisting of leucocytes that neutralize and phagocytose the organism and necrotic debris.

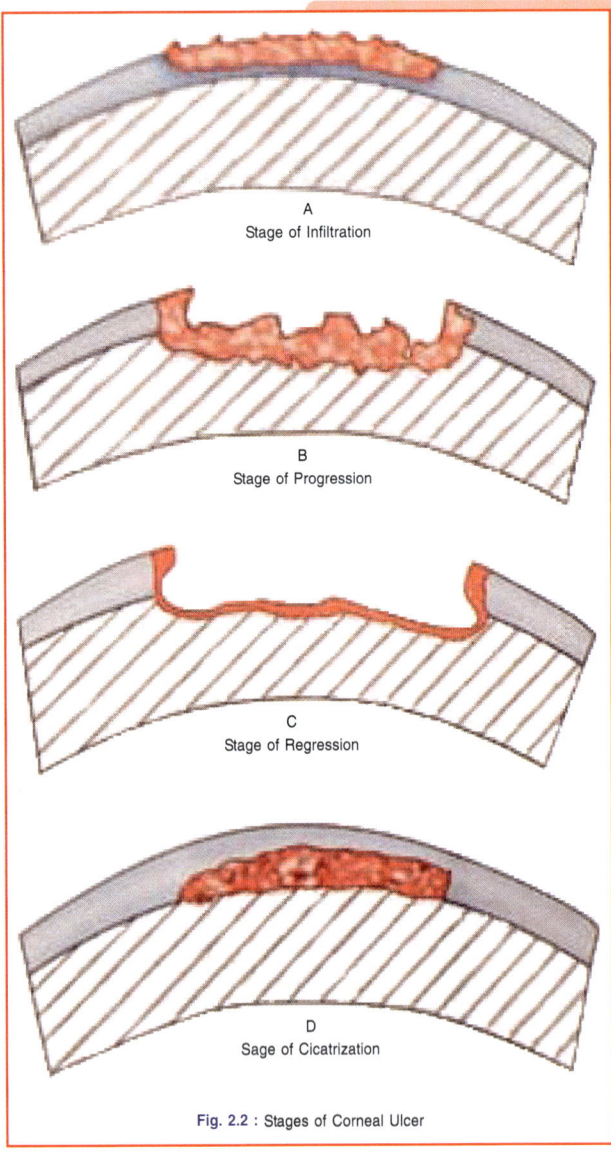

A
Stage of Infiltration

B
Stage of Progression

C
Stage of Regression

D
Sage of Cicatrization

Fig. 2.2 : Stages of Corneal Ulcer

➢ Ulcerated area becomes smooth & clear.

4) *Stage of Cicatrization :*

   ➢ Healing continues by epithelization which forms permanent covering. Beneath this is fibrous tissue laid down by the fibroblast.

   ➢ Stroma thickens and fills in the epithelium, pushing epithelial cells anteriorly.

   ➢ Degree of scarring from healing varies :

   a) superficial ulcer   : heals without opacity.

   b) BM & superficial stroma : Nebula damage

   c) 1/3rd & > 1/3rd of   : Macula, stroma damage   Leucoma.

(Fig. 2.3)

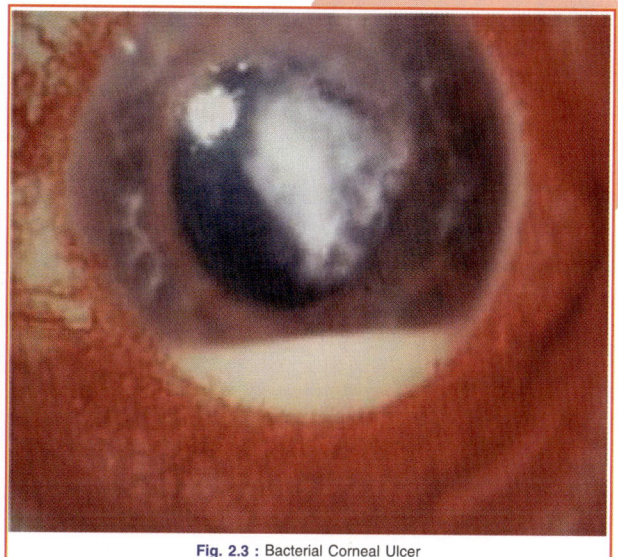

Fig. 2.3 : Bacterial Corneal Ulcer

Clinical features :

Symptoms :

1) Pain
2) Foreign body sensation
3) Lacrimation
4) Photophobia
5) Blurred vision
6) Redness of eye due to circumcorneal congestion.

Signs :

1) Swelling of lids
2) Blepharospasm
3) Conjunctival hyperaemia, chemosis
4) Corneal ulcer : yellowish white, oval/irregular.

   Margins : swollen & overhanging.

   Floor : Covered by necrosed material and presence of stromal edema around the ulcer.

5) Anterior chamber :

   may / may not show pus

   in bacterial corneal ulcer : Hypopyon is sterile

6) *Iris* : muddy colour
7) *Pupil :* may be small
8) ↑ IOP in some cases

Complications :

1) Corneal scarring :

   Slight blurring of vision to total blindness.

2) Perforation of Corneal ulcer :
   - Due to sudden strain of cough/sneeze
   - Can lead to :
     a) Iris prolapse
     b) Adherent leukoma
     c) Staphyloma
     d) Phthisis bulbi.
     e) Corneal fistula
     f) Endophthalmitis

3) Secondary Glaucoma
4) Toxic Iridocyclitis
5) Descemetocele :
   - Herniation of Descemet membrane

Management :

I) Clinical Evaluation :

1) *History Taking :* Mode of onset
2) General Examination
3) *Occular Examination :*
   - Diffuse light examination for lesions of lids, conjunctiva, cornea.
   - Regurgitation test to rule out lacrimal sac infection.
4) *Lab Investigations :*

   Routine : Hb, TLC, DLC, ESR, Blood sugar, urine, stool.

   Microbiological investigation

II) Treatment :

1) Of Uncomplicated ulcer :

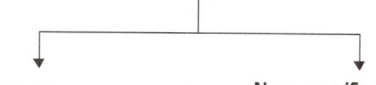

Specific Treatment	Non specific Treatment
a) Topical Antibiotics (to cover both gram positive & negative)	a) Cycloplegics
Any of the two :	1% Atropine to decrease ciliary muscle spasm & to prevent posterior synechiae formation
i) fortified cefazolin 5%	
ii) fortified Tobramycin 1.3%	
OR	b) Analgesics, Antiin-flammatory agents

fortified Vancomycin every 5 mins for 30 mins then

every 15 mins for 2 hrs then

every 1 hrly for 1st 48 hrs then

till healing { 2 hrly during the day &
is ensured { 4 hrly at night

then 4-6 hrly till occurance of healing.

b) Systemic Antibiotics : cepha-losporin/ciprofloxacin

c) Vitamins A, B, C

- **GENERAL MEASURES :**

    1) Hot fomentation (local heat application)

    2) Dark goggles use

    3) Rest, good diet, fresh air.

2) Of Non healing ulcer :

a) Removal of known cause of non healing ulcer (foreign body, inadequate therapy, wrong diagnosis, DM, Anemia, Malnutrition).

b) Mechanical debridement of ulcer :

    by scraping floor of ulcer with spatula.

c) Cauterization of ulcer :

    with pure carbolic acid.

d) Bandage / Soft contact lenses

e) Peritomy.

3) Of impending perforation :

a) No strain (avoid sneezing, coughing, straining during stool)

b) Pressure bandage.

c) Decrease IOP (Acetazolamide, mannitol)

d) Tissue adhesive glue

e) Bandage/soft contact lenses

f) Conjunctival flap

g) Amniotic membrane transplantation

h) Penetrating therapeutic keratoplasty.

4) Of perforation :

Urgent tectonic keratoplasty

+

(e) (f) (g) (h) from impending perforation.

❑ HYPOPYON CORNEAL ULCER : (Fig 2.4)

☞ Hypopyon is accumulation of polymorphonuclear leucocytes in the lower angle of anterior chamber.

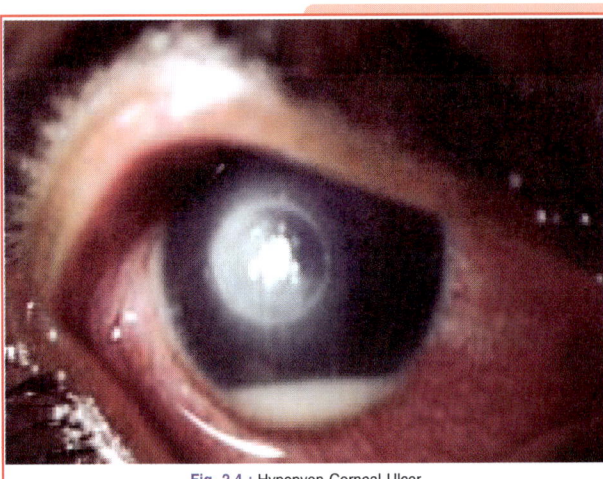

Fig. 2.4 : Hypopyon Corneal Ulcer

☞ Any corneal ulcer may be associated with hypopyon however it is customary to reserve the term 'Hypopyon corneal ulcer' for characteristic ulcer caused by 'Pneumococcus' and is known as 'Ulcus serpens'.

☞ Corneal ulcer with hypopyon is used for ulcer associated with hypopyon due to other causes such as :

a) Staphylococcus

b) Streptococcus

c) Gonococcus

d) Moraxella

e) Fungi

☞ Source of infection is mostly Chronic Dacryocystitis.

☞ It is yellowish white ulcer occuring near the centre of cornea, creep over the cornea in serpiginous fashion.

☞ Hypopyon in bacterial causes is sterile since outpouring of leucocytes is due to the toxin and not due to invasion by bacteria.

☞ On other hand, hypopyon in fungal (mycotic) ulcer is non-sterile as there is direct invasion by the fungi.

Clinical features ⎫ Same as Bacterial
Management   ⎬ Corneal Ulcer

❑ MYCOTIC (FUNGAL) CORNEAL ULCER :

Etiology :

1) Fungi :

    a) Filamentous :

        ➢ Aspergillus fumigatus (most common)

> ➤ Fusarium
> ➤ Alternaria
> ➤ Cephalosporium
> ➤ Penicillium
> ➤ Curvularia

b) *Yeast :*
> ➤ Candida albicans
> ➤ Cryptococcus

c) *Dimorphic :*
> ➤ Histoplasma
> ➤ Coccidioides
> ➤ Blastomyces

2) *Modes of infection :*

a) Injury by vegetative material such as crop leaf, branch of tree, wooden stick, hay.

Common sufferers are field workers during harvesting season

b) Injury by animal tail.

c) Secondary fungal ulcers are common in patients who are immunosuppressed systemically or locally.

3) *Role of antibiotics & steroids :*

Antibiotics disturb the symbiosis between bacteria & fungi and steroids make the fungi facultative pathogens which are otherwise symbiotic saprophytes.

Clinical features :

ᴦ Symptoms are similar to the bacterial corneal ulcer but in general are less marked than equal sized bacterial ulcer.

ᴦ Signs are more prominent than symptoms.

a) Greyish white dry looking ulcer with elevated rolled out feathery & hyphate margins. **(Fig. 2.5)**

b) Feathery finger like extension into surrounding stroma under intact epithelium.

c) Sterile immune ring (yellow line) of Wessely. **(Fig. 2.6)**

d) Multiple small satellite lesions. **(Fig. 2.5)**

e) Non-sterile (infected) hypopyon. **(Fig. 2.5)**

> *i.e.* pseudohypopyon containing the fungus.

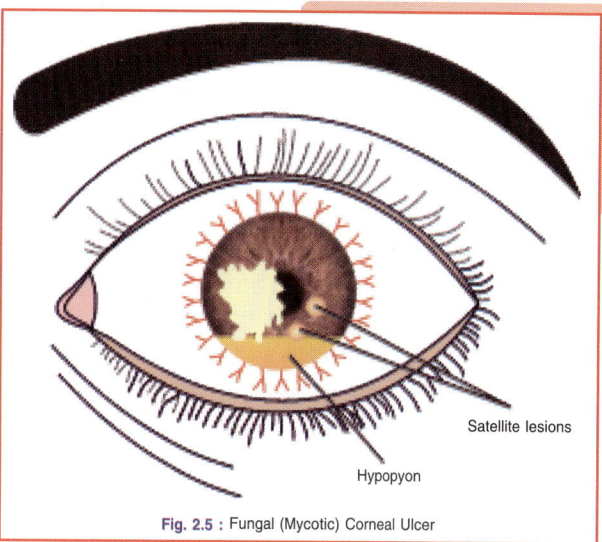

Satellite lesions

Hypopyon

Fig. 2.5 : Fungal (Mycotic) Corneal Ulcer

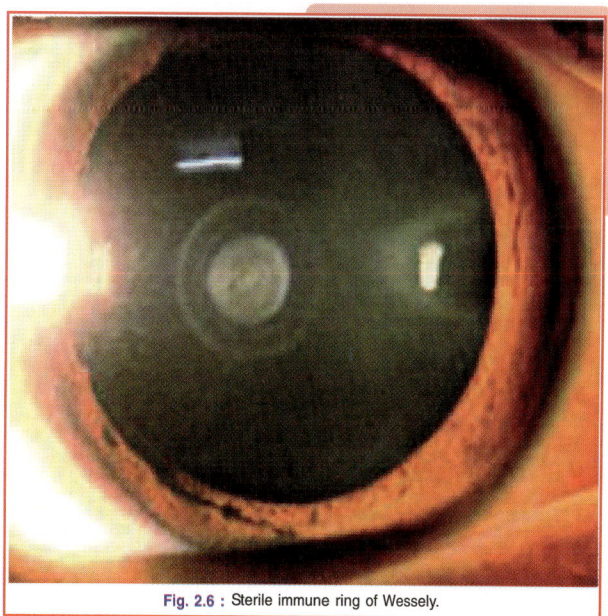

Fig. 2.6 : Sterile immune ring of Wessely.

f) Perforation is rare.

g) Corneal Vascularization is absent.

Diagnosis :

1) Clinical manifestations associated with history of injury by vegetative material.

2) Chronic ulcer worsening inspite of most efficient treatment.

3) Lab investigations :

Examination by wet KOH and culture on Sabouraud's agar reveals :

a) filamentous fungi – A. fumigatus, fusarium

b) Non-filamentous – Candida (yeast like)

4) Confocal microscopic examination.

5) PCR.

Treatment :

A) Specific :

i) Topical antifungals

> for filamentous fungi (Aspergillus, fusarium) : Natamycin eye drops 5% are DOC, every 1 hourly for 6-8 weeks. Miconazole ointment, Amphotericin B.

> for yeast (candida) : Amphotericin B. is DOC, Nystatin, flucytosine.

ii) Intracameral & intracorneal / intrastromal administration of voriconazole.

iii) Systemic antifungals :

Tab fluconazole, ketoconazole, voriconazole for 2-3 weeks.

B) Adjunctive :

Cycloplegic (1% Atropine ointment or drop is DOC) used to :

⌦ reduce ciliary muscle spasm.

⌦ prevent posterior synechiae formation.

⌦ reduce uveal inflammation.

C) Non-specific/General measures :

similar to bacterial corneal ulcer.

D) Therapeutic penetrating keratoplasty.

☞ Topical steroids enhances fungal replication and corneal invasion and are contraindicated during early therapy of fungal corneal ulcer.

☐ HERPES SIMPLEX CORNEAL ULCER (Keratitis) :

☞ Most common viral corneal ulcer.

Etiology :

1) HSV (Herpes simplex virus)

HSV-I : causes infection above the waist.

HSV-II : causes infection below the waist.

2) Mode of infection :

HSV-I : Kissing or close contact with patient suffering from herpes labialis.

HSV II : Transmitted to eyes of neonates through infected genitalia of mother.

Clinical features :

2 forms :

A) Primary Herpes :

Unilateral blepharoconjunctivitis characterized by vesicles on skin of lids, follicular conjunctivitis, preauricular lymphadenopathy, punctate keratitis (sometimes).

B) Recurrent ocular herpes :

After primary infection, recurrent disease involve any or all layers of cornea. Divided into :

a) Epithelial keratitis :

i) Corneal vesicles : vesicles coalesce & erupt to form dendritic/geographic ulcer.

ii) Superficial punctate keratitis.

iii) Dendritic ulcer : Typical lesion of herpes keratitis. There is associated marked diminution of sensation. **(Figs. 2.7 & 2.8)**

iv) Geographic (amoeboid) ulcer.

b) Stromal keratitis :

2 types :

i) Disciform keratitis : **(Fig. 2.9)**

due to the damage to endothelial cells as a result of hypersensitivity to HSV antigen.

ii) Diffuse stromal necrotic keratitis : due to active viral invasion & tissue destruction.

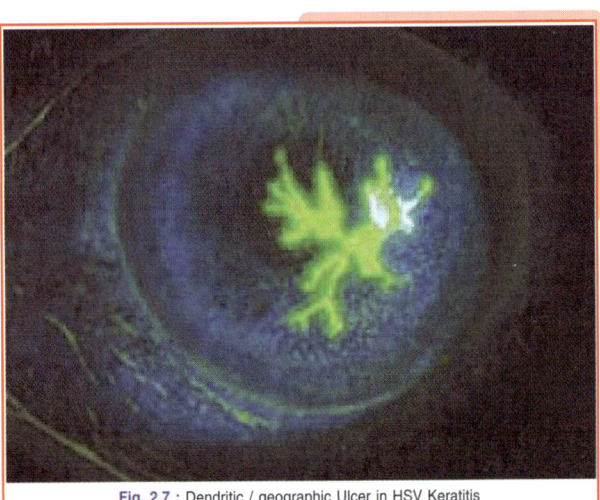

Fig. 2.7 : Dendritic / geographic Ulcer in HSV Keratitis

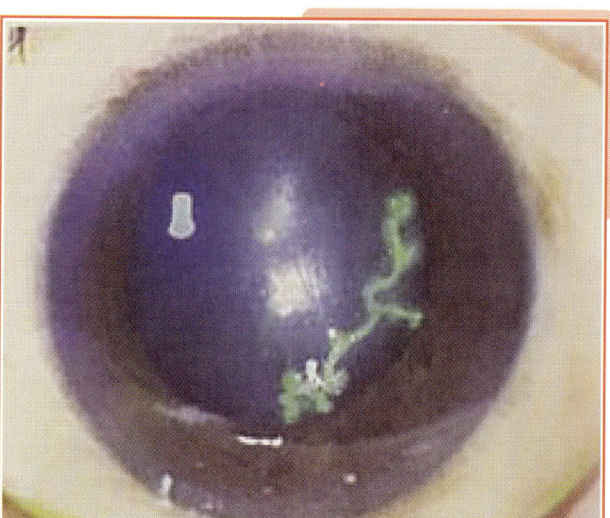

Fig. 2.8 : HSV Dendritic Keratitis

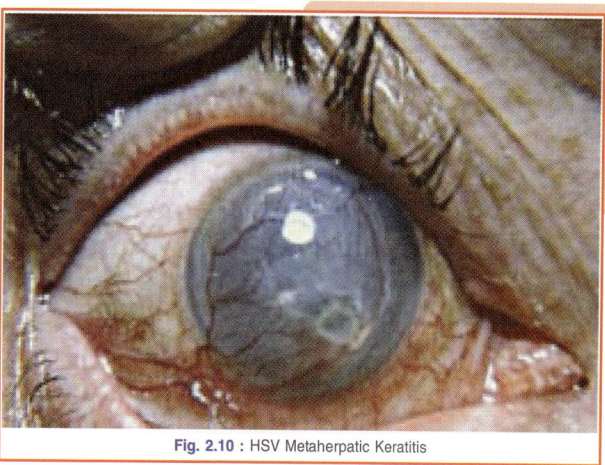

Fig. 2.10 : HSV Metaherpatic Keratitis

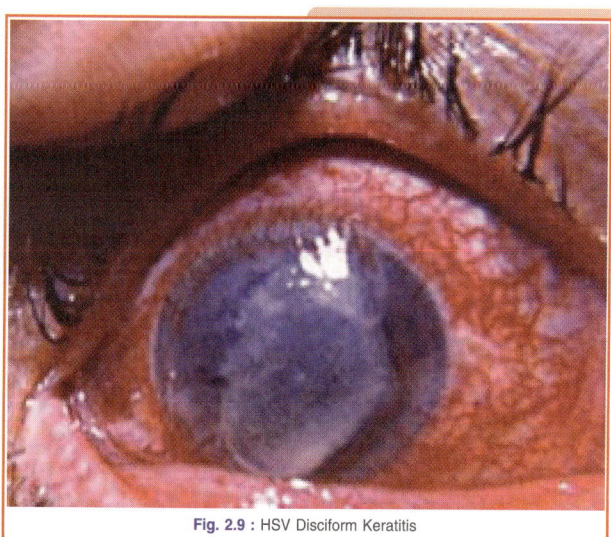

Fig. 2.9 : HSV Disciform Keratitis

c) *Metaherpatic keratitis (epithelial sterile trophic ulceration) :* **(Fig. 2.10)**

> ➢ not an active disease.

> ➢ it is mechanical healing problem at the site of previous herpetic ulcer.

> ➢ indolent linear/ovoid epithelial defect.

Treatment :

Depends upon the type of keratitis :

1) *Primary ocular herpes :*

Usually self limited, treatment is recommended to limit the corneal involvement :

- ✎ Topical trifluridine/vidarabine.

- ✎ Oral Acyclovir.

- ✎ Atropine may be added to reduce ciliary muscle spasm.

2) *Recurrent ocular herpes :*

a) *Epithelial (dendritic, geographic, punctate keratitis) :*

> ➢ Topical antivirals (Acyclovir, Gancyclovir, Triflurothymidine, Vidarabine, Idoxuridine are DOC). 5 times a day for 2-3 weeks.

> ➢ Topical steroids are contraindicated.

> ➢ Systemic antivirals (Acyclovir 3 times a day for 2-3 weeks).

> ➢ Mechanical debridement of infected epithelium.

> ➢ Non-specific/general measures as bacterial ulcer.

b) *Stromal (disciform/diffuse stromal necrotic) :*

> ➢ Topical steroids 4-5 times a day along with Topical/oral Acyclovir twice a day.

> ➢ Non-specific/general measures as bacterial ulcer.

c) *Metaherpetic keratitis :*

Neither topical steroids nor antivirals are used. Treatment is aimed at promoting the healing by :

i) use of lubricants (artificial tears).

ii) bandage / soft contact lens.

iii) Tarsorrhaphy (lid closure).

❑ CORNEAL OPACITIES :

⚘ Corneal opacity means loss of normal transparency of cornea due to scarring. **(Fig. 2.11)**

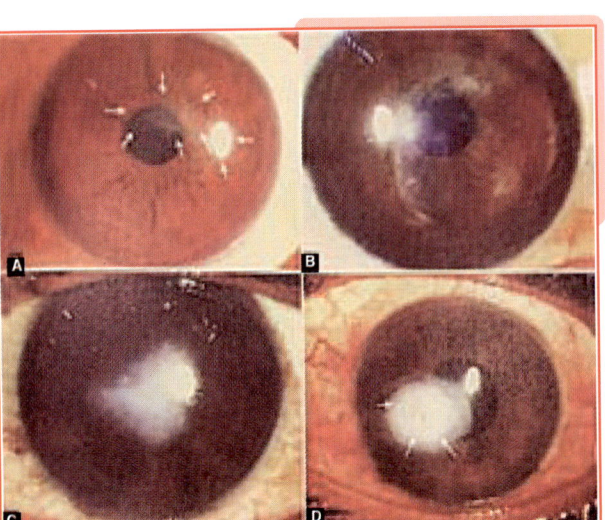

Fig. 2.11 : Corneal Opacity

A : Nebula   B : Macula   C : Leucoma   D : Adherent Leucoma

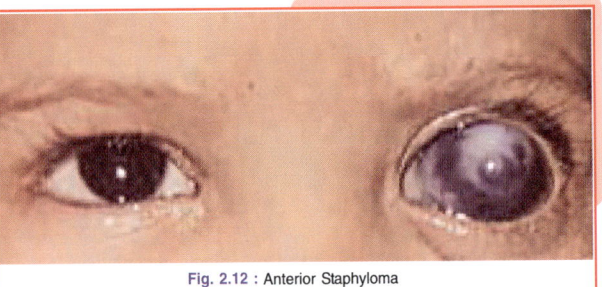

Fig. 2.12 : Anterior Staphyloma

S : Sclerocornea

T : Tear in Descemet's membrane : birth trauma

U : Ulcer (HSV, bacteria)

M : Metabolic (Mucopolysaccharidosis)

P : Posterior corneal defect (Peter's anomaly)

E : Endothelial dystrophy (congenital, hereditary)

D : Dermoid

Types :

1) *Nebula* : 'Very faint opacity' due to superficial scar involving Bowman's layer & superficial stroma.

2) *Macula* : 'Semi dense opacity' due to scar in about half of stroma.

3) *Leucoma* : 'Dense opacity' due to scarring in more than half of stroma.

4) *Adherent leucoma* : Occurs when healing occurs after perforation of cornea with incarceration of iris.

5) *Corneal facet* : Corneal surface is depressed at the site of healing.

6) *Kerectasia* : Corneal curvature is increased at the site of opacity.

7) *Anterior Staphyloma* : Ectasia of pseudocornea which results after total sloughing of cornea with iris plastered behind it is called Anterior staphyloma. **(Fig. 2.12)**

Causes :

1) Developmental anomalies or following birth trauma.

2) Healed corneal wounds.

3) Healed corneal ulcer.

Congenital opacities of cornea : 'STUMPED'

Classification

Treatment :

1) *Nebula :*

   a) Lamellar keratoplasty

   b) Phototherapeutic keratectomy with excimer laser (TOC)

2) *Macula/leucoma :*

   a) Keratoplasty

   b) Optical Iridectomy (TOC)

3) *Opacities with blind eye :*

   a) Cosmetic colored contact lens.

   b) Tattooing of scar by Indian black ink, Gold, Platinum.

◻ KERATOPLASTY :

- Also known as Corneal grafting or Corneal transplantation.

- It is an operation in which patient's diseased cornea is replaced by donor's healthy clear cornea, obtained from cadavers.

- Removed from cadaveric donors within 6 hours after death (Golden period), sometimes upto 12 hours after death in countries with cold climate.

- Cornea is transplanted immediately or is preserved in an eye bank by various preservation techniques :

   a) **Short term** : cornea is used within (in MK medium) **48-72 hours (max : 96 hours)**

b) Intermediate (in optisol 6S) : by organ culture methods, cornea is used **within 30 days**

c) Long term : by cryopreservation, cornea is used **within 1 year**

Types of corneal grafting :

1) Full thickness (penetrating) keratoplasty

2) Partial thickness (lamellar) keratoplasty

  ☙ Cornea is immunologically privileged organ hence corneal graft rejection is less common than that of other organs (as it is non vascular).

  ☙ Corneal graft diameter between '7 and 8.5 mm' has more chances of survival.

Penetrating keratoplasty steps :

1) Excision of donor corneal button.

2) Excision of recipient corneal button.

3) Suturing of corneal graft into the host bed.

Indications for penetrating keratoplasty :

1) Corneal edema after previous surgery is the most common indication.

2) Corneal scarring.

3) Corneal dystrophy

4) Corneal degeneration.

5) Corneal infections.

6) Corneal deposits.

7) Medically unresponsive conditions (due to fungi Acanthamoeba).

8) Bullous keratopathy.

9) Keratoconus.

Indications for lamellar keratoplasty :

1) Keratoconus.

2) Corneal ectasia.

3) Corneal dystrophy, degeneration that involves visual axis but spare Descemet's membrane.

4) Surgical induced abnormalities from Refractive Keratotomy or keratomileusis.

5) Tectonic lamellar keratoplasty.

  ☙ to restore normal peripheral corneal thickness that has been abnormally thinned e.g. in Terrien's marginal degeneration, Mouren's ulcer.

  ☙ to restore normal anatomical thickness after surgical excision of tissue from corneal surface such as in Pterygium, Dermoid.

Endothelial keratoplasty (EK) :

  ⚘ Third type of keratoplasty.

  ⚘ Newest form and is gaining widespread popularity.

  ⚘ New type of partial thickness corneal graft in which only inner endothelial layer is replaced, while healthy anterior part of patient's cornea is retained.

Types of EK :

1) DLEK (Deep lamellar EK) / PLK (Posterior lamellar)

2) DSAEK (Descemet stripping automated EK)

   if femto second laser is used : (FS DSΛEK)

3) DMEK (Descemet membrane EK).

  ☙ Speed and quality of visual recovery after EK is much better than the conventional keratoplasty.

Complications of EK :

1) Graft detachment/dislocation : Most common

2) Graft failure

3) Graft rejection

4) CME (Cystoid Macular Edema)

5) RD (Retinal Detachment)

Indications of EK :

1) Fuch's endothelial dystrophy.

2) Posterior polymorphous dystrophy.

3) Pseudophakic corneal edema.

4) Aphakic corneal edema.

5) Failed corneal graft.

6) Irido-corneal endothelium syndrome.

❑ DIFFERENTIAL DIAGNOSIS OF RED EYE :

I) **Conjunctiva :**

  1) Conjunctivitis.

  2) Subconjunctival hemorrhage

  3) Trauma

  4) Dry eye

II) Cornea :

1) Corneal ulcer   4) Laceration

2) Keratitis   5) Abrasion

3) Foreign body   6) Contact lens wear

III) Sclera :

1) Episcleritis

2) Scleritis

IV) Iris & ciliary body :

1) Iridocyclitis

2) Iritis

V) Anterior chamber :

1) Acute angle closure glaucoma

2) Hyphaema

VI) Eyelid :

1) Entropion

2) Ectropion

3) Trichiasis

VII) Orbit :

1) Orbital cellulitis

VIII) Lacrimal apparatus :

1) Acute dacryocystitis

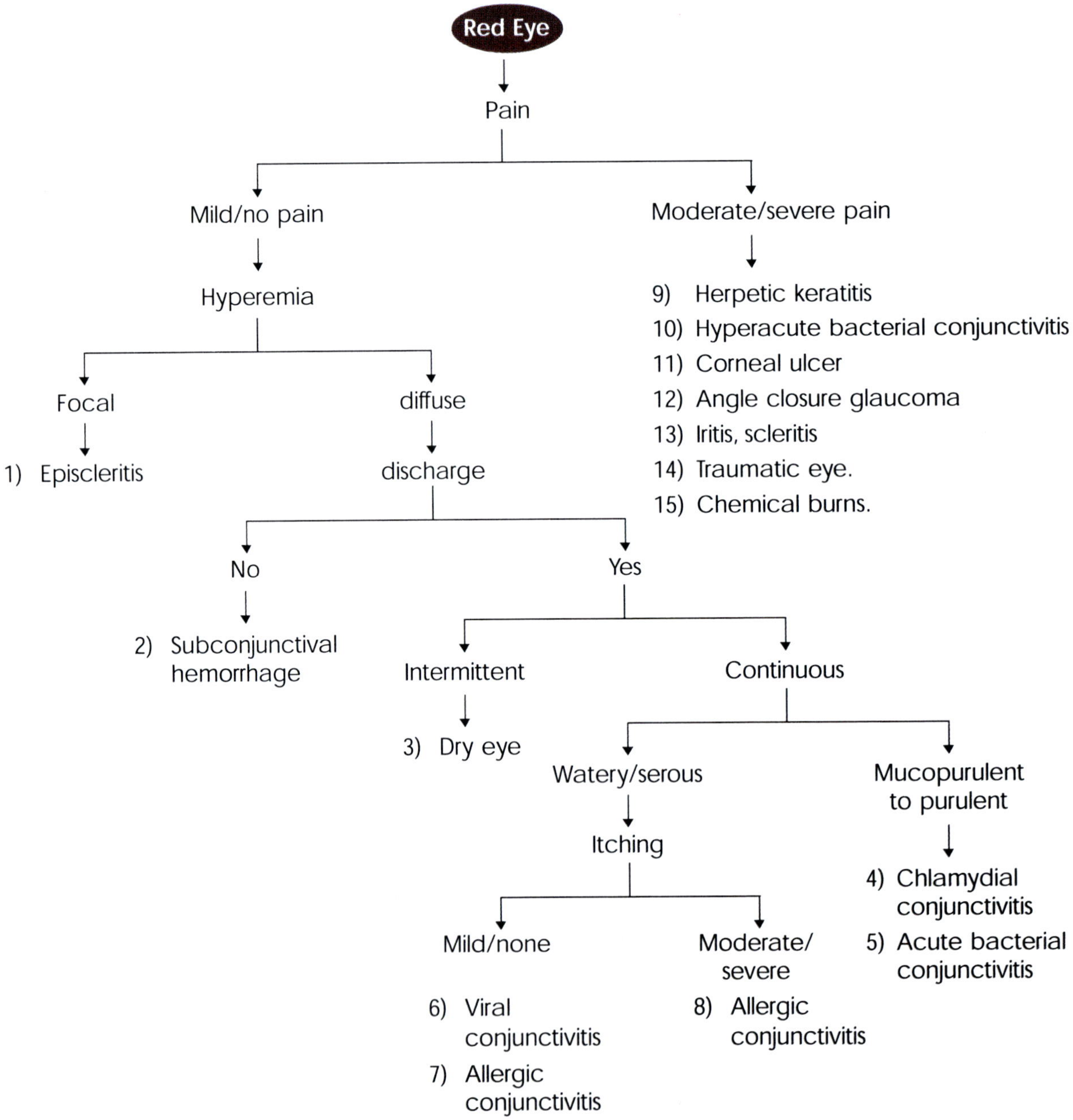

Red Eye

↓

Pain

Mild/no pain   Moderate/severe pain

↓   ↓

Hyperemia   9) Herpetic keratitis
                       10) Hyperacute bacterial conjunctivitis
                       11) Corneal ulcer
Focal   diffuse   12) Angle closure glaucoma
                       13) Iritis, scleritis
1) Episcleritis   14) Traumatic eye.
           discharge   15) Chemical burns.

No   Yes

↓

2) Subconjunctival
   hemorrhage   Intermittent   Continuous

                   ↓

               3) Dry eye   Watery/serous   Mucopurulent
                                                    to purulent
                                  ↓   ↓
                               Itching
                                              4) Chlamydial
                                                 conjunctivitis
               Mild/none   Moderate/   5) Acute bacterial
                              severe   conjunctivitis

            6) Viral   8) Allergic
               conjunctivitis   conjunctivitis

            7) Allergic
               conjunctivitis

☐ INTERSTITIAL KERATITIS :

- ✍ Inflammation of the corneal stroma with or without involvement of posterior corneal layers constitute Deep Keratitis.

- ✍ Deep Keratitis may be :

  a) Non suppurative :
  - ➤ Interstitial keratitis.
  - ➤ Disciform keratitis.
  - ➤ Keratitis profunda.
  - ➤ Sclerosing keratitis.

  b) Suppurative :
  - ➤ Central corneal abscess ⎫ metastatic
  - ➤ Posterior corneal abscess ⎭ in nature.

I) Interstitial keratitis :

- ✎ Inflammation of corneal stroma without primary involvement of epithelium or endothelium.

- ✎ Inflammation may be due to infectious process or due to immunologic response to foreign antigen in form of antigen antibody complex deposition, complement mediated, delayed hypersensitivity reaction.

Etiology :

1) *Viral* : HSV, Herpes zoster, EBV, Mumps, Measles.
2) *Bacterial* : TB, Syphilis, LGV, Leprosy, Lyme disease
3) *Others* : Sarcoidosis, Onchocerciasis, RA, Cogan's syndrome.

A) Syphilitic (Luetic) Interstitial Keratitis :

- ➤ 90% due to congenital syphilis.
- ➤ 10% due to acquired syphilis.

Clinical features :

- ➤ Triad of congenital syphilis is Hutchinson's triad :
  1) Interstitial keratitis.
  2) Hutchinson's teeth.
  3) Vestibular deafness.

- ➤ 3 Stages :
  1) *Initial progressive stage :*
     - ⇒ Keratic precipitates (KPs).

⇒ Pain, lacrimation, photophobia, blepharospasm, circumcorneal injection.

⇒ Diffuse corneal haze which gives ground glass appearance. **(Fig. 2.13)**

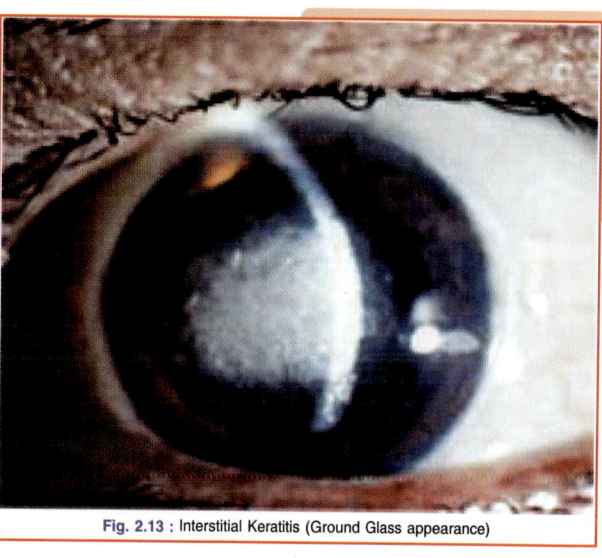

Fig. 2.13 : Interstitial Keratitis (Ground Glass appearance)

2) *Florid stage :*
   - ⇒ deep vascularization of cornea, consisting of radial bundle of brush like vessels.
   - ⇒ As these vessels are covered by hazy cornea, they look dull reddish pink which is called 'Salmon patch appearance'.

3) Regression stage :
   - ⇒ Resolution of lesion leaves behind some opacities and ghost vessels. **(Fig. 2.14)**

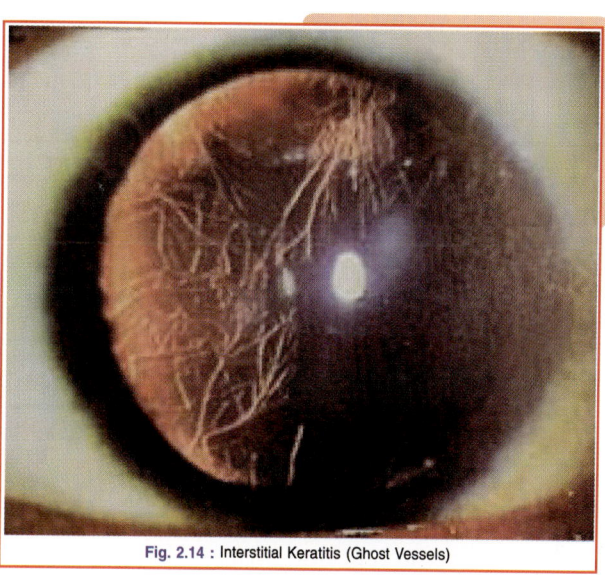

Fig. 2.14 : Interstitial Keratitis (Ghost Vessels)

Management :

Investigations :

1) Clinical examination.

2) VDRL test.

3) T. pallidum immobilization test.

Treatment :

1) <u>Local treatment</u> :
   - ⇨ Topical corticosteroids : dexamethasone every 2-3 hours.
   - ⇨ Atropine ointment 2-3 times a day.
   - ⇨ Dark goggles for photophobia.
   - ⇨ Keratoplasty for corneal opacities.

2) <u>Systemic treatment</u> :
   - ⇨ High dose penicillin.
   - ⇨ Systemic steroids.

B) <u>Tuberculous Interstitial Keratitis</u> :

➢ ***Clinical features*** similar to syphilitic Interstitial keratitis except that it is more frequently unilateral and sectorial (usually in lower sector of the cornea).

➢ ***Treatment :***
   1) Systemic antitubercular drugs.
   2) Topical steroids.
   3) Cycloplegics.

C) <u>Cogan's syndrome</u> :

➢ Comprises of Interstitial keratitis, Acute tinnitus, vertigo, deafness.

➢ ***Treatment :***
   1) Topical / Systemic corticosteroids.

☐ KERATOCONUS (Conical Cornea) :

✍ Keratoconus is a progressive, bilateral, non inflammatory ectatic corneal disease characterized by paraxial stromal thinning and weakening that leads to corneal surface distortion. **(Figs. 2.15 & 2.16)**

Etiology :

Still not clear. May be due to :

1) Developmental anomalies.

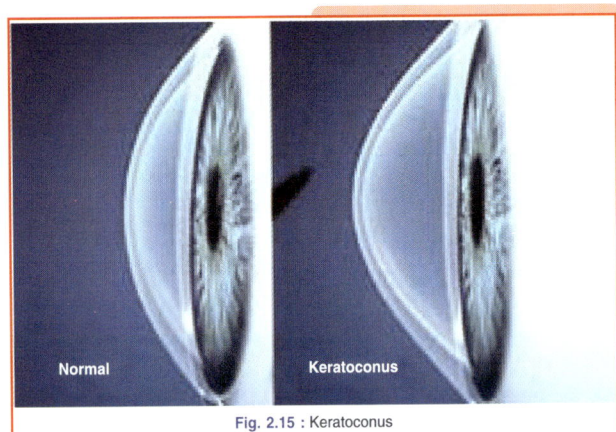
Fig. 2.15 : Keratoconus

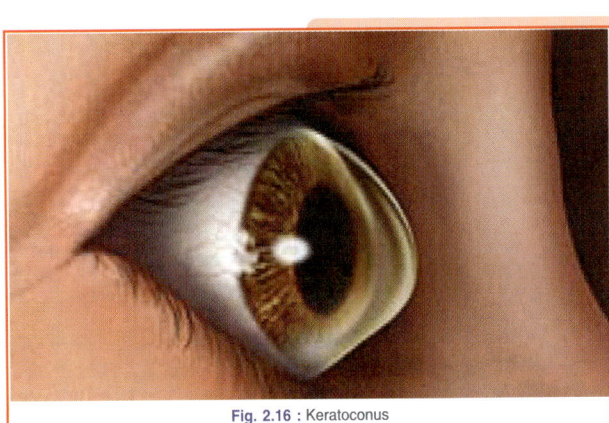
Fig. 2.16 : Keratoconus

2) Degenerative changes.

3) Hereditary dystrophy.

4) Endocrine anomaly.

Pathogenesis :

Defective mucopolysaccharide & collagen synthesis

↓

Progressive thinning and ectasia.

Clinical features :

A) *Symptoms :*

1) Begins as blurred vision with shadowing around the images.

2) Progressive blurring of vision and vision becomes distorted.

3) Glare.

4) Halos around the light.

5) Light sensitivity & ocular irritation.

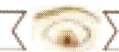
6) Visual loss occurs :

Primarily from : Irregular Astigmatism, Progressive Myopia.

Secondarily from : Corneal scarring.

B) Signs :

- ✎ Hallmark of keratoconus is :

    a) Central or paracentral stromal thinning.

    b) Apical protrusion of anterior cornea.

    c) Irregular Astigmatism.

- ✎ Examination findings :

    1) Distorted window reflex (corneal reflex).

    2) Placido disc examination shows irregularity of circles.

    3) Slit lamp examination shows :

        a) Thinning and ectasia of central cornea.

        b) Opacity at the apex.

        c) 'Fleischer's Ring' at the base of cone : Seen by using cobalt blue light. **(Fig. 2.17)**

        d) Folds in Descemet's & Bowman's membrane. **(Fig. 2.18)**

        e) Vogt lines (very fine, vertical, deep stromal stria) which disappear with external pressure on the globe. **(Fig. 2.19)**

    4) Retinoscopy :

        'Yawning reflex (Scissor reflex)' and high oblique or irregular Astigmatism.

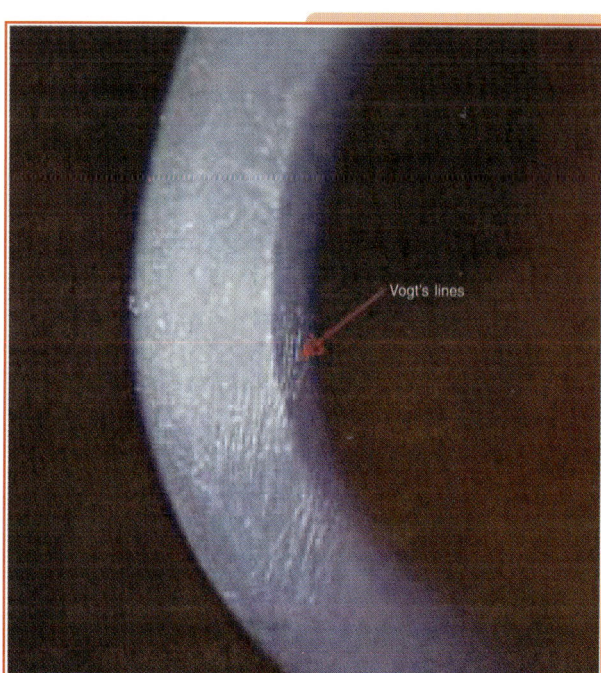

Fig. 2.18 : Folds in Descemet's & Bowman's Membrane

Vogt's lines

Fig. 2.19 : Vogt's lines (striae)

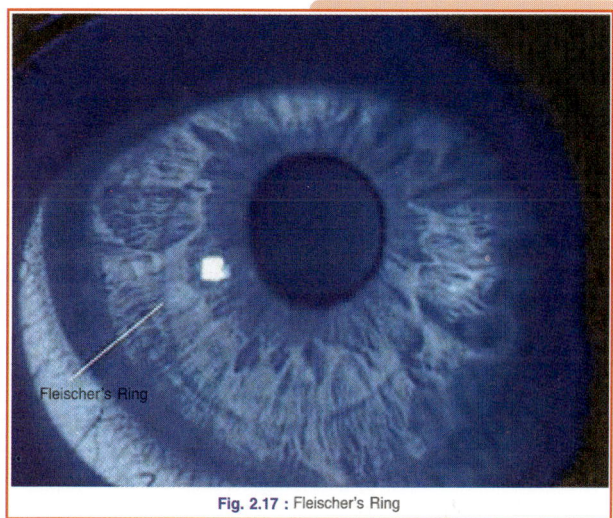

Fleischer's Ring

Fig. 2.17 : Fleischer's Ring

5) Distant direct ophthalmoscopy :

'Oil droplet reflex' *i.e.* an annular shadow which separates the central and peripheral areas of cornea.

6) Munson's sign : **(Fig. 2.20)**

Localized bulging of lower lid when patient looks down. It is a late sign.

7) Prominent corneal nerves.

8) Keratometry : Normal is 45D.

In keratoconus it is increased.

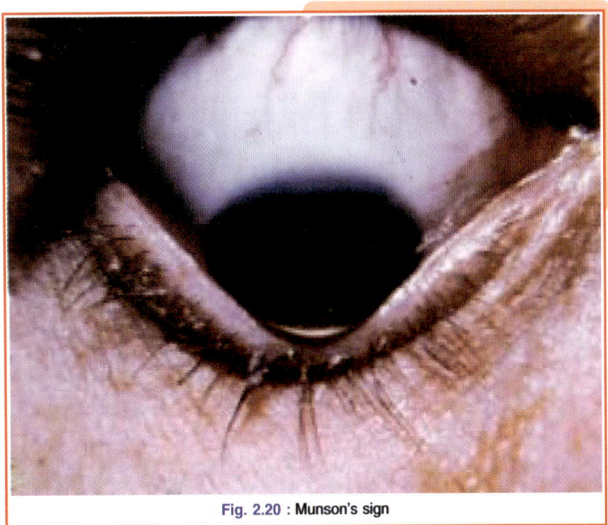

Fig. 2.20 : Munson's sign

$$\text{Grading of Keratoconus} \begin{cases} \text{Mild} & : < 48\ D \\ \text{Moderate} : 48\text{-}54\ D \\ \text{Severe} & : > 54\ D \end{cases}$$

9) Corneal Topography (study of shape of corneal surface) is most sensitive method for detecting keratoconus.

It can document presence of keratoconus even before keratometric or slit lamp findings becomes apparent.

'Forme fruste' : earliest subclinical form of keratoconus detected on topography.

Morphological classification of keratoconus :

Depending on the size and shape of the cone :

1) Nipple cone (< 5 mm, steep curvature).
2) Oval cone (5-6 mm, ellipsoid shape).
3) Globus cone (> 6 mm, globe like)

Complications :

1) *Acute hydrops :* **(Fig. 2.21)**

due to Descemet's rupture.

Associations :

1) *Ocular conditions :* ☺ **CLEVE(R) AF**

a) Congenital cataract.
b) Leber's congenital amaurosis.
c) Ectopia lentis.
d) VKC vernal keratoconjunctivitis.

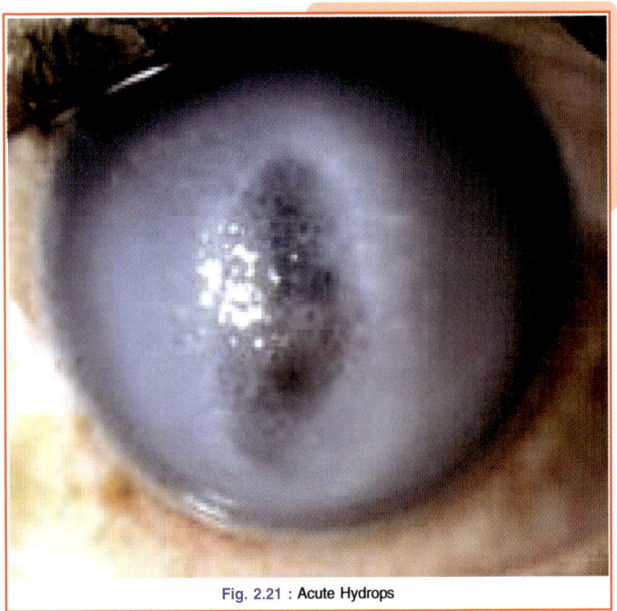

Fig. 2.21 : Acute Hydrops

e) Endothelial dystrophy of cornea.
f) Aniridia.
g) Floppy eyelid syndrome.

2) *Systemic conditions :* ☺ ODEMA

a) Osteogenesis imperfecta.
b) Down's syndrome.
c) Ehler's Danlos syndrome.
d) Marfan's syndrome.
e) Mitral valve prolapse.
f) Atopy.

(Fig. 2.22)

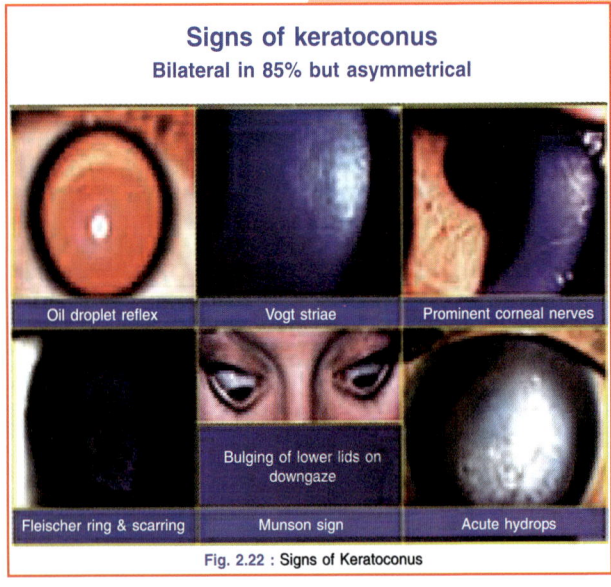

Signs of keratoconus
Bilateral in 85% but asymmetrical

Oil droplet reflex | Vogt striae | Prominent corneal nerves

Bulging of lower lids on downgaze

Fleischer ring & scarring | Munson sign | Acute hydrops

Fig. 2.22 : Signs of Keratoconus

Treatment :

1) Spectacles for regular or mild irregular Astigmatism.

2) Rigid gas permeable contact lens for higher Astigmatism.

3) Rose-K (scleral contact lens) in early to moderate cases, Intacs (intracorneal ring segments) can also be used in early to moderate cases.

4) Corneal collagen cross linking with Riboflavin (CXL or C3R) and UV-A rays slows the progression.

5) Epikeratoplasty in patient intolerant to lens and without significant corneal scarring.

6) DALK (Deep Anterior Lamellar Keratoplasty), PK (Penetrating Keratoplasty) if there is significant corneal scarring.

Chapter

3

Lens

Most Important (Must Read Topics)	Elective Topics
1) Senile cataract	1) Cosmetic contact lens
2) Congenital cataract	2) Ectopia lentis
3) Complicated cataract	3) Metabolic cataract
4) Rosette cataract	4) Blue dot cataract
5) Intra ocular lens	
6) Coronary cataract	
7) Hypermature/Morgagnian cataract	
8) Phacoemulsification	

☐ SENILE CATARACT :

Cataract is opacity (clouding) of the crystalline lens of the eye or in its envelope (capsule). **(Fig. 3.1)**

I. **Classification :**

A) *Etiological :* (☺ **STEM DOTS CR**)

1) Senile Cataract

2) Traumatic Cataract

3) Electric Cataract

4) Metabolic Cataract

5) Dermatogenic Cataract

6) Osseous diseases leading to Cataract

7) Toxic (corticosteroids, Miotics, Cu, Fe) Cataract

8) Syndromes (Treacher collins, Down's,

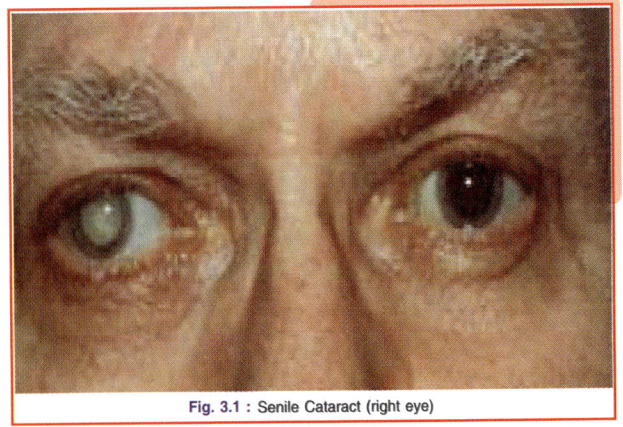

Fig. 3.1 : Senile Cataract (right eye)

Lowe, Dystrophia myotonica) leading to Cataract

9) Complicated cataract

10) Radiational cataract

B) *Morphological :*

1) *Capsular cataract :*
   ⇨ Anterior
   ⇨ Posterior

2) Subcapsular cataract
   ⇨ Anterior
   ⇨ Posterior

3) Cortical cataract

4) Supranuclear cataract

5) Nuclear cataract

6) Polar cataract :
   ⇨ Anterior
   ⇨ Posterior

II. Etiopathogenesis :

1) Hereditary

2) Diabetes Mellitus

3) UV Radiations

4) Nutritional deficiency (A.C.E.)

5) Age :
   ➢ Usually occurs after the age of 50 years.
   ➢ If it occurs before 45 years, it is called pre-senile cataract.

a) *Cortical cataract :*

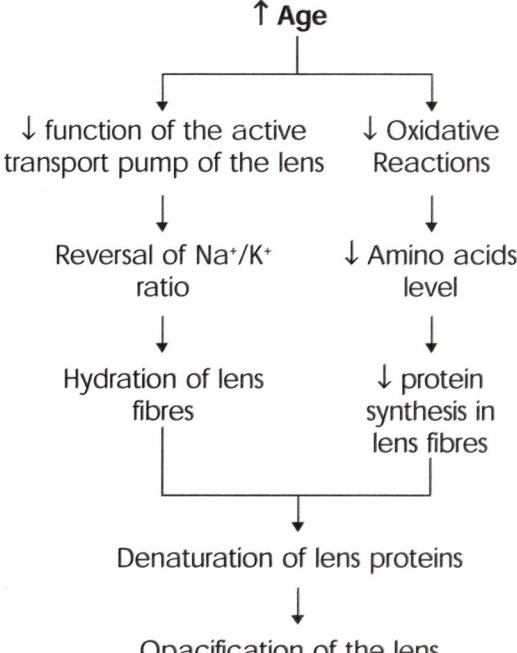

↑ **Age**

↓ function of the active transport pump of the lens → Reversal of Na⁺/K⁺ ratio → Hydration of lens fibres

↓ Oxidative Reactions → ↓ Amino acids level → ↓ protein synthesis in lens fibres

Denaturation of lens proteins

Opacification of the lens

b) *Nuclear cataract :*

Intensification of age related nuclear sclerosis
↓
Hydration & compaction of the lens nucleus
↓
Hard cataract

III. Stages of cataract :

a) *Cortical cataract :*

1) *Stage of lamellar seperation :*
   ⇨ demarcation of cortical fibres owing to the separation by fluid.
   ⇨ Reversible stage.

2) *Stage of Incipient cataract :*
   ⇨ Early detectable opacities with clear areas between them.

   a) Cuneiform cataract : **(Fig. 3.2)**
      ❏ Wedge shaped cataract with clear areas between them.
      ❏ Typical radial spoke like pattern of greyish white opacities.
      ❏ Starts at the periphery and extends centrally so visual disturbances are seen at later stages.

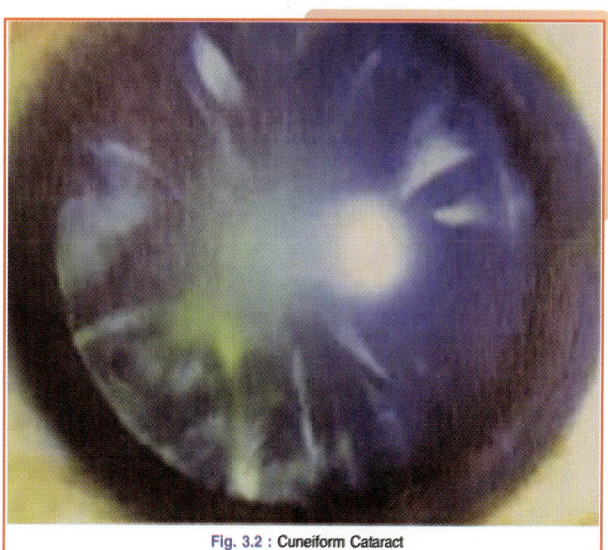

Fig. 3.2 : Cuneiform Cataract

b) <u>Cupuliform cataract</u> :

- ❑ Saucer shaped deformity below the capsule.
- ❑ Central part is affected first and than extends outwards so lies right in path of axial rays and thus early loss of visual acuity.

3) *Immature senile cataract :* **(Fig. 3.3)**

- ⇨ Lens appears 'greyish white'.
- ⇨ Opacification progresses further but clear cortex is visible.

      └⮞ So, Iris shadow is visible.

- ⇨ also called as 'Intumescent cataract'.
- ⇨ gives 'sectorial markings with mother of pearl appearance'.

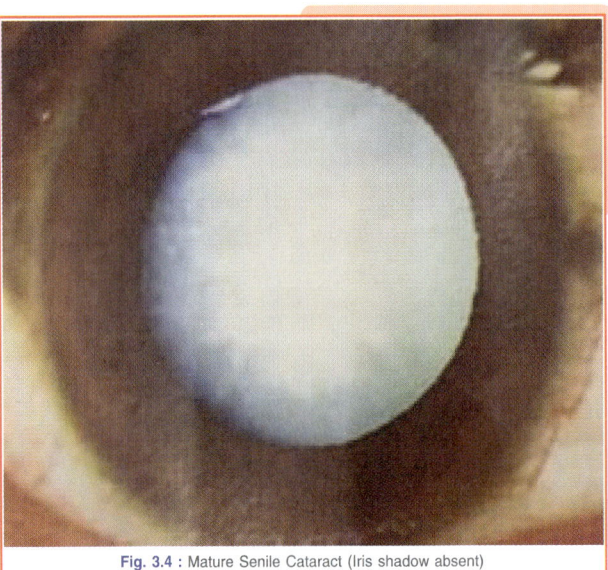
Fig. 3.4 : Mature Senile Cataract (Iris shadow absent)

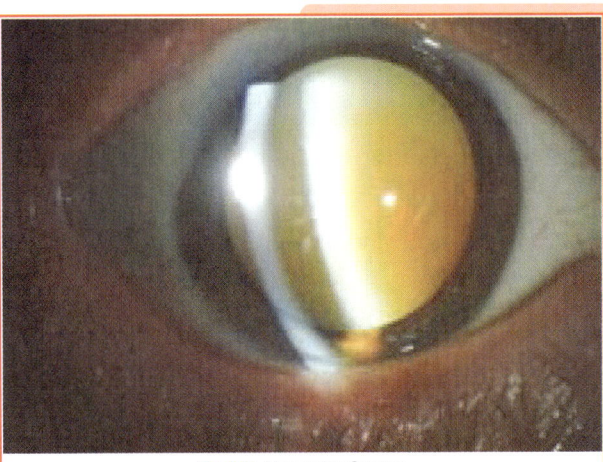
Fig. 3.5 : Morgagnian Cataract

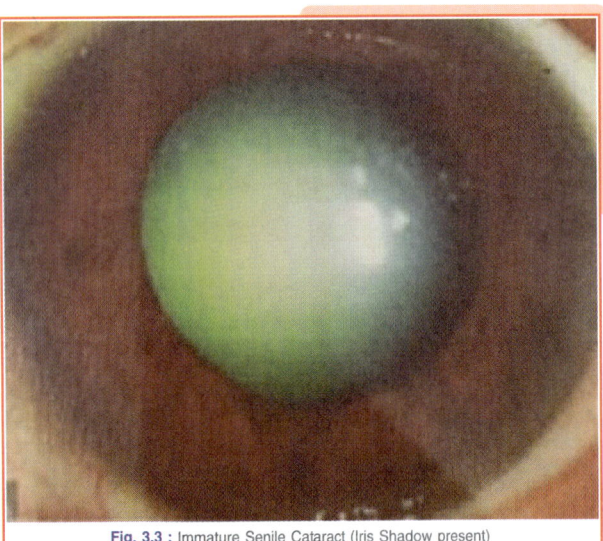
Fig. 3.3 : Immature Senile Cataract (Iris Shadow present)

4) *Mature senile cataract :* **(Fig. 3.4)**

- ⇨ Opacification is complete
- ⇨ Lens appears 'pearly white'.
- ⇨ Whole of cortex is involved
- ⇨ Iris shadow is not visible
- ⇨ also called as 'Ripe cataract'.

5) *Hypermature cataract :*

a) <u>Morgagnian cataract</u> : **(Fig. 3.5)**

- ❑ Whole of the cortex liquifies

- ❑ Lens is converted into a bag of milky fluid.
- ❑ Small brownish nucleus settles in the bottom, altering its position with the change of position of head.
- ❑ Calcium deposits may also be seen on the capsule

b) <u>Sclerotic cataract</u> : **(Fig. 3.6)**

- ❑ Cortex is disintegrated and lens is shrunken due to the leakage of water.
- ❑ Iridodonesis occurs.

b) *Nuclear cataract :*

- ➤ Nuclear sclerosis → renders the lens

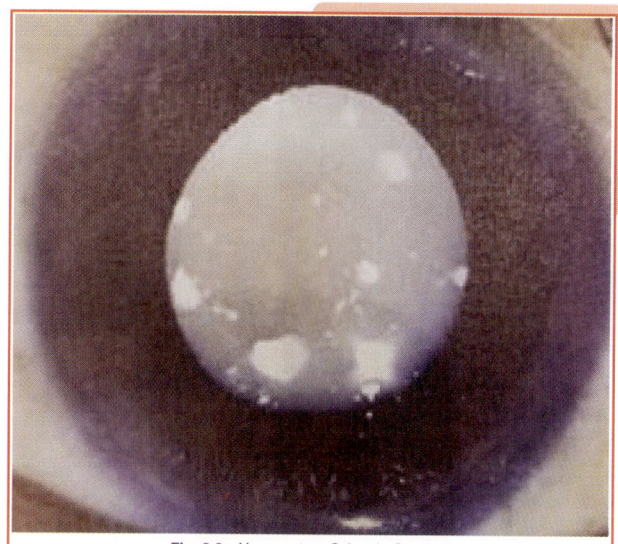

Fig. 3.6 : Hypermature Sclerotic Cataract

inelastic & hard → ↓ ability to accommodate and thus obstruct the light rays.

➤ Central to peripheral involvement.

➤ Nucleus becomes greyish yellow to black due to deposition of pigments, so known as 'Pigmented Nuclear Cataract'.

➤ If colour is :

i) *Brown* : Cataracta brunescens **(Fig. 3.7)**

ii) *Black* : Cataracta nigra **(Fig. 3.8)**

iii) *Reddish* : Cataracta rubra

IV. Symptoms :

1) Gradual, painless, progressive loss of vision

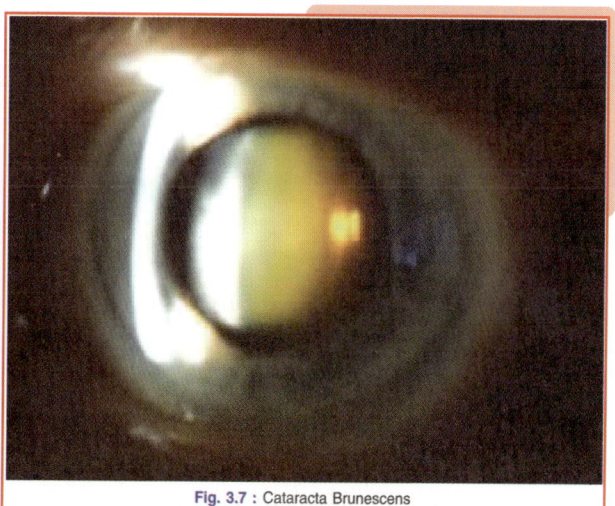

Fig. 3.7 : Cataracta Brunescens

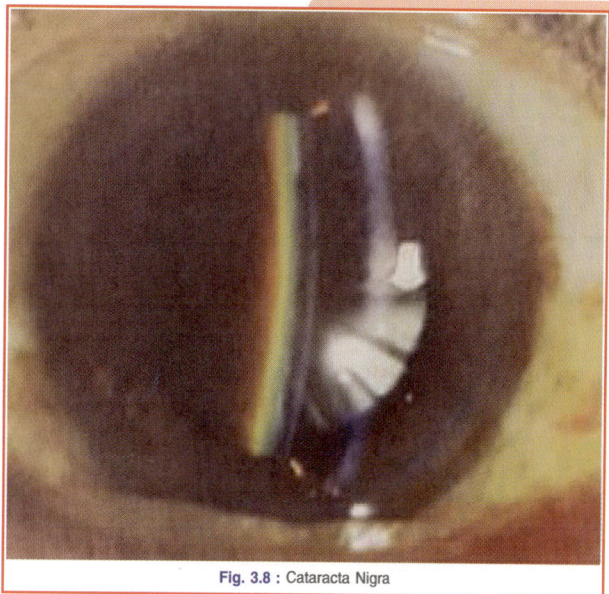

Fig. 3.8 : Cataracta Nigra

2) Visual field loss.

3) Frequent change of glasses

4) Monocular polyopia / diplopia

5) Colored halos.

6) Dark (black) spots infront of the eye.

7) Color shift

8) Glare

9) Loss of contrast sensitivity

10) Second shift/myopic shift

11) Index myopia

12) Index hypermetropia

13) Night blindness

14) Day blindness

Signs :

1) Visual acuity changes.

2) Oblique Illumination :

Color of the lens depends upon the stages.

3) Iris shadow :

In Immature senile cataract.

V. Complications of cataract :

1) Lens Induced Glaucoma :

a) Phacomorphic glaucoma :

➤ Lens swell up by absorbing the fluid resulting in shallow anterior chamber. Angle closes, blocking trabecular meshwork and thus ↑ IOP.

⇨ Type of secondary angle closure glaucoma.

⇨ Most common type of lens induced glaucoma.

⇨ Seen in intumescent stage of senile cataract.

⇨ Also seen in subluxation / dislocation of lens & spherophakia.

b) *Phacolytic Glaucoma :*

⇨ In hypermature stage, lens proteins leak into the anterior chamber and are engulfed by macrophages.

⇨ Leads to clogging of trabecular meshwork → ↑ IOP.

⇨ Type of secondary open angle glaucoma.

c) *Phacotopic Glaucoma :*

⇨ Hypermature lens subluxation / dislocation causes glaucoma by blocking the angle of anterior chamber and pupil.

2) *Lens Induced Uveitis :*

➤ Lens proteins are sequestered antigens. When they leak into the anterior chamber they are treated as foreign, inciting a immune reaction.

➤ Results in anterior uveitis.

➤ Characterised by ciliary congestion, aqueous flare.

3) *Subluxation / Dislocation of Lens :* (Figs. 3.9, 3.10 & 3.11)

➤ In hypermature stage, zonules of the lens may weaken and break. Leads to :

i) Subluxation (when some zonules are still intact and part of lens lies in patellar fossa).

ii) Dislocation (when all zonules are broken and no part of lens lies in patellar fossa).

VI. Management :

A) *Non surgical measures :*

1) Treatment of the cause of cataract

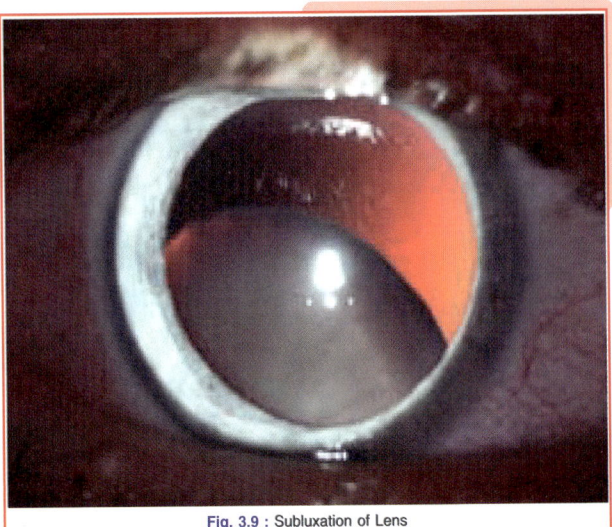

Fig. 3.9 : Subluxation of Lens

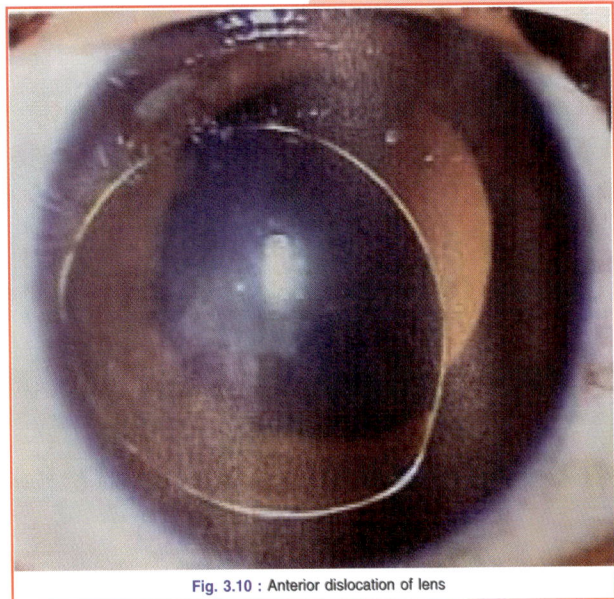

Fig. 3.10 : Anterior dislocation of lens

(DM, Drug removal, Irradiation removal).

2) To delay the progression :

⇨ Topical iodide salts of Ca^{2+}/K^+, Vit. E, Aspirin.

3) To improve the vision in Incipient/ Immature stage :

⇨ Prescription of Refractive glasses.

B) *Surgical Measures :*

➤ *Investigations :*

1) Clinical history

❏ DM/HTN/COPD/UTI etc.

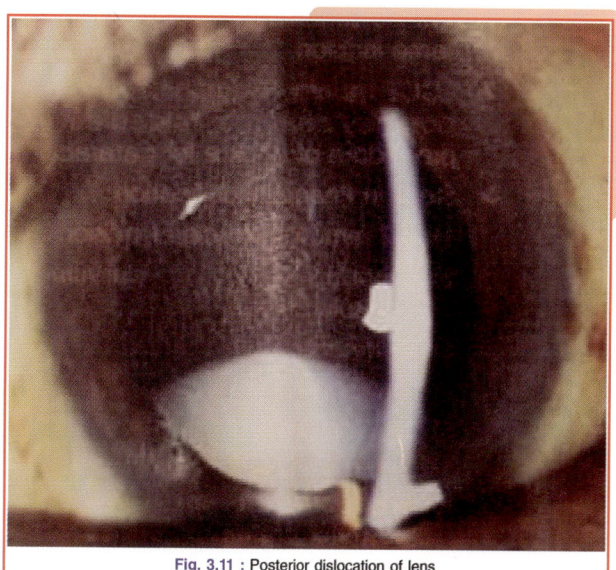

Fig. 3.11 : Posterior dislocation of lens

2) General examination

3) Ophthalmological :

   a) <u>Visual acuity</u> : (Snellen's chart):

      ✦ With unaided, best corrected, pin hole.

      ✦ PL/PR is noted.

   b) <u>Cornea</u> :

      ✦ Keratometry

      ✦ Corneal topography.

   c) <u>Pupil</u> :

      ✦ Apparent pupillary defect.

      ✦ Pupillary reflexes (swinging flash light test, Marcus-Gunn pupil).

   d) <u>Conjunctiva, lids, lacrimal apparatus</u> :

      ✦ In chronic dacryocystitis : DCT/DCR is performed before cataract surgery.

      ✦ ROPLAS (Regurgitation on pressure over lacrimal apparatus and sac).

   e) <u>Anterior chamber</u> :

      ✦ Corneal scarring, KP's (keratic precipitates).

   f) <u>IOT</u> :

      ✦ Tonometry (Digital, schiotz)

      ✦ Gonioscopy.

   g) <u>Slit lamp biomicroscopy</u> :

      ✦ for anterior segment evaluation.

   h) <u>B scan USG</u> :

      ✦ for posterior segment / fundus evaluation.

   i) <u>Contrast sensitivity functions</u> :

      ✦ FACTS (Functional acuity contrast testing).

      ✦ Vision contrast test system.

      ✦ Pelli Robston contrast test.

   j) <u>Retinal / Macular function tests</u> :

      ✦ Light perception

      ✦ Maddox Rod test

      ✦ Color perception

      ✦ Laser inferometry

      ✦ Entoptic visualization

      ✦ ERG (electroretinogram)

      ✦ EOG (electrooculogram)

      ✦ VER (Visual evoked Response)

   k) <u>IOL power calculation</u> :

      ✦ By SRK formula.

      SRK formula, Power of IOL = A-2.5L - 0.9K.

      K : Keratometry.

      L : Axial length of eyeball (Biometry).

      A : Constant.

Pre-operative preparations :

1) <u>Consent</u> :

   Information about the procedure, risk involved, expected outcome.

2) Scrub bath, care of hair, marking of eye.

3) <u>Pre operative antibiotics & disinfectants</u> :

   ➢ Topical Moxifloxacin / Gatifloxacin

   ➢ Povidone Iodine (10% or 5%).

4) IOP lowering

5) <u>Mydriasis</u> :

   ➢ Topical tropicamide

6) <u>Anaesthesia</u> :

General / Local (Local is preferred).

Operative Techniques :

1) ECCE (Extra Capsular Cataract Extraction) :

➢ Nucleus, cortex, central part of the anterior capsule is removed.

➢ Leaving behind intact posterior capsule, peripheral part of the anterior capsule and zonules.

➢ Presently, ECCE with posterior chamber IOL is surgery of choice for all types of cataract.

➢ Only contraindication of ECCE :

Subluxation / Dislocation of lens.

➢ Techniques of ECCE :

1) Conventional ECCE.

2) Manual SICS (Small Incision Cataract Surgery)

3) Phacoemulsification.

2) ICCE (Intra Capsular Cataract Extraction) :

➢ Lens is removed in toto as single piece.

➢ Nucleus, cortex is removed with the capsule after breaking the zonules.

➢ So, no support is left for posterior chamber IOL, only Anterior Chamber IOL can be implanted.

➢ Only Indication for ICCE :

Markedly subluxated / dislocated lens in which zonules are already broken, so ECCE cannot be done.

➢ Contraindication :

In young (< 40 years) because zonules are too strong.

3) Phacoemulsification :

➢ It is an advancement in doing ECCE.

➢ Nucleus is converted into pulp or emulsified using high frequency sound waves and then sucked out of the eye through small (3.2 mm) sclerocorneal junction incision.

➢ Special foldable IOL is inserted into the posterior chamber through the same incision.

➢ ECCE by phacoemulsification with posterior chamber foldable IOL is procedure of choice for cataract.

➢ Steps in Phacoemulsification :

1) 3.2 mm corneoscleral incision.

2) Continuous curvilinear capsulorrhexis.

3) Hydrodissection.

4) Hydrodilineation.

5) Emulsification & Aspiration of the nucleus and then the cortex.

6) Foldable IOL implantation in posterior chamber.

➢ Recovery with phacoemulsification is fastest as incision is very small and no sutures are taken.

Post operative management :

1) Patient is asked to lie down on the back for about 2-3 hours and advised to take nil orally.

2) Diclofenac Na for mild to moderate post operative pain injection.

3) Next morning bandage/eye patch is removed and eye is inspected for any complications (post operative complications).

4) Antibiotic eye drops 4 times a day for 2 weeks.

5) Topical steroids.

6) Topical NSAIDs (Ketorolac).

7) Topical Timolol.

8) Topical Cycloplegic-mydriatic (Homatropine).

9) After 2 months, sutures (SICS, CS) are removed if applied.

10) Spectacles are prescribed :

after 8 weeks in SICS.

after 4 weeks in phacoemulsification.

VII. Complications of cataract surgery :

A) Preoperative complications.

B) Operative complications.

C) Early post operative complications.

D) Late post operative complications.

E) IOL Related complications.

A) Pre-operative complications :

1) **Anxiety :**
   - ⇨ due to fear, apprehension of operation
   - ⇨ Diazepam 2-5 mg bed time may be given.

2) **Nausea, Gastritis :**
   - ⇨ Due to pre operative medications such as acetazolamide.
   - ⇨ Oral antacids or omission of further dose may be prescribed.

3) **Allergic / Irritative conjunctivitis :**
   - ⇨ Due to pre operative topical antibiotics.
   - ⇨ Postpone the operation for 2 days, withdrawl of drugs is required.

4) **Corneal abrasion :**
   - ⇨ During Schiotz tonometry.
   - ⇨ Patching with antibiotic ointment for a day, postpone the operation for 2 days.

5) **Due to local anaesthesia :**
   - ⇨ Subconjunctival, Retrobulbar hemorrhage.
   - ⇨ Occulocardiac reflex (due to retrobulbar block).
   - ⇨ Perforation of the globe.

B) Operative complications :

1) **Superior Rectus laceration :**
   - ⇨ While applying bridle suture in conventional ECCE, SICS.

2) **Excessive bleeding :**
   - ⇨ During incision in Anterior chamber.
   - ⇨ Cauterization of bleeding vessels must be done.

3) **Incision Related Complications :**
   - ⇨ In conventional ECCE : irregular incision.
   - ⇨ In manual SICS, phacoemulsification :
     - a) button holing of anterior wall of the tunnel.
     - b) premature entry into the anterior chamber.
     - c) scleral disinsertion.

4) Injury to cornea (Descemet's membrane), iris, lens.

5) Iridodialysis (tear of iris from the root).

6) **Due to Anterior Capsulorrhexis :**
   - ⇨ Escaping capsulorrhexis.
   - ⇨ Small capsulorrhexis.
   - ⇨ Very large capsulorrhexis.
   - ⇨ Eccentric capsulorrhexis.

7) **Posterior capsule Rupture (PCR) :**
   - ⇨ leads to nuclear drop into the vitreous.

8) **Vitreous loss :**
   - ⇨ due to the rupture of posterior capsule.

9) Zonular dehiscence.

10) Expulsive choroidal hemorrhage.

11) Posterior loss of lens fragments due to PCR.

12) Nucleus drop into the vitreous cavity.

C) Early post operative complications : (till 4 W)

1) **Hyphaema :**
   - ⇨ Collection of blood in the anterior chamber from conjunctival / scleral vessels.
   - ⇨ Most hyphaema absorb spontaneously, needs no treatment.
   - ⇨ If hyphaema is large, associated with ↑ IOP, acetazolamide must be given.
   - ⇨ If not absorbed within a week : Paracentesis must be done to drain the blood.

2) **Iris Prolapse :**
   - ⇨ due to inadequate suturing after ICCE or conventional ECCE.
   - ⇨ must be reposited back and sutured if there is small prolapse.
   - ⇨ for large prolapse : Abscission & suturing.

3) *Striate keratopathy :*

⇨ mild corneal edema with Descemet's fold.

⇨ Rx : Instillation of 5% NaCl along with steroids.

4) *Flat (shallow) anterior chamber :*

⇨ due to wound leak, pupillary block.

5) *Post operative anterior uveitis :*

⇨ due to the trauma by instruments.

⇨ Rx : Use of topical steroids, cycloplegics, NSAID's.

6) *Bacterial endophthalmitis :*

⇨ most dreaded complication.

⇨ due to contaminated solutions, instruments, surgeon's hands, patients own flora from conjunctiva, eyelids, airborne bacteria.

⇨ Rx : Antibiotics, steroids, cycloplegics are given.

7) *TASS (Toxic anterior segment syndrome).*

D) *Late post operative complications : (4W - 1 year)* ☺ A B C D E F G

1) *After cataract :*

⇨ also called as secondary cataract.

⇨ It is opacity which persists or develops after extracapsular lens extraction.

⇨ most common complication of ECCE.

⇨ Cause :

a) Residual opaque lens matter.

b) Proliferative type of cataract.

⇨ Clinical features : **(Fig. 3.12)**

a) Thickened posterior capsule.

b) Dense membranous after cataract

c) Soemmering's Ring :

thick ring of after cataract behind the iris enclosed between two layers of the capsule.

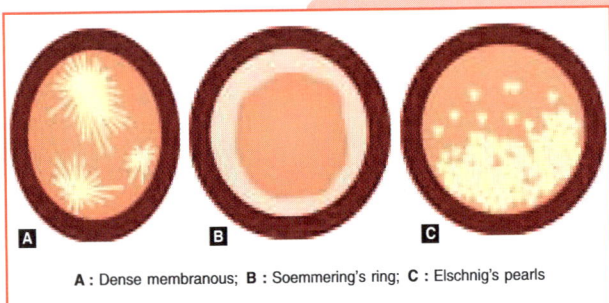

A : Dense membranous; **B :** Soemmering's ring; **C :** Elschnig's pearls

Fig. 3.12 : After Cataract : Clinical features

d) Elschnig's pearls :

vacuolated epithelial cells are clustered like soap bubbles along the posterior capsule.

⇨ Treatment :

a) if thin : Nd:YAG laser capsulotomy, discission with cystitome or Zieglar's knife.

b) thick membranous : Surgical membranectomy.

c) Soemmering's ring, with clean posterior capsule : no treatment.

d) Elschnig's pearls : Nd YAG laser capsulotomy.

2) *Bullous Keratopathy :*

⇨ due to surgical, chemical injury to the cornea.

⇨ Rx : Penetrating keratoplasty is done.

3) *Cystoid macular edema (CME) :*

⇨ Collection of fluid in Henle's layer of macula.

⇨ On fundoscopy : Honeycomb appearance.

⇨ On fluoroscein angiography : Flower petal pattern.

⇨ Causes :

a) vitreous incarceration in wound

b) due to prostaglandins.

⇨ Treatment :

Anterior vitrectomy with steroids, Anti prostaglandins.

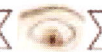

4) *Retinal Detachment :*

more common in aphakics and in ICCE.

5) *Delayed chronic post operative endophthalmitis :*

⇨ when organism of low virulence (propionobacterium acne, staph epidermidis) is trapped in capsular bag.

⇨ Fungal endophthamitis characterized by 'Puff ball vitreous exudates'.

⇨ <u>Treatment</u> : Pars plana vitrectomy, Antifungal drugs.

6) *Epithelial Ingrowth :*

⇨ conjunctival epithelium invade the anterior chamber through defect in incision.

⇨ grows, lines back of the cornea and trabecular meshwork leading to Glaucoma.

7) *Fibrous Downgrowth :*

⇨ into the anterior chamber, cause secondary glaucoma.

8) *Glaucoma in aphakia/pseudophakia.*

E) IOL Related Complications :

1) Complications like corneal endothelial damage, uveitis, CME, secondary glaucoma :

mostly with iris supported IOL.

2) *UGH syndrome :*

Uveitis, Glaucoma, Hyphaema :

mostly with rigid type of IOL.

3) *TASS (Toxic anterior segment syndrome) :*

Uveal inflammation by ethylene gas which is used to sterile the IOL (in early case), or by lens material (in late case).

4) Pupillary capture of IOL.

5) *Malpositioning of IOL :*

a) Sunset syndrome (inferior dislocation)

b) Sunrise syndrome (superior dislocation)

c) Lost lens syndrome (complete dislocation into the vitreous cavity).

d) Windshield wiper syndrome :

❑ when very small IOL is placed vertically in the sulcus.

❑ superior loop moves left and right with movements of the head.

◘ CONGENITAL CATARACT :

⬨ Occurs due to the disturbances in development and growth of the lens. **(Fig. 3.13)**

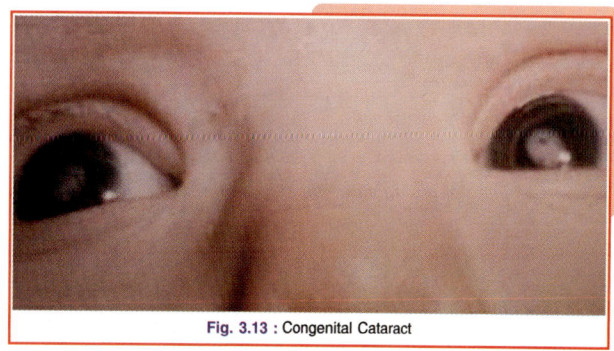

Fig. 3.13 : Congenital Cataract

⬨ It may be :

a) Congenital cataract.

b) Developmental cataract.

a) **Congenital cataract :**

➢ Present at birth.

➢ Opacity is limited to embryonic or foetal nucleus.

b) **Developmental cataract :**

➢ from infancy to adolescence.

➢ Opacity involves infantile or adult nucleus, deeper parts of the cortex, capsule.

Etiology :

1) *Idiopathic :* 1/3ʳᵈ of total congenital cataract.

2) *Hereditary :* 1/3ʳᵈ of total congenital cataract.

✎ Chromosomal (Trisomy 21)

✎ Skeletal (stickler syndrome).

➢ CNS (Cerebro-oculo-facial syndrome).

➢ Renal (Lowe's syndrome)

Common familial cataract :

a) cataracta pulverulenta.

b) zonular cataract.

c) coronary cataract & total soft cataract.

3) *Other* : Maternal & foetal/infantile factors-1/3rd of total congenital cataract.

Maternal : a) Malnutrition

b) Infection (Rubella, CMV)

c) Drugs (Thalidomide, steroids)

d) Radiation

Foetal/ : a) Anoxia
Infantile
b) Birth trauma

c) Metabolic disorders

d) Congenital (Lowe's)

e) Ocular diseases (PHPV)

f) Malnutrition

Types :

I) *Congenital capsular cataract :*

➢ Anterior

➢ Posterior

II) *Polar cataract :*

➢ Anterior

➢ Posterior

III) *Congenital nuclear cataract :*

➢ Cataracta pulverulenta.

➢ Lamellar (Zonular) cataract

➢ Sutural & Axial cataract :

➢ Floriform

➢ Coralliform

➢ Spear shaped

➢ Dendritic sutural

➢ Anterior axial embryonic

➢ Total nuclear

IV) *Generalized cataract :*

➢ Coronary cataract

➢ Blue dot cataract

➢ Total congenital

➢ Congenital membranous cataract

Following are most common :

1) *Anterior capsular (polar) :* **(Fig. 3.14)**

➢ involves central part of the anterior capsule.

Causes :

a) developmental delay in the formation of anterior chamber.

b) corneal perforation (penetrating injury, ophthalmia neonatorum).

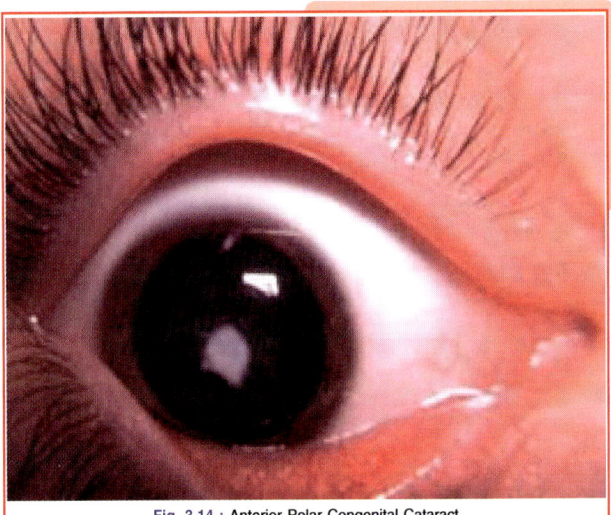

Fig. 3.14 : Anterior Polar Congenital Cataract

Types :

a) Thickened white plaque.

b) Anterior pyramidal cataract : cone shaped

c) Reduplicate (double) cataract.

➢ Transparent zone between two opacities (one on the capsule, other on the cortex).

➢ Buried opacity is called Imprint.

➢ and two together constitute Reduplicate cataract.

2) *Posterior capsular (polar) :* **(Fig. 3.15)**

➢ due to the presence of posterior part of vascular sheath of the lens.

3) *Cataracta centralis pulverulenta :* **(Fig. 3.16)**

➢ 'Powdery fine white dots' within the embryonic/foetal nucleus.

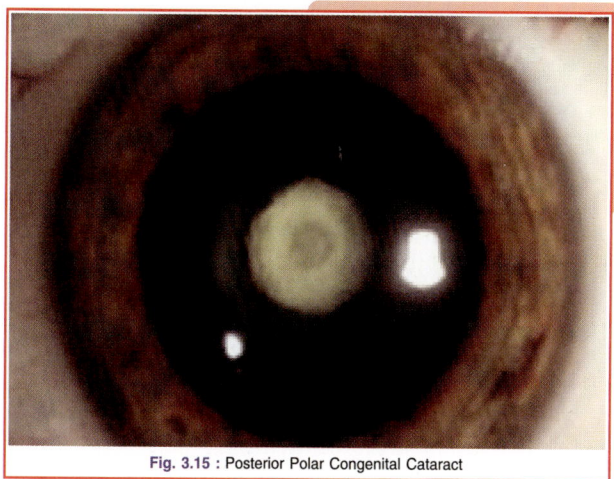

Fig. 3.15 : Posterior Polar Congenital Cataract

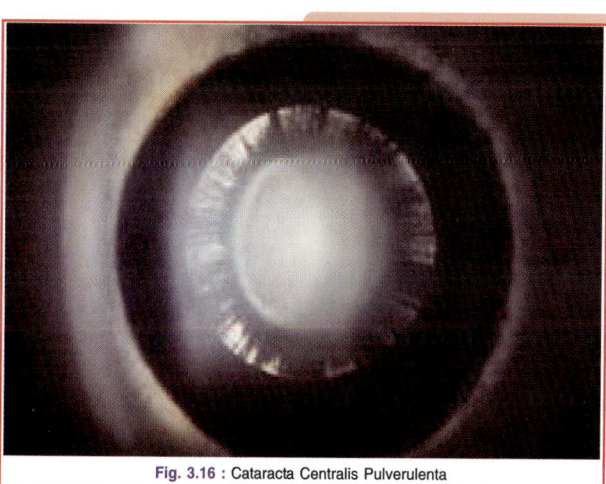

Fig. 3.16 : Cataracta Centralis Pulverulenta

4) Lamellar (Zonular) cataract : (Fig. 3.17)

- 50% of all visually significant congenital cataract.

- Zone around the foetal/embryonic nucleus is opacified.

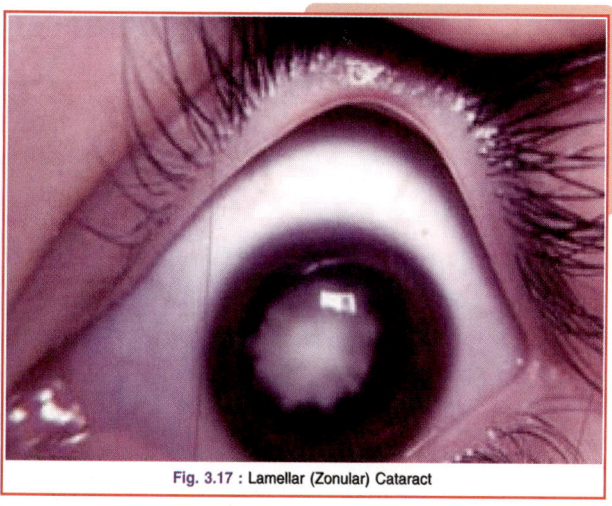

Fig. 3.17 : Lamellar (Zonular) Cataract

Etiology :

a) Lack of vit. D is a potent factor, evidence of Rickets is found in affected children.

b) Hypoparathyroidism (hypocalcemia) during pregnancy.

c) Maternal rubella infection.

Characteristic feature :

Area of lens within and around the opaque zone is clear, although linear opacities like 'spokes of wheel (rider)' may run towards the equator. **(Fig. 3.18)**

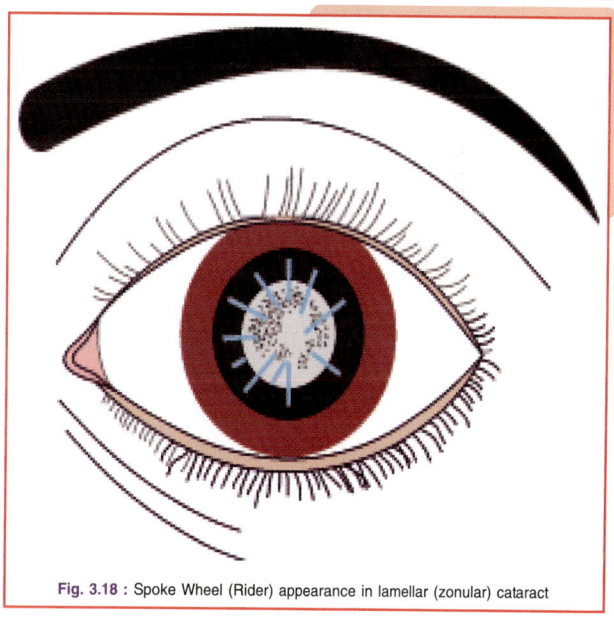

Fig. 3.18 : Spoke Wheel (Rider) appearance in lamellar (zonular) cataract

5) Sutural & axial cataract : (Fig. 3.19)

➤ Opacities occur in Y-suture of fetal nucleus.

➤ Individual opacities have distinct pattern :

   a) Anterior axial embryonic cataract : fine dot near anterior Y suture of the fetal nucleus.

   b) Dendritic sutural cataract : fine dots along the dendritic suture.

   c) Spear shaped cataract : heaps of scattered crystalline needles.

   d) Floriform cataract : like the petals of flower.

   e) Coralliform cataract :

      ❑ also known as fusiform, spindle shaped cataract.

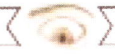

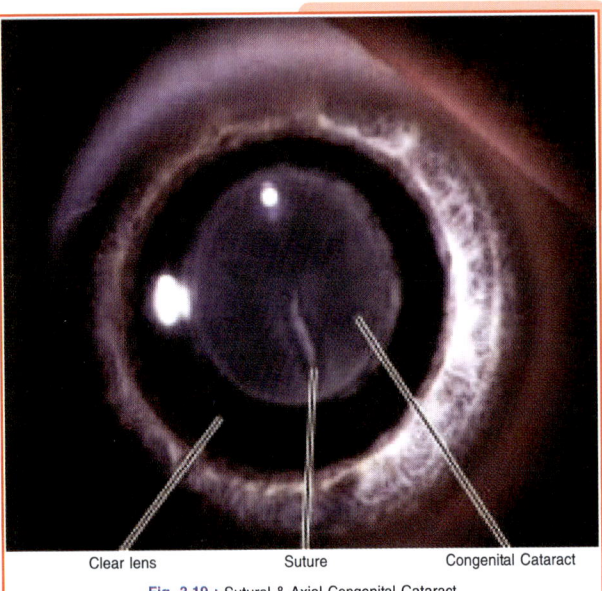

Clear lens   Suture   Congenital Cataract

Fig. 3.19 : Sutural & Axial Congenital Cataract

❑ Anteroposterior spindle shaped opacity with offshoots giving an appearance resembling a coral.

6) Total Nuclear Cataract : (Fig. 3.20)

➢ Involves embryonic & foetal nucleus as it is because of disturbances in development at a very early stage.

➢ Dense chalky white central opacity seriously impairing the vision.

➢ Associated with Rubella infection in mother.

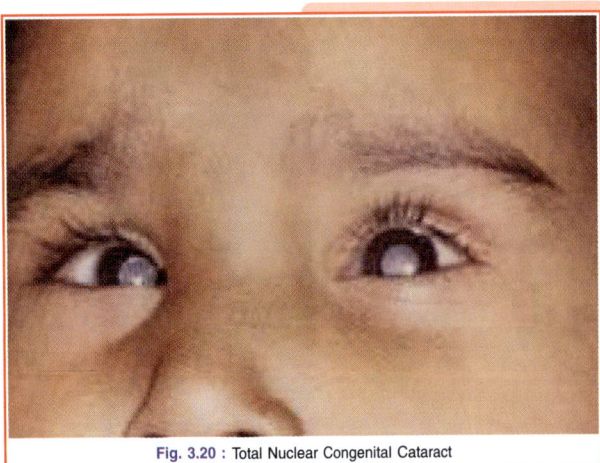

Fig. 3.20 : Total Nuclear Congenital Cataract

7) Coronary Cataract : (Fig. 3.21)

➢ Common form of developmental cataract occuring about in puberty.

➢ Adolescent nucleus or deeper layer of cortex is involved.

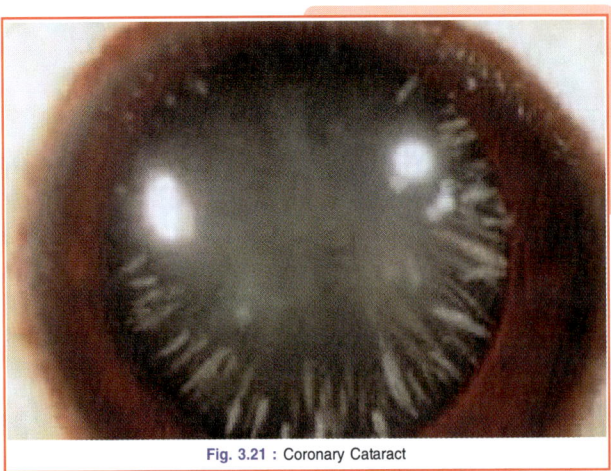

Fig. 3.21 : Coronary Cataract

➢ Opacities are hundreds in number & have regular radial distribution in periphery of the lens (corona of club shaped opacities).

➢ Opacities are peripheral, so vision is usually unaffected.

8) Blue Dot Cataract : (Fig. 3.22)

➢ Most common congenital cataract.

➢ Small opaque tiny blue dots, multiple in number are scattered all over the lens.

➢ also known as cataracta coerulea / punctata

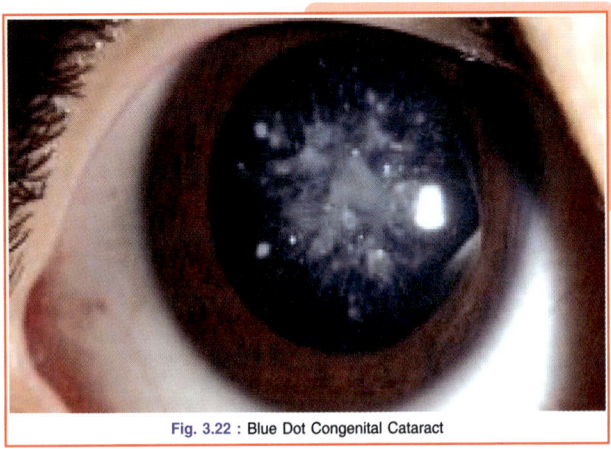

Fig. 3.22 : Blue Dot Congenital Cataract

9) Total congenital cataract : (Fig. 3.23)

Etiology :

a) Hereditary

b) Maternal Rubella

└▸known as 'Rubella Cataract'.

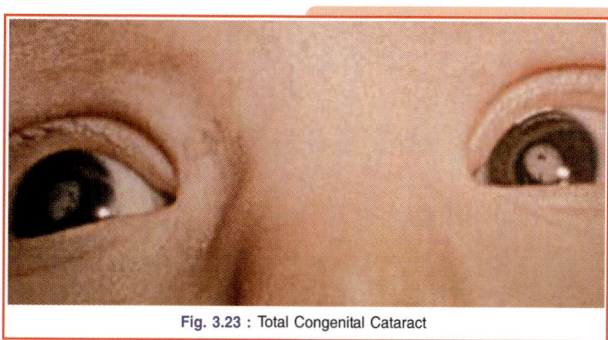

Fig. 3.23 : Total Congenital Cataract

Characteristic :

a) Child is born with 'pearly white' nuclear cataract.

b) Lens matter may be soft or liquefied (congenital Morgagnian Cataract).

10) *Congenital membranous cataract :* **(Fig. 3.24)**

➢ There occurs total or partial absorption of congenital cataract, leaving behind thin membranous cataract.

➢ Rarely there is complete disappearance of all the lens fibres. Such a patient may be misdiagnosed as Congenital aphakia. Associated with Hallermann-Streiff-Francois syndrome.

Management :

A) *Clinical –* Investigative work up :

1) *Ocular examination :*

➢ Density and morphology of cataract.

➢ Assessment of visual function : difficult in infants, small children.

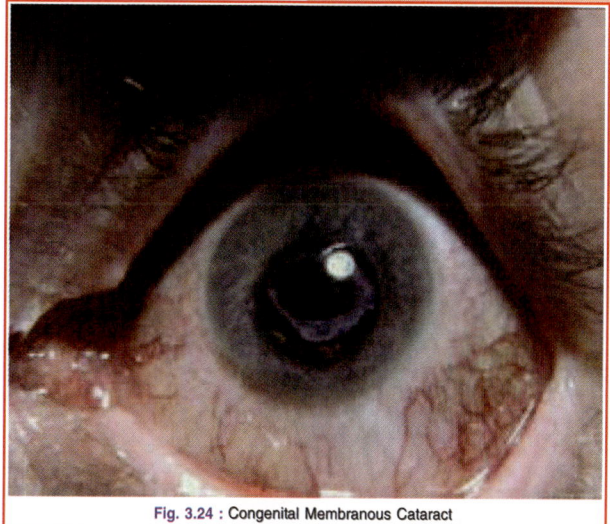

Fig. 3.24 : Congenital Membranous Cataract

Special tests :

a) fixation reflex

b) forced choice preferential looking

c) VEP (Visually evoked potential)

d) OKN (Optic kinetic nystagmus)

➢ Associated ocular defects must be noted.

2) *Lab Investigations :*

➢ Intrauterine infections.

➢ Urine test for Galactosemia

➢ Urine chromatography for Lowe's syndrome.

➢ Blood sugar for hyperglycemia.

➢ Serum calcium for hypocalcemia.

B) *Indications & Timing of Paediatric Cataract Surgery :*

1) *Partial and small central cataract which are visually insignificant :* Non surgical treatment with pupillary dilatation by mydriatics with careful follow-up till puberty.

2) *Large and dense opacity :*

➢ ECCE is TOC.

➢ ICCE is contraindicated in children.

3) *Timing of Surgery :*

➢ Critical period for development of fixation reflex in both unilateral and bilateral visual deprivation disorders is between '2-4 months of age'. Any cataract dense enough to impair the vision must be dealt before this age.

➢ Timing depends whether cataract is unilateral/bilateral and opacity is partial/dense.

a) Bilateral Cataract :

i) Dense : 4-6 weeks of age.

ii) Partial : No surgery.

b) Unilateral cataract :

i) Dense : Urgent within days followed by aggressive antiamblyopic therapy.

ii) Partial : No surgery, mydriatics are given.

C) Surgical Procedures :

- 'ECCE by Phacoemulsification' is surgery of choice.
- ICCE is contraindicated because of vitreous traction and loss at Weiger capsulohyaloid ligament.
- *Methods for ECCE :*
  i) Posterior capsulectomy & Anterior vitrectomy (Procedure of choice) via limbal or pars plana approach.
  ii) Lens aspiration.
  iii) Lensectomy.
- Traditional treatment of needling or discission are absolete now.

D) Correction of Paediatric aphakia :

i) if child is < 2 years : Contact lens.
ii) if child is > 2 years : PC IOL implantation

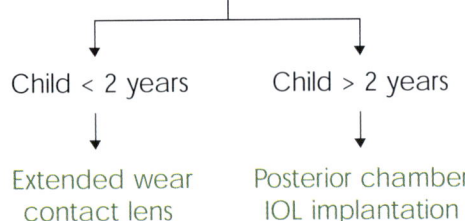

Congenital / Developmental Cataract
↓
ECCE by Phacoemulsification (Posterior capsulectomy & Anterior vitrectomy)

Child < 2 years → Extended wear contact lens

Child > 2 years → Posterior chamber IOL implantation

◻ COMPLICATED CATARACT :

- Also known as secondary cataract.
- It is opacification of the lens secondary to some other intraocular disease.

Etiology :

1) Inflammatory conditions :
   - Anterior uveitis (most common cause)
   - Iridocyclitis
   - Endophthalmitis
   - Hypopyon corneal ulcer.
2) Degenerative conditions :
   - Retinal dystrophy
   - Retinitis pigmentosa

3) Retinal Detachment
4) Glaucoma (Primary/Secondary)
5) Intraocular tumors
   - Retinoblastoma, Melanoma.

Clinical features :

- Starts as posterior subcapsular cortical cataract.
- On slit lamp examination, opacities are :
  a) 'Bread-crumb' in appearance. **(Fig. 3.25)**
  b) 'Polychromatic lustre' : Characteristic sign. Appearance of red, green, blue particles.
  c) Diffuse yellow haze in adjoining cortex.
  d) Chalky white appearance of lens as opacity spreads in rest of the cortex.
  e) Deposition of Ca^{2+} in later stages.

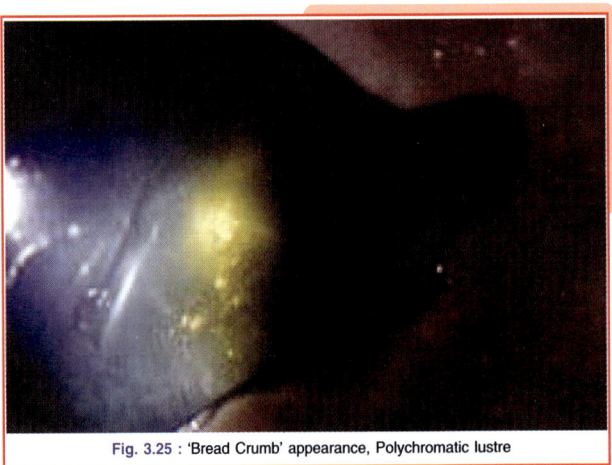

Fig. 3.25 : 'Bread Crumb' appearance, Polychromatic lustre

- It may be also because of drugs, Drug Induced Cataract.
  1) Corticosteroid induced.
     ➤ in posterior capsule, so posterior subcapsular opacities.
  2) Miotics induced.
     ➤ anterior subcapsular cataract.
  3) Others :
     ➤ Amiodarone, chlorpromazine, busulphan, Gold, Allopurinol.

◻ ROSETTE CATARACT : (Traumatic Cataract) : (Fig. 3.26)

- It occurs following trauma to the eye.
- also known as concussion cataract.

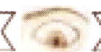

⚙ Trauma causes mechanical injury to the lens fibres.

⚙ 2 types :

   i)   Early Rosette cataract

   ii) Late Rosette cataract

   i)   Early Rosette Cataract :

   'feathery lines of opacities' along star shaped sutural lines, usually in posterior cortex.

   ii) Late Rosette cataract :

     ➢ in posterior cortex, develops 1-2 years after the injury.

     ➢ Sutural extensions are shorter and more compact than early rosette cataract.

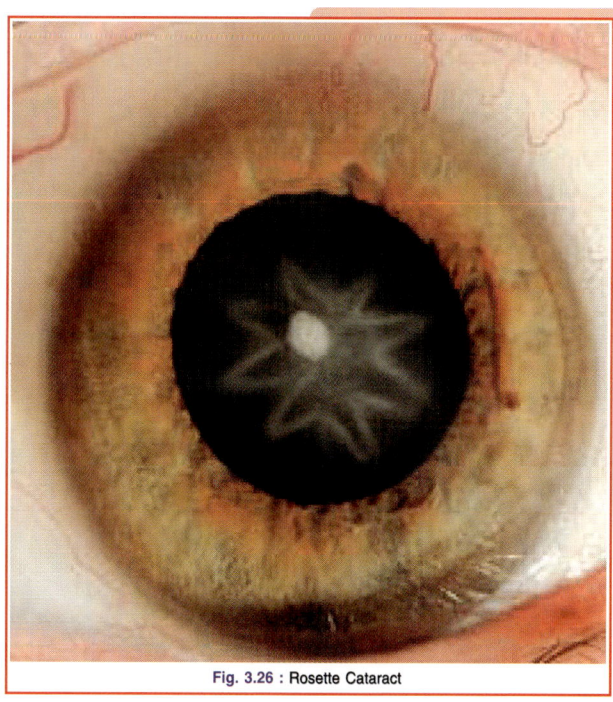

Fig. 3.26 : Rosette Cataract

⬛ INTRA OCULAR LENS : (Fig. 3.27)

⚙ IOL implantation is method of choice for correcting aphakia.

⚙ IOL is artificial lens which the surgeons implant to replace the eye's crystalline lens.

⚙ Best position of IOL is within the capsular bag in posterior chamber.

⚙ Other sites :

   i)   Anterior chamber (in front of the iris).

   ii) Iris supported (with sutures).

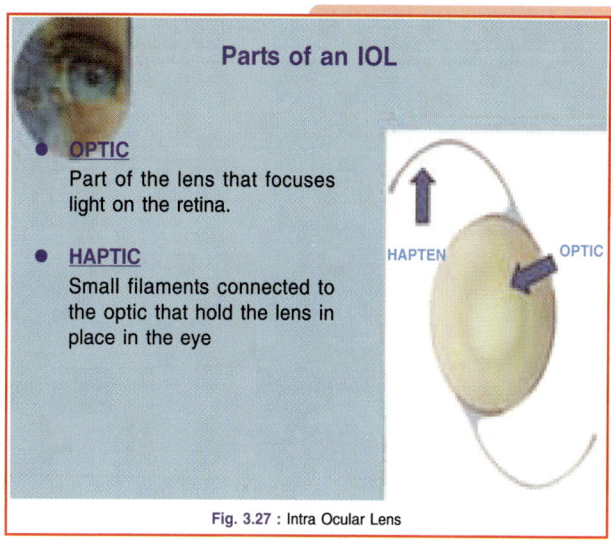

Parts of an IOL

● **OPTIC**
Part of the lens that focuses light on the retina.

● **HAPTIC**
Small filaments connected to the optic that hold the lens in place in the eye

HAPTEN   OPTIC

Fig. 3.27 : Intra Ocular Lens

Types of IOL :

A) Based on method of fixation :

   I)   Anterior chamber IOL (AC-IOL) :

     ➢ infront of the iris, used only when it is not possible to use PC-IOL.

     ➢ Kelman multiflex type of AC-IOL is used commonly.

   ii) Iris supported lens :

     ➢ fixed on the iris with help of sutures, loops or claws.

     ➢ Singh & Worst's Iris claw lens.

   iii) PC-IOL :

     ➢ in the capsular bag.

     ➢ Modified C loop & quadriloop.

B) Based on material of manufacture :

   i)   Rigid IOL :

     ➢ made from PMMA (Polymethyl methacrylate).

   ii) Foldable IOL :

     ➢ used after phacoemulsification.

     ➢ Made from silicone, acrylic, hydrogel, collamer.

   iii) Rollable IOL :

     ➢ used after Phokonit technique (microincision 1 mm).

     ➢ made from hydrogel.

C) Based on focusing ability of IOL :

i) Unifocal IOL

➢ most commonly used.

➢ They can make patient emmetropic, myopic, hypermetropic.

ii) Multifocal IOL :

➢ focuses both on distance and near.

➢ so, also known as simultaneous vision lenses.

➢ 2 types : Refractive & Diffractive type.

➢ Also called pseudoaccommodative IOL.

iii) Accommodative IOL :

➢ improve near vision.

➢ crystalens & synchrony lens.

D) Special function IOL :

i) Toric IOL :

➢ correct Astigmatism.

ii) Aspheric IOL :

➢ reduce spherical aberrations.

iii) Aniridia IOL :

➢ cover the defects of aniridia or partial iris loss in trauma.

E) Aphakic & phakic Refractive IOL.

Calculation of IOL power (Biometry) :

By SRK (Sanders, Retzlaff, Kraff) formula :

P = A - 2.5L - 0.9K

P : Power of lens.

A : Constant for each lens type.

L : Axial length of eyeball in mm, determined by A scan.

K : Corneal curvature, determined by keratometry.

☐ COSMETIC CONTACT LENS :

✍ It is an artificial device whose front surface substitutes anterior surface of the cornea.

✍ So in addition to the correction of refractive errors, irregularities of front surface of the cornea can also be corrected by contact lens.

Types of contact lens :

1) Hard lens :

✎ made from PMMA (polymethyl methacrylate)

✎ being hard, can cause corneal abrasions.

✎ Impermeable to O_2 thus restricting the tolerance.

2) RGP lens :

✎ Rigid gas permeable lens, permeable to O_2.

✎ They are also hard, made from :

a) Silicone acrylate (copolymer of PMMA).

b) CAB (Cellulose acetate butyrate).

3) Soft lens : (most frequently prescribed) :

✎ made of HEMA (hydroxyethyl methacrylate).

✎ soft, O_2 permeable.

✎ most comfortable, well tolerated.

✎ But have problems of wettability, proteinaceous deposits, gets cracked, limited life, inferior optical quality.

Indications :

1) Optical Indications :

✎ Refractive error for cosmetic purposes.

✎ Absolute indications :

i) Anisometropia.

ii) Unilateral aphakia.

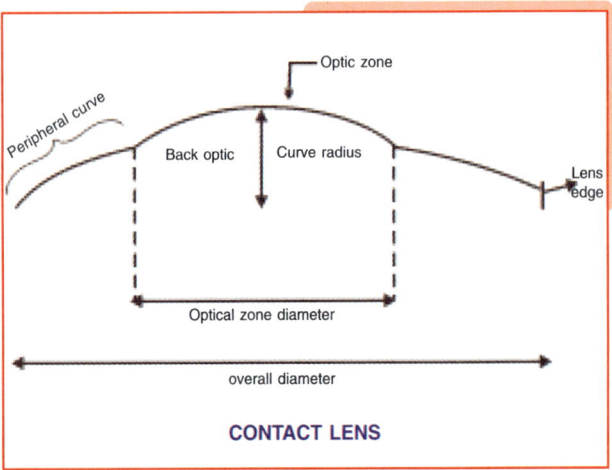

CONTACT LENS

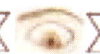
iii) High myopia.

iv) Keratoconus.

v) Irregular astigmatism.

2) *Therapeutic Indications :*

i) Corneal diseases (non healing corneal ulcer, bullous keratopathy)

ii) Iris diseases (Aniridia, Coloboma).

iii) Glaucoma (as a vehicle for drug delivery).

iv) Amblyopia

v) Bandage soft contact lens following keratoplasty.

3) *Preventive Indications :*

i) Symblepharon.

ii) Exposure keratitis.

iii) Trichiasis.

4) *Diagnostic Indications :*

i) Gonioscopy

ii) ERG

iii) Examination of fundus

iv) Fundus Photography.

v) Goldmann's 3 mirror examination.

5) *Operative Indications :*

i) Goniotomy

ii) Vitrectomy

iii) Endocular photocoagulation.

6) *Cosmetic Indications :*

i) unsightly corneal scar (color contact lens).

ii) ptosis (haptic contact lens).

iii) Phthisis bulbi (cosmetic scleral lens).

7) *Occupational indications :*

i) Sportsmen.

ii) Pilot.

iii) Actors

Contraindications :

i) Mental incompetance, poor motivation.

ii) Chronic dacryocystitis.

iii) Dry eye syndromes.

iv) Chronic conjunctivitis.

v) Corneal dystrophy, degeneration.

vi) Episcleritis, scleritis, Iridocyclitis.

ECTOPIA LENTIS :

It is lens displacement from its normal position (patellar fossa) due to the partial or compete rupture of lens zonules. **(Fig. 3.28)**

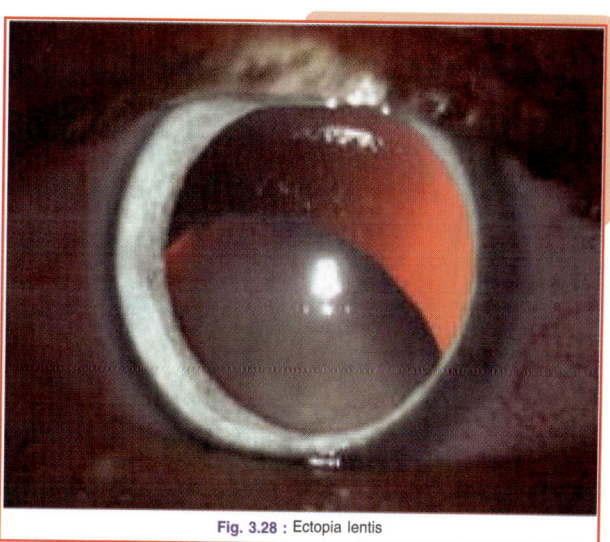

Fig. 3.28 : Ectopia lentis

Types :

1) *Simple ectopia lentis (AD) :*

   - displacement is bilaterally symmetrical and usually upwards.

2) *Ectopia lentis et pupillae (AR) :*

   - displacement of lens is associated with slit shaped pupil which is displaced in opposite direction.

3) *Ectopia lentis with systemic lens anomalies :*

   i) Marfan's syndrome (upwards).

   ii) Homocystinuria (inferior & nasally).

   iii) Weill Marchesani syndrome (forward).

   iv) Ehlers Danlos syndrome (subluxation).

   v) Hyperlysinemia (laxity of ligaments).

   vi) Stickler syndrome.

   vii) Sulphite oxidase deficiency. (here ectopia lentis is universal feature).

METABOLIC CATARACT :

Metabolic cataract is due to endocrine disorders and biochemical abnormalities.

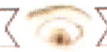

✐ <u>Few types</u> are :

1) Diabetic cataract.
2) Galactosaemic cataract.
3) Hypocalcaemic (Tetanic) cataract.
4) Cataract due to the error of copper metabolism.
5) Cataract due to Lowe's syndrome.

I) Diabetic Cataract :

<u>2 types</u> :

1) Senile cataract in diabetics :
   ⇨ appears at an early stage and has rapid progression.

2) True diabetic cataract : **(Fig. 3.29)**
   ⇨ also known as :

       'Snowflake cataract' or

       'Snowstorm cataract'.

   ⇨ Glucose

   NADPH +   Aldol Reductase

   Sorbitol

   Overhydration of lens, fluid vacuoles appears underneath the anterior and posterior capsules (bilateral snowflake-like white opacities) in the cortex.

II) Galactosaemic cataract :

   ✎ due to inborn error of galactose metabolism.

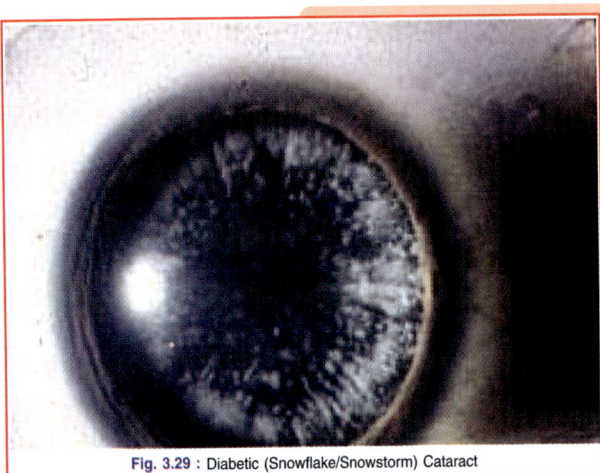

Fig. 3.29 : Diabetic (Snowflake/Snowstorm) Cataract

<u>2 types</u> :

1) Classical galactosaemia :
   ⇨ due to GPUT (Galactose-1-phosphate uridyl transferase) deficiency.

2) Related disorder :
   ⇨ due to GK (galactokinase) deficiency.

Characteristic features :

➢ 'Oil droplet like central lens opacities'. **(Fig. 3.30)**

➢ They are bilateral.

➢ Galactosaemic cataract can be prevented by eliminating milk and milk products from the diet when diagnosed early.

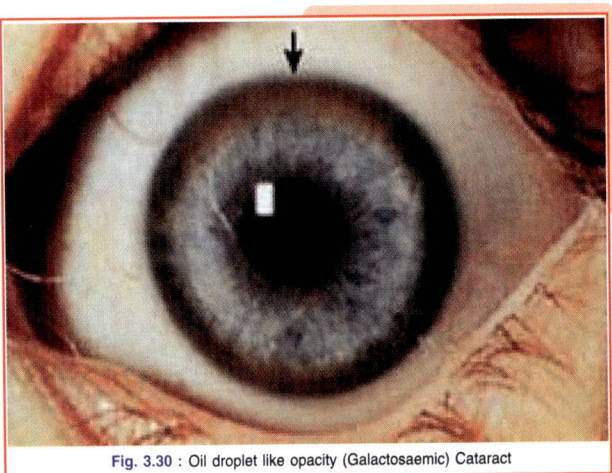

Fig. 3.30 : Oil droplet like opacity (Galactosaemic) Cataract

III) Hypocalcaemic (Tetanic cataract) :

➢ due to parathyroid tetany caused by atrophy or inadvertent removal (during thyroidectomy) of parathyroid gland.

➢ characteristic : multicoloured crystals or small white flecks of opacities in the cortex.

➢ zonular cataract occurs in infants with hypocalcemia.

IV) Cataract due to error of copper metabolism :

➢ as seen in Wilson's disease.

➢ Characteristic features :

   a) Sunflower cataract *i.e.* yellowish

brown dots due to cuprous oxide deposition in the anterior lens capsule and cortex in stellate pattern.

b) Kayser-Fleischer Ring *i.e.* golden ring due to copper deposition in the periphery of Descemet membrane in cornea, more common in Wilson's disease. **(Fig. 3.31)**

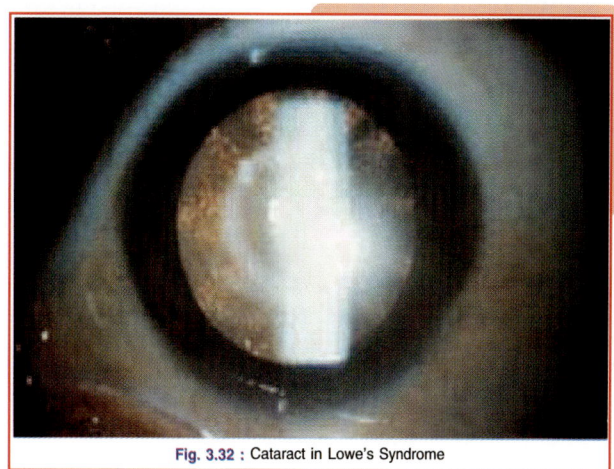

Fig. 3.32 : Cataract in Lowe's Syndrome

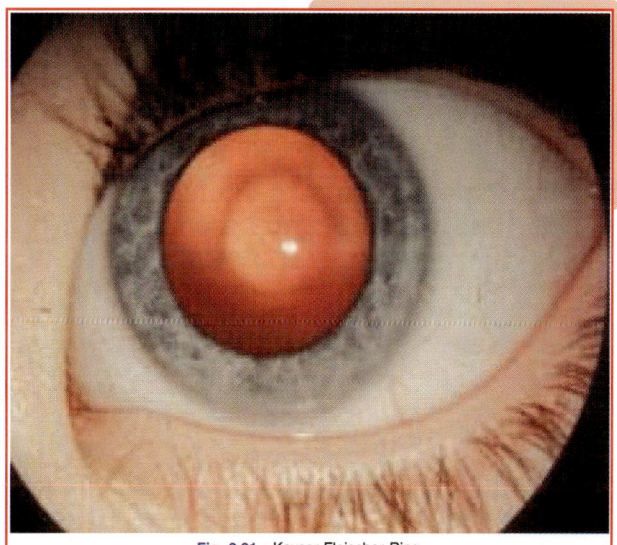

Fig. 3.31 : Kayser-Fleischer Ring

V) Cataract in Lowe's syndrome : (Fig. 3.32)

➤ Lowe's syndrome (oculo-cerebral-renal) is due to inborn error of amino acid metabolism.

➤ Ocular features : **BCG**

1) Blue sclera

2) Congenital cataract

3) Glaucoma

➤ Systemic features :

1) Mental retardation & dwarfism.

2) Frontal prominence

3) Muscular hypotonia

4) Osteomalacia.

▢ **CORONARY CATARACT**
▢ **BLUE DOT CATARACT**
} discussed in congenital cataract

▢ **HYPERMATURE CATARACT/ MORGAGNIAN CATARACT**
▢ **PHACOEMULSIFICATION**
} discussed in senile cataract

Chapter

4

Glaucoma

Most Important (Must Read Topics)	Elective Topics
1) Causes of Loss of Vision	1) Rubeosis Iridis
2) Glaucoma, classification	2) Trabeculectomy
3) Primary Open Angle Glaucoma	3) Fincham Test
4) Primary Angle Closure Glaucoma	4) Diurnal test of IOP variation
5) Buphthalmos	

☐ LOSS OF VISION (LOV) :

✐ It is absence of vision where it existed before.

✐ It may be sudden or gradual loss of vision.

A) Sudden LOV causes :

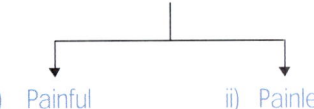

i) Painful
1) Acute congestive (angle closure) Glaucoma
2) Acute Iridocyclitis (Uveitis)
3) Endophthalmitis
4) Optic neuritis

ii) Painless
1) Central Retinal Artery occlusion (CRAO)
2) Central Retinal Vein Occlusion (CRVO)
3) Macular edema
4) Retinal Detachment
5) 'Exudative' Age related macular degeneration (ARMD)

6) Vitreous & Retinal hemorrhage
7) Subluxation/ Dislocation of lens.
8) Methyl alcohol amblyopia

B) Gradual LOV Causes :

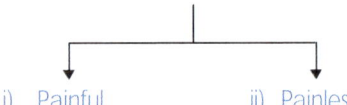

i) Painful
1) Corneal ulcer
2) Chronic simple Glaucoma
3) Chronic Iridocyclitis (Uveitis)

ii) Painless
1) Cataract (Senile & developmental)
2) 'Dry type' age related macular degeneration (ARMD)
3) Diabetic Retinopathy
4) Refractive errors
5) Progressive pterygium

6) Corneal dystrophy

7) Corneal degeneration

8) Chorioretinal degeneration

9) Presbyopia

GLAUCOMA : DEFINITION, CLASSIFICATION :

- Glaucoma is not a single disease process but group of disorders characterised by chronic progressive optic Neuropathy resulting in characteristic appearance of optic disc and specific pattern of irreversible visual field defects that are associated frequently but not invariably with raised Intraocular pressure (IOP). **(Fig. 4.1)**

- Raised IOP without optic Neuropathy is simply called Ocular Hypertension.

- Glaucoma with normal IOP (upto 20 mmHg) is called Normal or low tension Glaucoma.

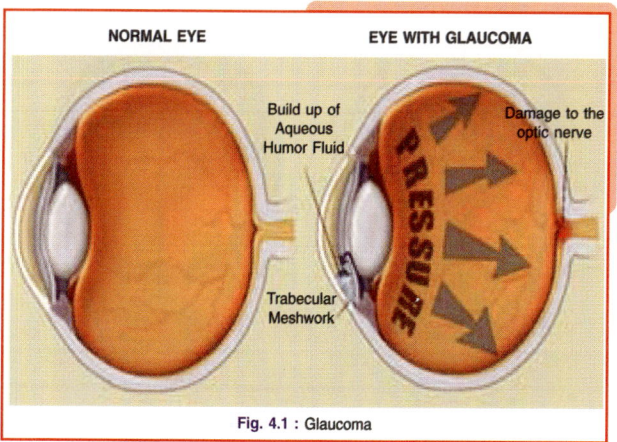

Fig. 4.1 : Glaucoma

Classification :

A) Primary Adult Glaucomas :

1) Primary Open Angle Glaucoma.

2) Primary Angle Closure Glaucoma.

3) Primary mixed mechanism glaucoma.

B) Secondary Glaucoma :

1) Lens induced

2) Pigmentory

3) Steroid induced

4) Neovascular

5) Traumatic

6) Introcular tumors

7) Aphakic

8) Pseudoexfoliative

C) Congenital/Developmental Glaucoma :

1) Primary Congenital/Developmental
   ➤ Congenital
   ➤ Infantile
   ➤ Juvenile

2) Developmental associated with ocular anomalies.

PRIMARY OPEN ANGLE GLAUCOMA/ CHRONIC SIMPLE GLAUCOMA :

- Characterized by :

1) Slowly progressive raised IOP (> 21 mmHg).

2) Open normal appearing anterior chamber angle.

3) Characteristic optic disc cupping.

4) Specific visual field defects.

- Most common form, 10 times more common than angle closure glaucoma.

I) Etiology :

1) Increased IOP.

2) *Hereditary :* due to following genes :
   ➤ Myocilin C (MYOC)
   ➤ Optineurin (OPTN)
   ➤ WD repeat domain 36 (WDR 36).

3) *Age :* increasing age at around 5th, 7th decade of life.

4) *Race :* more severe in black than white.

5) Myopes

6) Thinner Central corneal thickness (CCT).

7) Diabetics.

8) Cigarette smoking.

9) High BP   } not associated with ↑ IOP

10) Thyrotoxicosis } but prevalence is higher

11) Corticosteroids.

II) Pathogenesis :

- Rise in IOP occurs due to the decrease in aqueous outflow facility due to increase resistance to aqueous outflow.

This is because of :

1) Age related thickening and sclerosis of trabecular meshwork.

2) Absence of vacuoles in cells lining canal of schlemm.

3) Narrowing of intertrabecular spaces.

4) Deposition of amorphous material in juxtacanalicular space.

III) Clinical Features :

Symptoms :

1) Usually asymptomatic, until it has caused significant loss of visual field.

2) Headache.

3) Eye ache.

4) Frequent change in presbyopic correction.

5) Scotoma (defect in visual field).

6) Difficulty in dark adaptation.

7) Significant loss of vision and blindness.

Signs :

A) *Anterior segment :*

Normal or low central corneal thickness (CCT).

B) *IOP changes :*

➤ Initially IOP is normal, but there is exaggeration of normal diurnal variation. So, Diurnal variation test is done. (IOP is checked every 3-4 hrs for 24 hrs.)

➤ Variation in IOP of :

> 5 mmHg (Schiotz) → Suspicious

> 8 mmHg → Diagnostic

➤ In later stages, IOP is permanently > 21 mmHg (30-45 mmHg)

C) *Visual field Defects :* **(Fig. 4.2)**

1) Isopteric contraction :

⇨ Earliest visual field defect but is not specific.

⇨ Generalised constriction of central and peripheral field.

2) Baring of blind spot :

⇨ Exclusion of blind spot from central field.

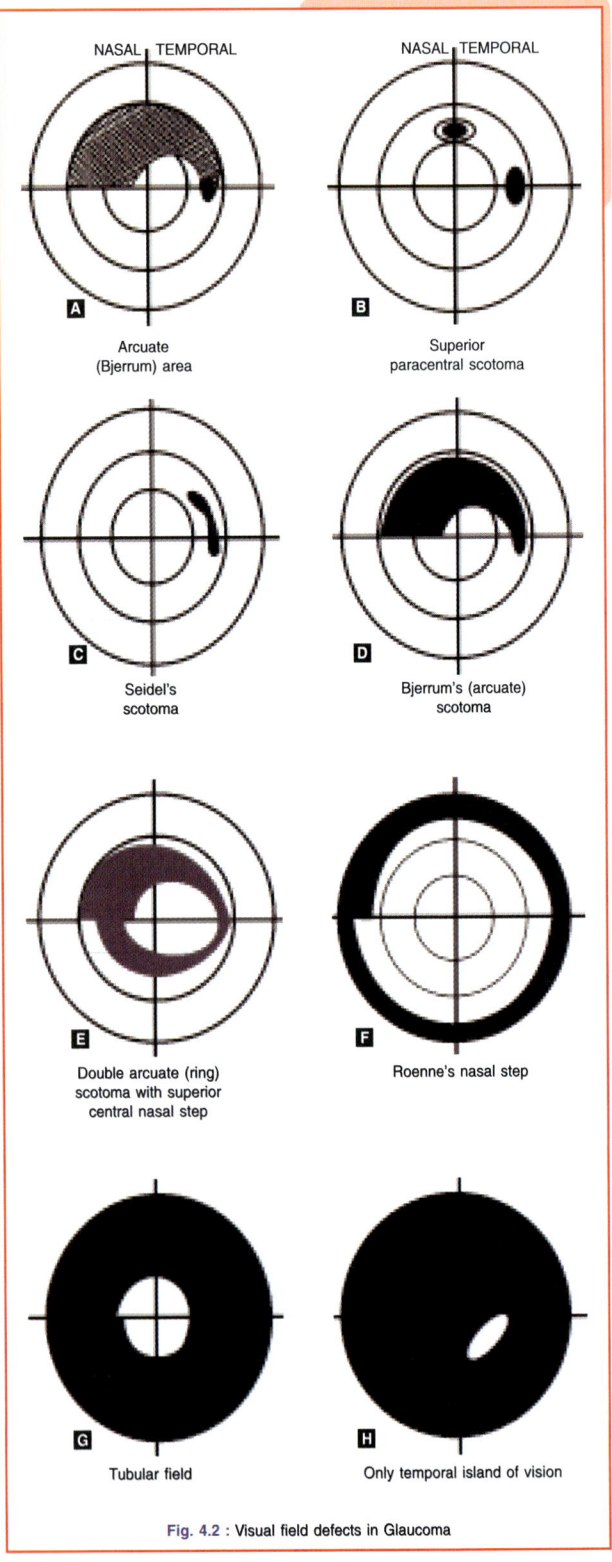

Fig. 4.2 : Visual field defects in Glaucoma

3) Paracentral scotoma :

⇨ Earliest clinically significant field defect.

⇨ Either below or above the blind spot in Bjerrum's area.

4) <u>Siedel's scotoma</u> :

⇨ Paracentral scotoma joins the blind spot to form sickle shape (Siedel's scotoma).

5) <u>Arcuate or Bjerrum's scotoma</u> :

⇨ Extension of Siedel's scotoma in the area above or below the fixation point.

6) <u>Ring or double Arcuate Scotoma</u> :

⇨ Two arcuate scotoma joins together.

7) <u>Roenne's central nasal step</u> :

⇨ Two arcuate scotoma runs in different arcs and meet to form sharp right angle defect.

8) <u>Tubular vision</u>.

D) *Optic Nerve Head Changes :* **(Figs. 4.3 & 4.4)**

<u>Early Glaucomatous changes</u> :

1) Vertically Oval Cup **(Fig. 4.5)**

2) Asymmetry of Cup **(Fig. 4.6)**

3) Large cup with cup disc ratio > 0.5 (Normal : 0.3-0.4) **(Fig. 4.7)**

4) Atrophy of Retinal nerve fibre layer. **(Fig. 4.8)**

5) Pallor on the disc. **(Fig. 4.9)**

6) Splinter hemorrhages. **(Fig. 4.10)**

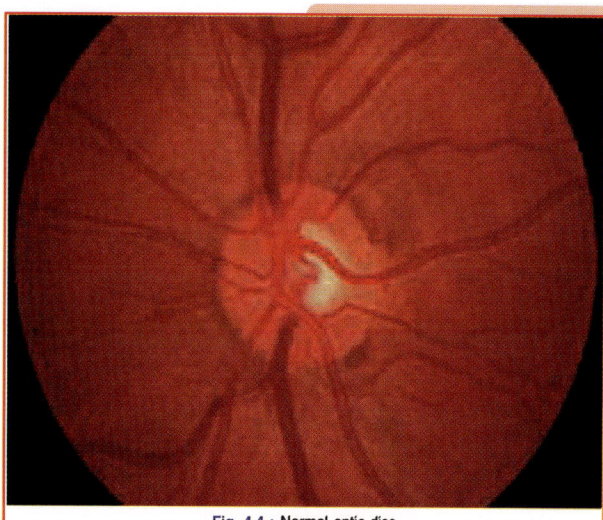

Fig. 4.4 : Normal optic disc

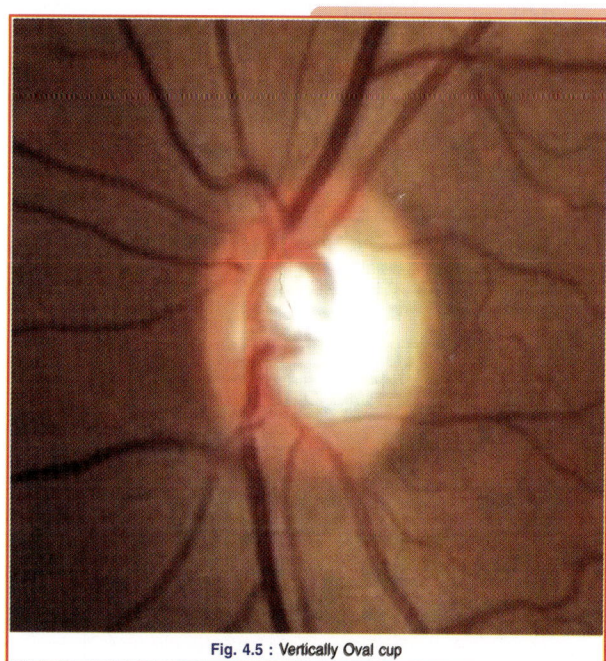

Fig. 4.5 : Vertically Oval cup

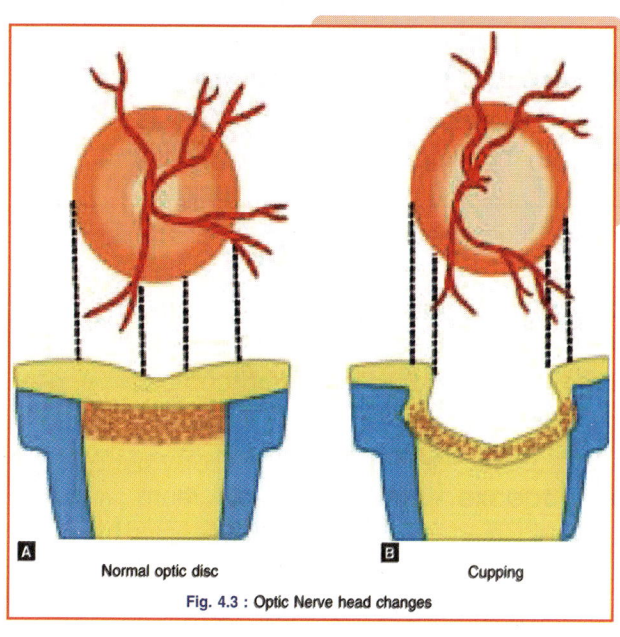

Normal optic disc   Cupping

Fig. 4.3 : Optic Nerve head changes

<u>Late Glaucomatous changes</u> :

1) Marked cupping (Cup : Disc 0.7-0.9)

2) Total bean pot cupping.

3) Thinning of neuroretinal rim. **(Fig. 4.11)**

4) Bayonetting sign (Nasal shifting of retinal vessels with broken appearance at disc margin). **(Fig. 4.12)**

5) Lamellar dot sign (pores in lamina cribrosa). **(Fig. 4.13)**

6) Pulsation of retinal arterioles at disc margin (Pathognomic).

7) Total disc pallor.

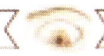

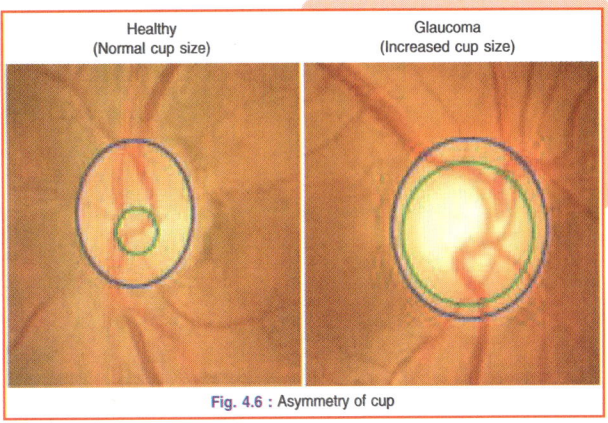

Healthy
(Normal cup size)

Glaucoma
(Increased cup size)

Fig. 4.6 : Asymmetry of cup

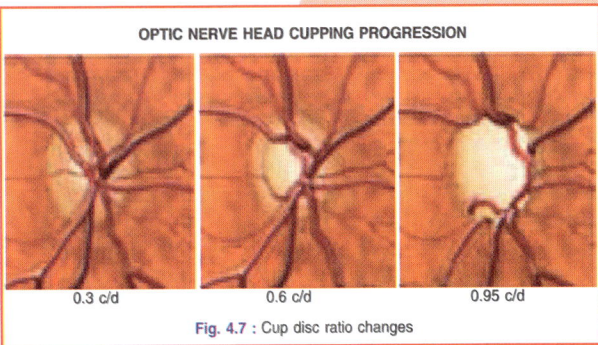

OPTIC NERVE HEAD CUPPING PROGRESSION

0.3 c/d   0.6 c/d   0.95 c/d

Fig. 4.7 : Cup disc ratio changes

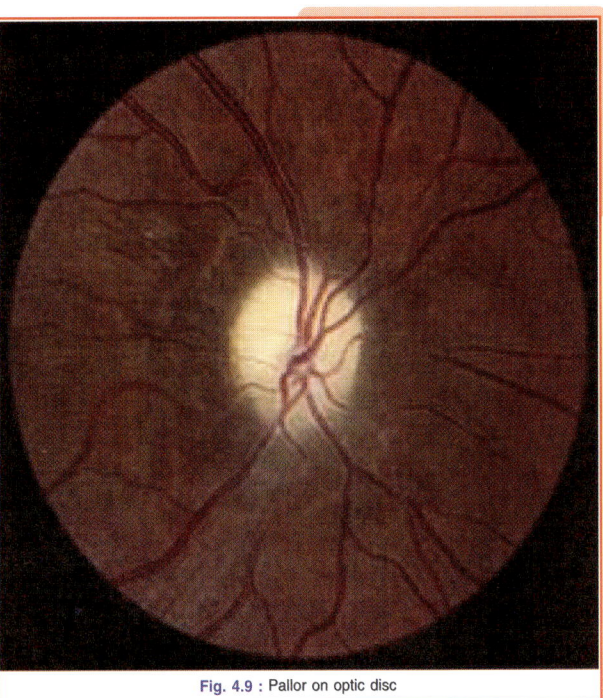

Fig. 4.9 : Pallor on optic disc

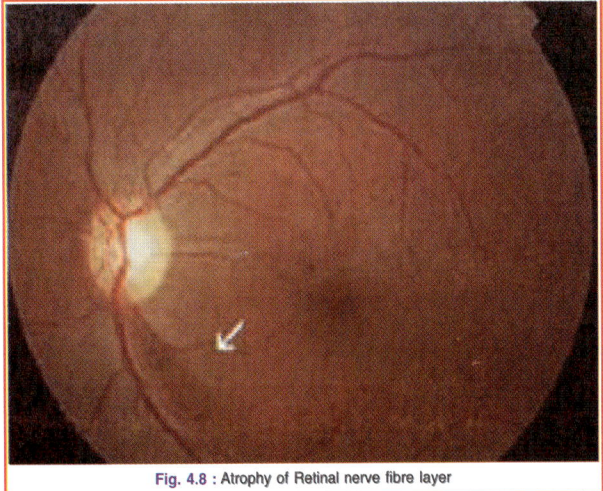

Fig. 4.8 : Atrophy of Retinal nerve fibre layer

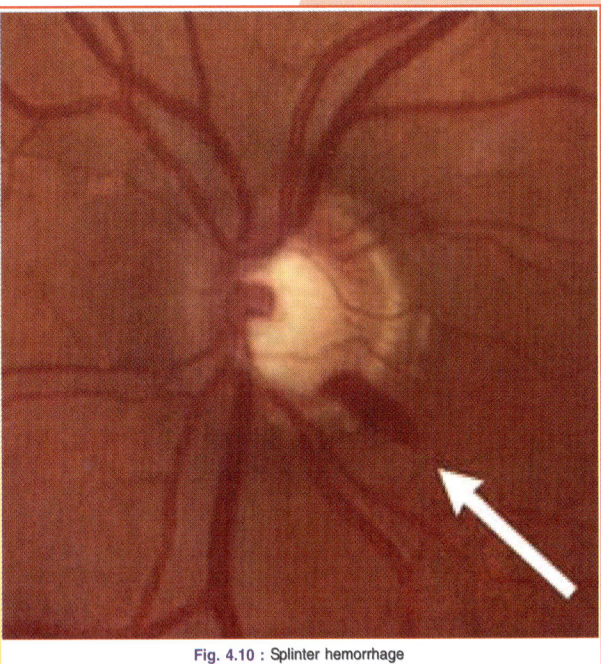

Fig. 4.10 : Splinter hemorrhage

IV) Diagnosis :

Atleast 2 of the following first three findings must be present to make the diagnosis of POAG, in presence of Normal Open Angle confirmed by Gonioscopy.

1) IOP > 21 mmHg on more than one occasion and variation of > 8 mmHg measured by Schiotz tonometry.

2) Glaucomatous changes in disc/optic nerve head as seen by :

   i)   Direct Ophthalmoscopy.

   ii) Indirect Ophthalmoscopy.

   iii) Slit lamp biomicroscopy using Hruby or Goldmann contact lens.

3) Typical visual field changes : as seen in Perimetry.

4) Defects in nerve fibre layer.

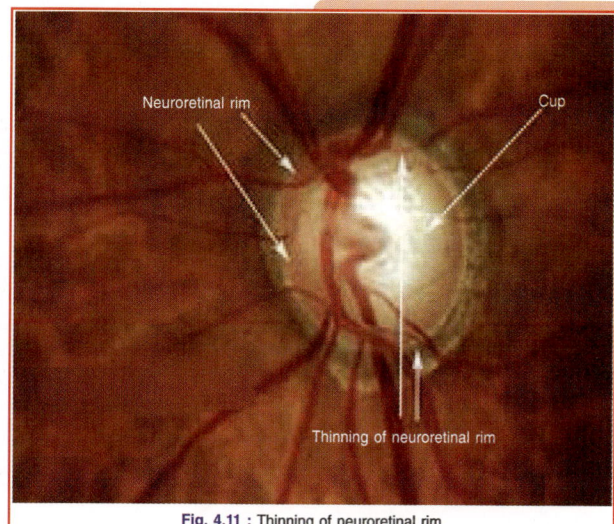

Fig. 4.11 : Thinning of neuroretinal rim

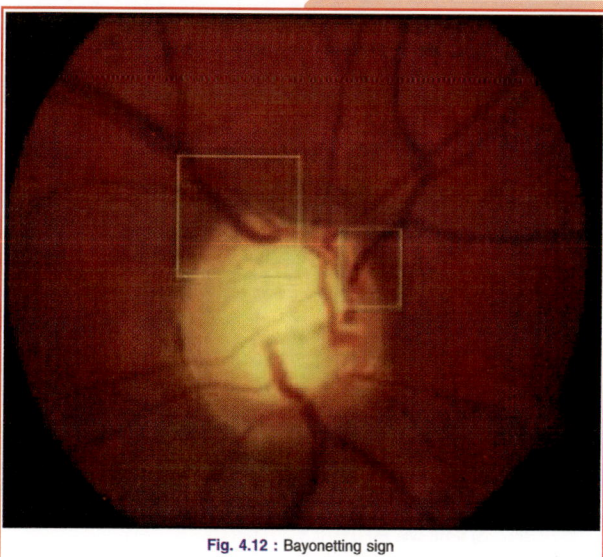

Fig. 4.12 : Bayonetting sign

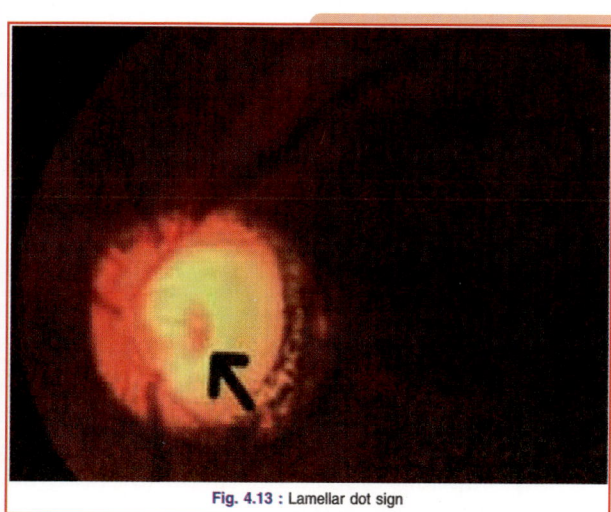

Fig. 4.13 : Lamellar dot sign

V) Treatment :

A) Investigations :

1) *Tonometry :*

   Applanation is preferred over Schiotz.

2) Central corneal thickness (CCT) :

   low CCT (< 545 microns)

3) Diurnal variation test.

4) Gonioscopy : wide open angle of AC.

5) Optic Disc changes.

6) Slit lamp examination.

7) Perimetry.

8) NFLA (Nerve fibre layer analyzer).

9) Provocative tests.

B) Medical Therapy :

➢ Medical Therapy is Treatment of choice for POAG.

➢ Topical β-blockers (Timolol, Betaxolol, Levobunolol, Carteolol) are DOC.

➢ Topical prostaglandin analogues (Latanoprost, Bimatoprost, Travoprost) are second DOC.

➢ *Other topical drugs :*

   i) α–agonists :

   non selective : Dipivefrine

   Selective α_2 : Apraclonidine, Brimonidine

   ii) Carbonic anhydrase inhibitors :

   Dorzolamide, Brinzolamide

   iii) Miotics :

   Pilocarpine, Physostigmine

➢ *Approach to the treatment :*

1) Start monotherapy with topical β-blocker / latanoprost.

2) If target IOT is not attained, either change over to alternative drug or use both of the above concurrently.

3) Brimonidine/Dorzolamide/Dipivefrine are used in Refractory cases

4) Topical miotics / Oral Acetazolamide are added only as last resort.

➢ *Systemic therapy :* last resort.

Drugs used are :

i) carbonic anhydrase inhibitors (Acetazolamide)

ii) osmotic agents (Mannitol, glycerol)

➢ α-agonists
β-blockers
Carbonic anhydrase inhibitors ⎫ decreases aqueous Secretion

➢ Prostaglandin analogues, Miotics ⎱ increases aqueous, uveoscleral outflow

➢ Osmotic agents : Reduce vitreous volume

C) *Argon or diode laser Trabeculoplasty :*

➢ It is done when IOP is not controlled despite of proper medical therapy or when patient is non compliant to medical therapy.

D) *Filteration surgery :*

➢ It is done when IOP is not controlled despite of proper medical therapy & trabeculoplasty or when patient is non compliant to medical therapy, but trabeculoplasty is not available.

➢ Trabeculectomy is done.

➢ POAG is bilateral but asymmetrical (IOP is different in both the eyes).

Treatment is started in eye with higher IOP and eye with relatively lower IOP acts as reference to *see* treatment response.

➢ If both the eyes have same IOP, treatment is started simultaneously in both the eyes.

It is worth noting that,

in POAG : Management of fellow eye is part of treatment.

in Angle closure Glaucoma : Management of fellow eye is part of prevention.

◻ PRIMARY ANGLE CLOSURE GLAUCOMA / ACUTE CONGESTIVE GLAUCOMA / NARROW ANGLE GLAUCOMA :

⚘ Type of primary glaucoma where rise in IOP occurs due to the blockage of aqueous outflow caused by the closure of narrower angle of anterior chamber.

⚘ Characterised by apposition of peripheral iris against the trabecular meshwork.

⚘ 2nd most common type of Glaucoma after POAG.

⚘ Females are affected more than males (4:1) **(Fig. 4.14).**

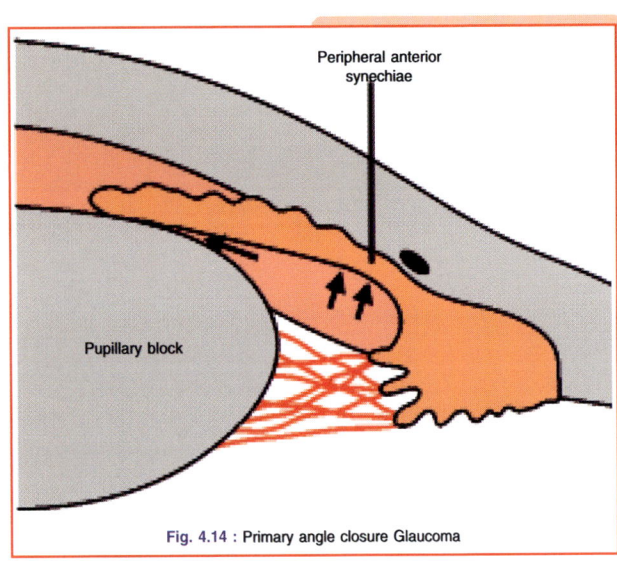

Fig. 4.14 : Primary angle closure Glaucoma

I) **Etiopathogenesis :**

Predisposing factors :

1) *Age* : 6th and 7th decade of life

2) *Gender :* Female : Male (4:1)

3) *Rare* : Common in Caucasians, Chinese

4) Shallow Anterior Chamber

5) Short eye

6) Hypermetropic eye

7) Large lens (older cataractous lens)

8) Anterior location of Iris Lens Diaphragm

9) Smaller Corneal Diameter.

Precipitating factors :

1) Dim light.

2) Emotional stress.

3) Use of mydriatics (Atropine)

Pathogenesis :

Increase in IOP is due to :

1) Pupillary block mechanism (mid dilated pupil). **(Fig. 4.15)**

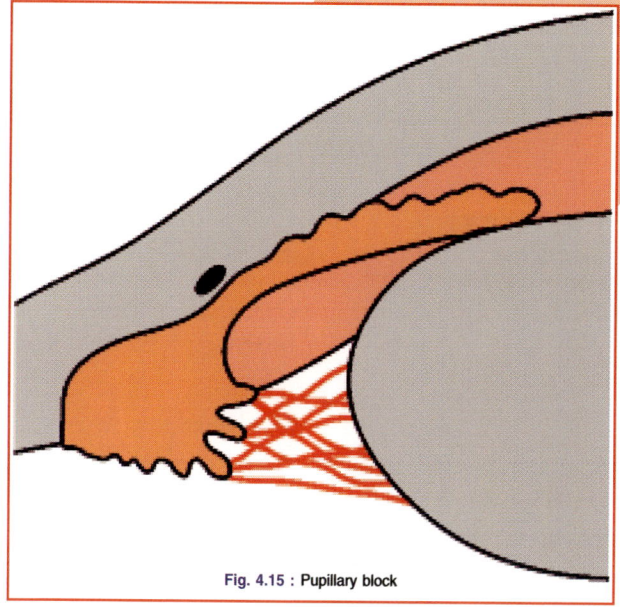

Fig. 4.15 : Pupillary block

2) Plateau iris configuration.

3) Phacomorphic mechanism.

Pupillary block :

Due to precipitating factors there occurs mid dilation of pupil → resulting in relative pupillary block.

↓

Then Iris bombe formation occurs.

↓

Angle closure due to Iridocorneal contact.

II) Classification :

A) ISEGO Classification :

1) PACS (Primary angle closure suspect).

2) PAC (Primary angle closure)

3) PACG (Primary angle closure glaucoma).

B) Clinical Classification :

PACS can be considered analogous to term 'Latent PACG' of this clinical classification.

1) Latent PACG (PACS) :

⇨ Shallow Anterior Chamber.

⇨ No symptoms except for occasionally :

a) halos around the light.

b) transient haziness of vision.

⇨ Only gonioscopic finding is : narrow angle < 20^0.

⇨ IOP is normal.

⇨ <u>Two provocative tests</u> :

a) Prone darkroom provocative test :

❑ Best physiological test.

❑ Patient is made to lie in dark room. There is increase in IOP > 8 mmHg.

b) Mydriatic / Cycloplegic provocative test :

❑ not preferred as it is not physiological.

❑ Mydriatic dilates the pupil → increase in IOP > 8 mmHg.

2) Subacute/Intermittent PACG :

⇨ Shallow anterior chamber.

⇨ Physiological factors like dim light or watching a movie in darkened cinema hall precipitate pupillary block and there occurs rise in IOP.

⇨ <u>Symptoms</u> :

a) Transient blurring of vision.

b) Colored halos around the light.

c) Headache

d) Browache.

e) Eyeache.

⇨ <u>Signs</u> :

eye is white but not congested.

⇨ Provocative tests are positive.

3) Acute PACG : (Congestive Glaucoma) **(Fig. 4.16)**

⇨ Characterised by sudden occlusion of entire angle with resultant acute rise of IOP to extremely high level.

⇨ <u>Symptoms</u> :

a) Sudden painful LOV :

Which radiates along branches of Vth nerve and is

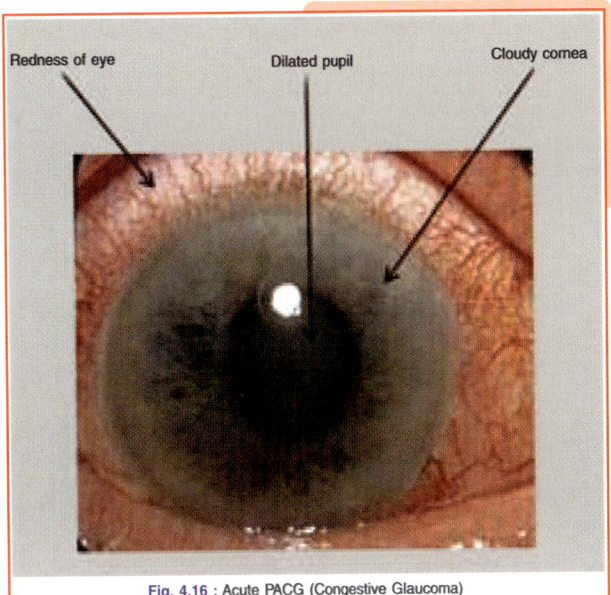

Redness of eye   Dilated pupil   Cloudy cornea

Fig. 4.16 : Acute PACG (Congestive Glaucoma)

associated with
↓

b) Nausea, Vomiting, Prostrations.

c) Colored halos.

d) Redness,   Photophobia,
   Lacrimation.

⇨ Signs :

   a) Shallow Anterior Chamber.

   b) Semidilated, vertically oval, fixed
      pupil, non reactive to both
      light and accommodation.

   c) IOP is increased (40-70 mmHg)

   d) Lid edema.

   e) Conjunctiva is chemosed,
      congested, red.

   f) Cornea is edematous,
      insensitive, cloudy.

   g) Iris is discolored.

   h) Angle of AC is closed.

   i) Optic disc is edematous,
      hyperaemic.

   j) Fellow eye : shallow AC,
      narrow angle.

4) *Chronic PACG :*

   ⇨ Constantly elevated IOP.

   ⇨ Decreased visual acuity.

   ⇨ Visual field defects like POAG.

   ⇨ Eyeball is white & not congested.

5) *Absolute   PACG   (Absolute
   Glaucoma) :* (Fig. 4.17)

   ⇨ If chronic PACG is untreated,
      patient passes into final phase *i.e.*
      'Absolute Glaucoma'.

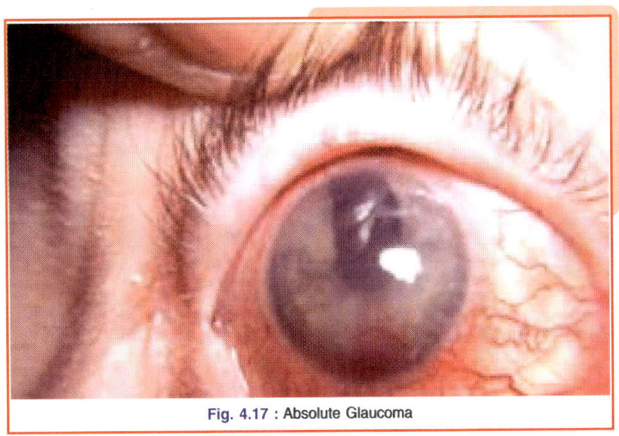

Fig. 4.17 : Absolute Glaucoma

Clinical features :

a) Painful blind eye, and is irritable.

b) Perilimbal Reddish blue zone.

c) Caput medusae (prominent
   enlarged vessel).

d) Hazy cornea with bullous keratopathy or filamentary keratitis.

e) Atrophic Iris.

f) Stony hard eyeball.

g) Raised IOP.

h) Fixed dilated pupil.

i) Optic disc atrophy.

It is worth noting that above phases does
not necessarily progress from one phase
to next in an orderly sequence.

e.g. eye may develop an acute PACG
from subacute PACG (or) directly
from subacute PACG it may pass to
chronic PACG without passing
through acute PACG.

Post Congestive ACG :

It refers to the clinical status of eye after an
attack of Acute Congestive PACG, with or
without treatment.

1) Post surgical post congestive Glaucoma :

   ➢ clinical status of eye after laser
      peripheral iridotomy for acute attack
      of PACG.

2) <u>Spontaneous angle opening</u> :

➤ Very rarely angle opens spontane-ously, and acute PACG subsides.

3) <u>Chronic congestive Angle closure Glaucoma</u> :

➤ Occur when acute PACG is not treated or when laser iridotomy is unsuccessful.

➤ It is worth noting that chronic congestive Angle Closure Glaucoma is different (eye is permanently congested & irritable) from chronic PACG (eye is painless, white but not congested).

4) <u>Ciliary body shut down</u> :

➤ Temporary cessation of aqueous secretion due to ischaemic damage to ciliary epithelium.

➤ Clinical features are similar to PACG except that IOP is low, pain is markedly reduced.

5) <u>Vogt's Triad</u> :

➤ Seen in any type of post congestive Glaucoma.

➤ i) Glaucomflecken (anterior subcapsular lenticular opacity). **(Fig. 4.18)**

ii) Patches of Iris Atrophy.

iii) Slightly dilated non reacting pupil.

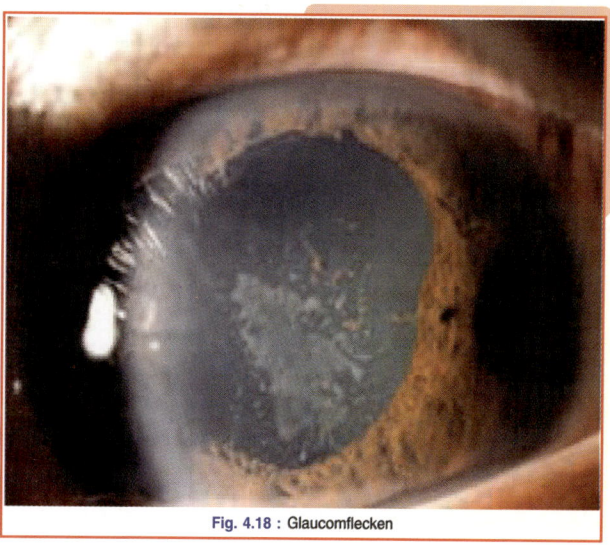
Fig. 4.18 : Glaucomflecken

III) **Differential Diagnosis of colored Halos in PACG :**

🐚 Colored halos in PACG are due to the accumulation of fluid in cornea (corneal edema). This can be differentiated from halos found in immature cataract and mucopurulent conjunctivitis.

🐚 In mucopurulent conjunctivitis, halos can be eliminated by irrigating the eye.

🐚 'Fincham's test' is used to differentiate halos of PACG and immature cataract.

🐚 Stenopic slit is passed accrossed the pupil : If

a) Halos are intact : Glaucoma.

b) Halos are broken : Immature into segments cataract

IV) **Treatment : (for acute congestive phase of PACG) :**

🐚 Definitive treatment (Treatment of choice) is surgery.

However initially, drugs are used to lower IOP during acute attack.

🐚 *Approach of treatment :*

a) Start iv acetazolamide / iv mannitol.

b) When IOT starts falling, start topical pilocarpine or Timolol.

c) Apraclonidine / Latanoprost may be added.

d) Once IOT is reduced, surgery is done.

'Topical pilocarpine 2% is preferred Antiglaucomatous drug'.

🐚 *Definitive management of choice :*

a) Laser (Nd:YAG) peripheral Iridotomy.

b) If laser is not available :

Surgical peripheral Iridectomy.

c) Other procedures :

i) Trabeculotomy

ii) Deep sclerotomy⎫ Filtration surgeries

iii) Viscoanulostomy⎭

🐚 Symptomatic treatment during an attack includes analgesics, antiemetics, topical steroids to reduce the inflammation.

🐚 Mydriatics (Atropine) are contraindicated as they precipitate Glaucoma.

- Prophylactic Peripheral laser iridotomy should be performed in fellow eye as PACG is bilateral disease.

- For latent stage (PACG suspect), subacute, chronic PACG :
  - ➤ Peripheral laser Iridotomy is treatment of choice.
  - ➤ Trabeculectomy is done when laser is not available or that fails.

- *For Absolute Glaucoma :*
  - i) Retrobulbar alcohol injection for pain relieve.
  - ii) Destruction of ciliary epithelium by cyclocryotherapy, cyclodiathermy, cyclophotocoagulation.
  - iii) Enucleation when pain is severe and is not controlled by conservative means.

☐ CONGENITAL/DEVELOPMENTAL GLAUCOMA (BUPHTHALMOS) :

- Congenital glaucoma is due to the failure or abnormal development of trabecular meshwork.

- Iris may not be completely separated from the cornea so that angle remains closed by persistent embryonic tissue (Barkan's membrane).

- It may or may not be associated with other syndrome.

Types :

A) *Primary congenital/developmental glaucoma :*

- Except for glaucoma, no other ocular or systemic anomaly is present.
- a) *Congenital* : at birth or within one month.
- b) *Infantile* : 1 m to 3-4 years of age.
- c) *Juvenile* : 4-10 years of age.

B) *Secondary Congenital Glaucoma :*

- Glaucoma with associated ocular/ systemic syndrome.
- Aniridia, Iridocorneal dysgenesis, Struge-Weber Syndrome, Lowe's syndrome, Von-Recklinghausen's neurofibromatosis, congenital microcornea, Rubella.

When disease manifest prior to the age of 3 years, eyeball enlarges and is bull like.

- bull like eyes → Buphthalmos **(Fig. 4.19)**

  ↓

- due to retention → Hydrophthalmos of aqueous humor

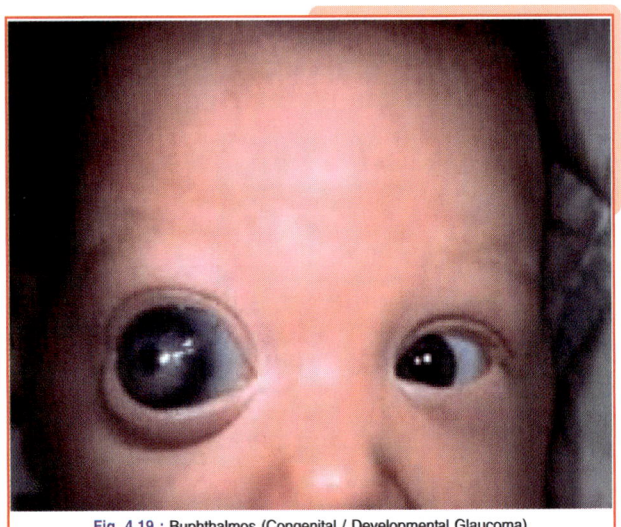

Fig. 4.19 : Buphthalmos (Congenital / Developmental Glaucoma)

Clinical Features :

- Bilateral, boys are affected more.

<u>Symptoms</u> :

- Classical Triad of : a) Lacrimation
  Buphthalmos   b) Photophobia
  c) Blepharospasm

- Eye Rubbing.

<u>Signs</u> :

1) Cornea :
   - ➤ Corneal edema – first sign.
   - ➤ Hazy cornea with 'frosted glass appearance'. **(Fig. 4.20)**
   - ➤ Corneal enlargement.
   - ➤ 'Haab striae' (discrete corneal opacities as lines with double contour due to Descemet's tear) **(Fig. 4.21)**

2) Sclera : thin & blue.

3) Anterior chamber : 'Deep'.

4) Iris : Iridodonesis, Iris atrophy.

5) Lens : anteroposteriorly flat, subluxated backwards.

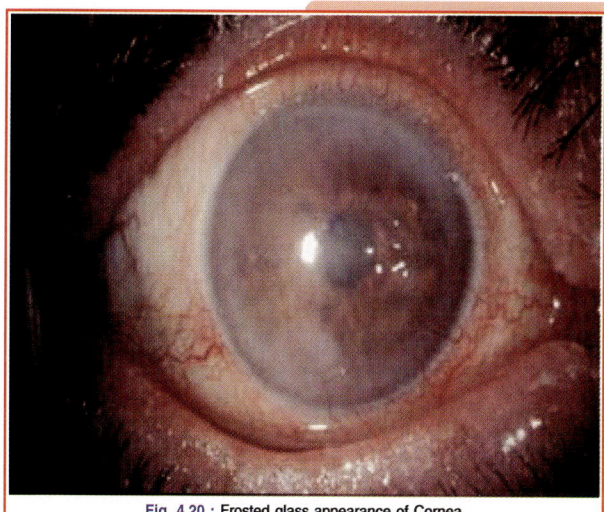

Fig. 4.20 : Frosted glass appearance of Cornea

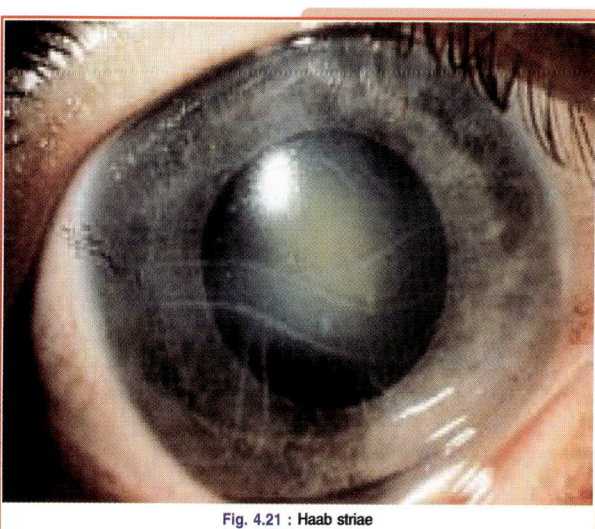

Fig. 4.21 : Haab striae

6) Large eye (Buphthalmos / Hydrophthalmos).

7) IOP is raised.

8) Optic disc cupping & atrophy.

9) Axial myopia due to increased axial length → Anisometropic amblyopia.

Management :

Investigations :

1) IOP measurement (Schiotz / Applanation).

2) Corneal diameter measurement by callipers.

3) Slit lamp examination.

4) Ophthalmoscopy for optic disc evaluation.

5) Gonioscopy for angle of anterior chamber.

Treatment :

☞ Unlike adult glaucoma, Initial treatment for congenital glaucoma → Surgical

↓

'Drainage angle surgery'.

☞ Surgical procedures :

  a) Goniotomy.

  b) Trabeculotomy : performed with corneal clouding.

  c) Trabeculectomy.

  d) Combined trabeculotomy and trabeculectomy.

☞ Glaucoma drainage devices (GDD) are used.

☞ Medications are not effective, however IOP is lowered by osmotic agents, acetazolamide, beta blockers till surgery is taken up. Miotics are of no use.

❑ RUBEOSIS IRIDIS (Neovascular Glaucoma) (NVG) :

It is a secondary angle closure glaucoma which results due to formation of neovascular membrane over the iris (Fig. 4.22).

Etiology :

i) Common causes :

  ❧ Proliferative Diabetic Retinopathy (most common).

  ❧ Central retinal vein occlusion (CRVO).

  ❧ Eale's disease.

  ❧ Sickle cell retinopathy.

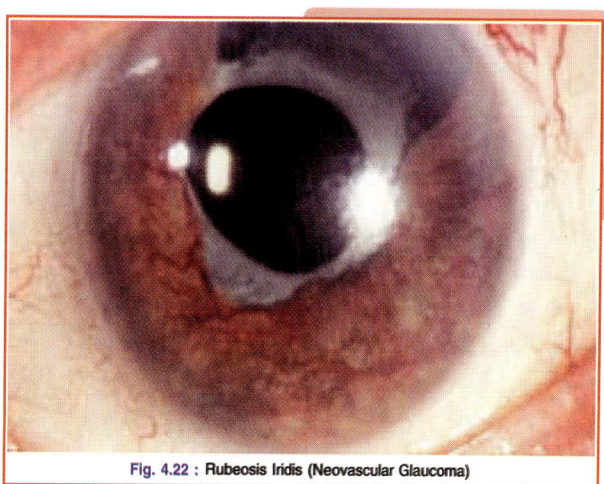

Fig. 4.22 : Rubeosis Iridis (Neovascular Glaucoma)

ii) Rare causes :

- Central retinal artery occlusion (CRAO).
- Uveitis (intraocular inflammation).
- Fuch's heterochromic iridocyclitis.
- Intraocular tumors (Retinoblastoma, choroidal melanoma)
- Radiation retinopathy
- Ocular ischaemic syndrome (carotid artery disease, carotid cavernous fistula)

In CRVO, glaucoma manifests about 100 days after thrombosis of central vein, so also called '100 days Glaucoma'.

Pathogenesis :

Most widely accepted theory for neovascularization is hypoxic retina producing diffusible angiogenic factor (VEGF) that stimulates new vessel formation.

Clinical stages :

1) *Pre glaucomatous stage :*
   - Stage of Rubeosis iridis.
2) *Open angle glaucoma stage :*
   - due to pretrabecular neovascular membrane formation.
3) *Secondary angle closure glaucoma :*
   - due to contracture of neovascular membrane (zipper angle closure) leads to goniosynechiae formation.

Treatment :

1) Panretinal photocoagulation is treatment of choice as it terminates the angiogenic stimulus for neovascularization of retina.
2) Glaucoma drainage devices *i.e.* artificial filtration shunt (Seton operation) may control the IOP.

◘ TRABECULECTOMY :

- It is an external filtration surgery.
- Most commonly done filtering surgery.
- Done when extensive peripheral synechiae are present (> 50% angle closure).

Indications :

1) *Primary angle closure glaucoma :*
   - when synechiae involves > 270^0 angle or if medical treatment fails, peripheral Iridectomy fails.
2) *Primary open angle glaucoma :*
   - if medical treatment fails.
3) Congenital & Developmental Glaucoma.
4) Secondary Glaucoma

Surgical Technique :

1) Initial steps :
   - Anaesthesia, cleansing, draping, exposure of eyeball, fixing with superior rectus suture.
2) Conjunctival flap is dissected.
3) Scleral flap is dissected and reflected down.
4) Excision of trabecular tissue.
5) Peripheral Iridectomy at 12 o'clock position.
6) Closure by suturing the scleral and conjunctival flap.
7) Subconjunctival injection of dexamethasone and gentamicin are given.
8) Patching the eye with sterile eye pad and bandage.

Complications :

1) Postoperative shallow anterior chamber.
2) Hyphaema.
3) Iritis.
4) Cataract due to accidental injury to lens.
5) Endophthalmitis.

- Sutureless Trabeculectomy is also done nowadays.

◘ FINCHAM TEST :

- discussed in Primary Angle closure Glaucoma.

◘ DIURNAL TEST OF IOP VARIATION :

- discussed in Primary Open Angle Glaucoma.

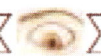

Chapter

5

Uveal Tract

Most Important (Must Read Topics)	Elective Topics
1) Iridocyclitis	—
2) Iris Bombe	
3) KP's	
4) Festooned Pupil	
5) Seclusio/occlusio Pupillae.	

❏ IRIDOCYCLITIS (Anterior Uveitis) :

It is the inflammation of Iris and pars plicata of ciliary body.

A) Etiology :

1) Infections :

- ➤ may be exogenous (from outside),

    endogenous (through blood stream),

    secondary (keratitis, scleritis etc.)

- ➤ Bacterial : TB, leprosy, syphilis.
- ➤ Viral : Herpes simplex, CMV, Herpes Zoster
- ➤ Fungal : Aspergillosis, candidiasis.
- ➤ Parasitic : Toxoplasmosis, Toxocariasis
- ➤ Ricketssial : Scrub typhus, epidemic typhus.

2) Immune Related :

- ➤ Microbial allergy.
- ➤ Anaphylactic uveitis
- ➤ Atopic uveitis.
- ➤ Autoimmune :

    Juvenile Rheumatoid Arthritis (JRA)

    Ankylosing Spondylitis (HLA-B27).

    Reiter's Syndrome (HLA-B27)

    Behcet's disease (HLA-B5)

    Vogt Koyanagi Harada (HLA-DR4)

    Lens induced, Psoriasis, IBD.

3) Traumatic :

- ➤ accidental / operative injuries to uveal tissue.

4) Toxic :

- ➤ from endotoxins / endocular / exogenous source

5) Non infective systemic diseases

➤ Sarcoidosis, PAN, DLE, DM, Psoriasis

6) Malignancy :

➤ Retinoblastoma, Leukemia, Lymphoma, Melanoma.

7) Idiopathic :

➤ Fuch's heterochromic Iridocyclitis.

B) Clinical Features :

Symptoms :

1) Pain

2) Redness

3) Photophobia

4) Lacrimation

5) Blepharospasm.

6) Defective vision

due to ciliary spasm, corneal haze (edema, KP's), aqueous turbidity.

(Fig. 5.1)

Signs :

1) Lid edema.

2) Circumcorneal ciliary congestion which has violaceous hue **(Fig. 5.2)**

3) *Cornea :*

i) Corneal edema.

ii) Keratic precipitates (KP's) :

⇨ Proteinaceous cellular deposits at the back of cornea on endothelium.

⇨ They are aggregation of polymorphonuclear cells, lymphocytes, epitheloid cells.

Types of KP's :

a) Mutton fat KP's : (Fig. 5.3)

❑ large, yellowish.

❑ characteristic of granulomatous uveitis.

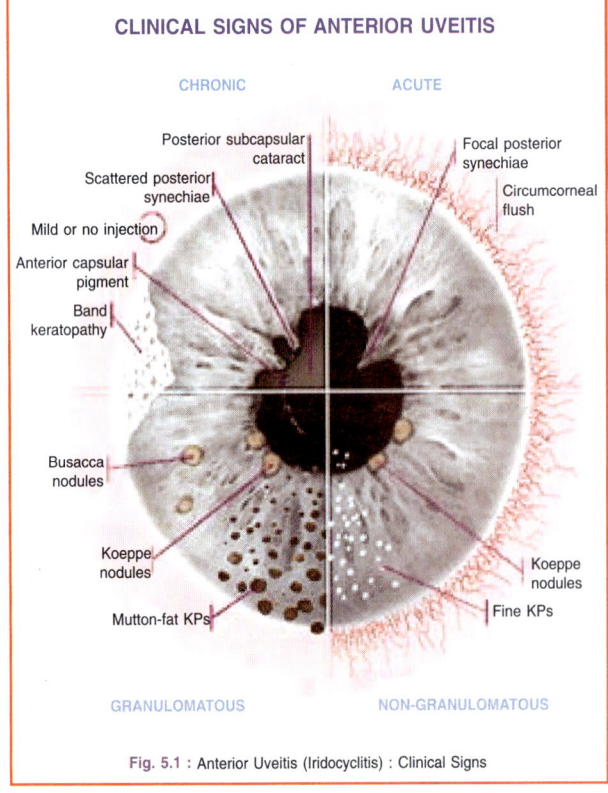

CLINICAL SIGNS OF ANTERIOR UVEITIS

CHRONIC   ACUTE

Posterior subcapsular cataract

Scattered posterior synechiae

Mild or no injection

Anterior capsular pigment

Band keratopathy

Busacca nodules

Koeppe nodules

Mutton-fat KPs

Focal posterior synechiae

Circumcorneal flush

Koeppe nodules

Fine KPs

GRANULOMATOUS   NON-GRANULOMATOUS

Fig. 5.1 : Anterior Uveitis (Iridocyclitis) : Clinical Signs

Circum corneal congestion (CCC)

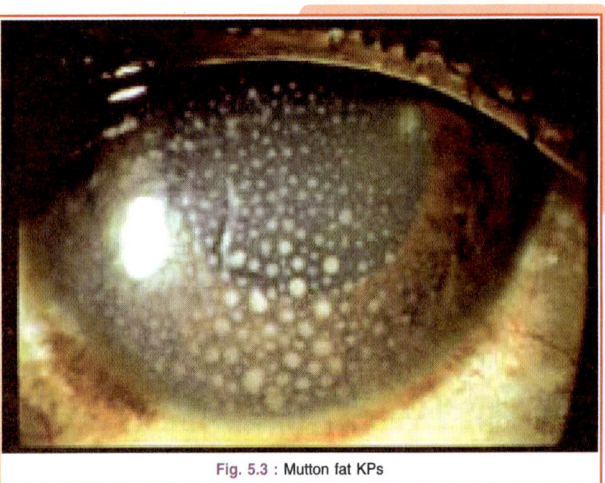

Fig. 5.2 : Circumcorneal Ciliary Congestion

Fig. 5.3 : Mutton fat KPs

- ❑ composed of epitheloid cells, macrophages.
- ❑ large, thick fluffy, lardaceous, having greasy/waxy appearance.

b) Small & medium KP's : (Fig. 5.4)

- ❑ granular KP's.
- ❑ characteristic of non-granulomatous uveitis.
- ❑ composed of lymphocytes.
- ❑ small, round, whitish precipitates.

c) Fine KP's : (Fig. 5.5)

- ❑ also called Stellate KP's.
- ❑ characteristic of Fuch's heterochromic iridocyclitis, herpetic iritis, CMV retinitis.

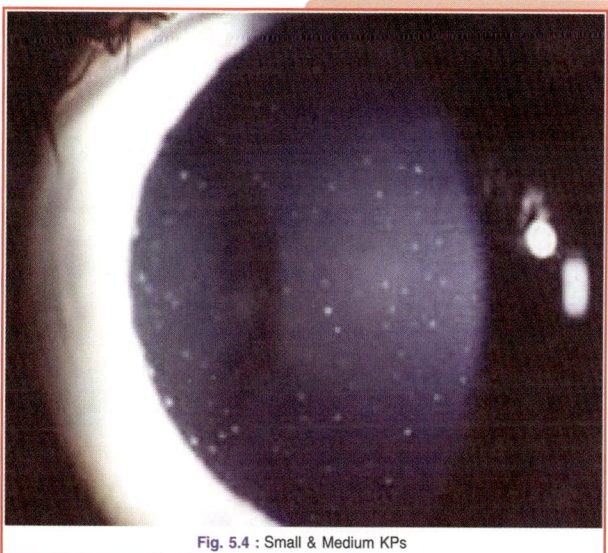

Fig. 5.4 : Small & Medium KPs

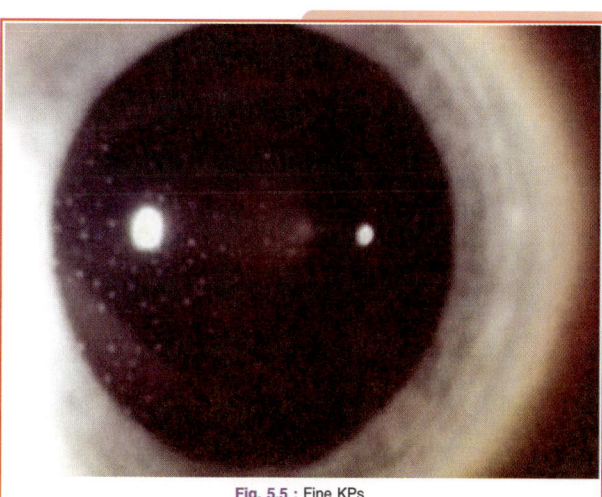

Fig. 5.5 : Fine KPs

d) Red KP's :

- ❑ composed of RBC, inflammatory cells.
- ❑ characteristic of hemorrhagic uveitis.

e) Old KP's :

- ❑ Characteristic of healed uveitis.
- ❑ have ground glass appearance due to hyalinization.

iii) Posterior corneal opacities.

4) *Anterior chamber signs :*

- i) Aqueous flare : earliest sign of anterior uveitis. **(Fig. 5.6)**
- ii) Deep anterior chamber (if posterior synechiae occurs).
- iii) Aqueous cells.
- iv) Hypopyon
- v) Hyphaema (in hemorrhagic uveitis)

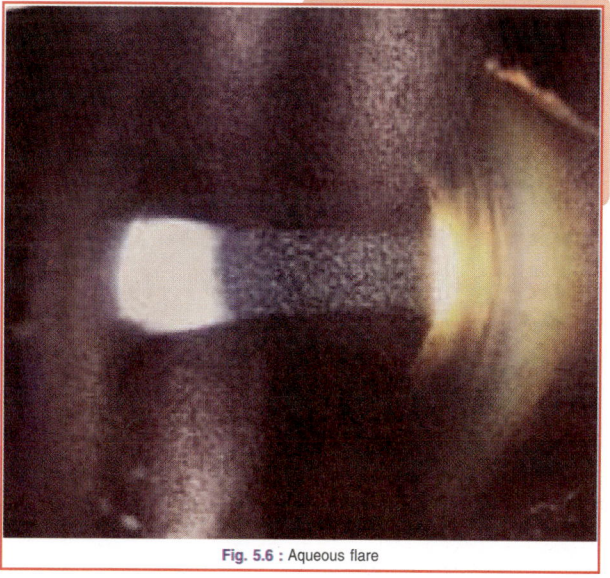

Fig. 5.6 : Aqueous flare

5) *Iris signs :*

- i) Muddy Iris (blurred, indistinct)
- ii) Iris atrophy.
- iii) Iris nodules. **(Fig. 5.7)**
    - a) at pupillary margin : Koeppe's nodules
    - b) at periphery of iris : Busacca's nodules.

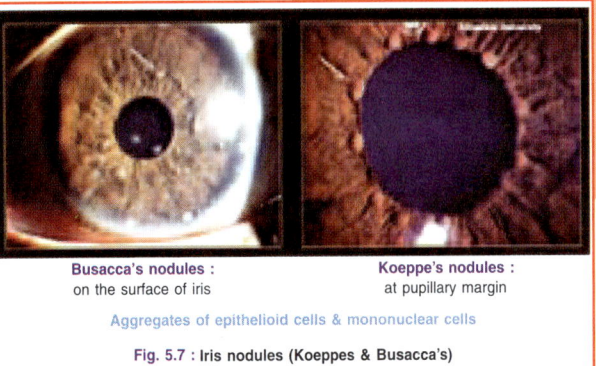

Busacca's nodules :
on the surface of iris

Koeppe's nodules :
at pupillary margin

Aggregates of epithelioid cells & mononuclear cells

Fig. 5.7 : Iris nodules (Koeppes & Busacca's)

c) Tubercular nodules.

d) Syphilitic nodules.

e) Sarcoid nodules.

iv) Posterior synechiae :

⇨ Adhesions between the iris (posterior surface) and anterior capsule of lens.

⇨ Depending on the portion of iris involved :

a) Segmental   posterior synechiae:

↣ adhesion to the lens at some points.

↣ dilatation of the pupil with segmental posterior synechiae causes intervening portions of the circle of pupil to dilate → 'Festooned appearance of pupil'. **(Fig. 5.8)**

b) Annular posterior synechiae : **(Fig. 5.9)**

↣ 360^0 adhesions of pupillary margin to the anterior capsule of lens.

↣ So, aqueous is unable to pass from posterior chamber to anterior chamber and collects behind the iris, which becomes bowed forwards like a sail, called 'Iris bombe'. **(Fig. 5.10)**

↣ Also known as Seclusio pupillae/Ring synechiae.

↣ AC from front is funnel shaped.

v) Rubeosis iridis (neovascularization of iris).

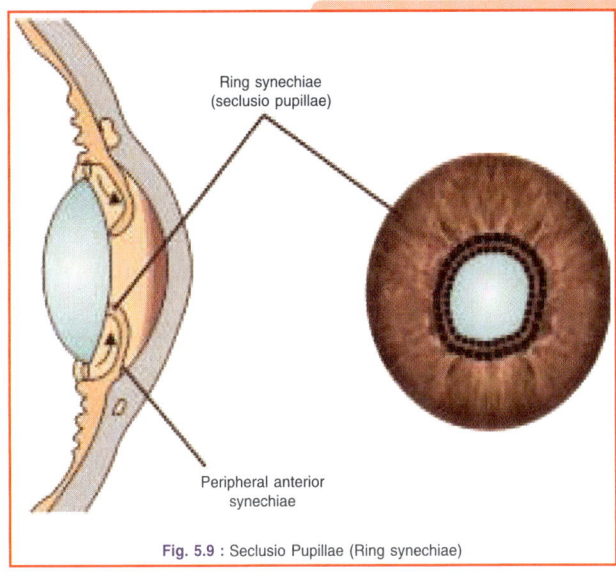

Ring synechiae
(seclusio pupillae)

Peripheral anterior
synechiae

Fig. 5.9 : Seclusio Pupillae (Ring synechiae)

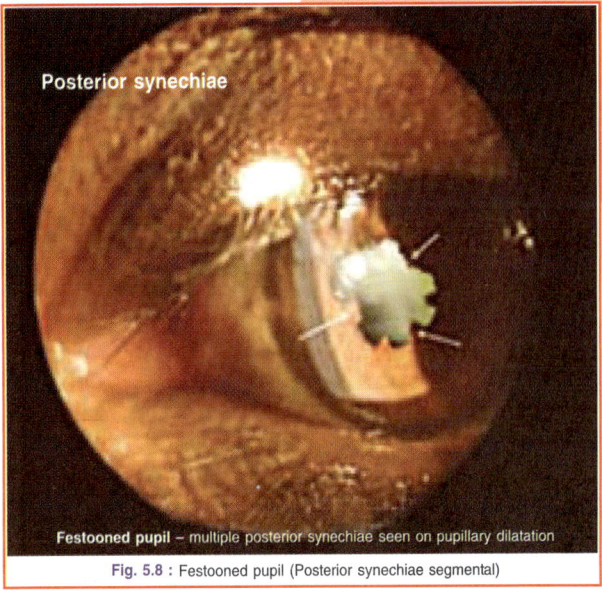

Posterior synechiae

Festooned pupil – multiple posterior synechiae seen on pupillary dilatation

Fig. 5.8 : Festooned pupil (Posterior synechiae segmental)

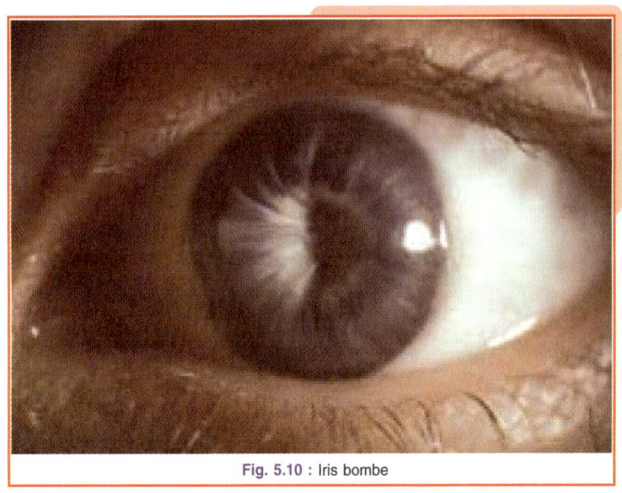

Fig. 5.10 : Iris bombe

vi) Anterior synechiae (adhesion of iris to cornea). **(Fig. 5.11)**

6) *Pupillary signs :*

i) narrow miotic pupil.

ii) Irregular pupil : festooned pupil due to segmental posterior synechiae.

iii) Sluggish pupillary reaction.

iv) ectropion pupillae.

v) Occlusio pupillae :

pupil is occluded due to organisation of exudates across the entire pupil.

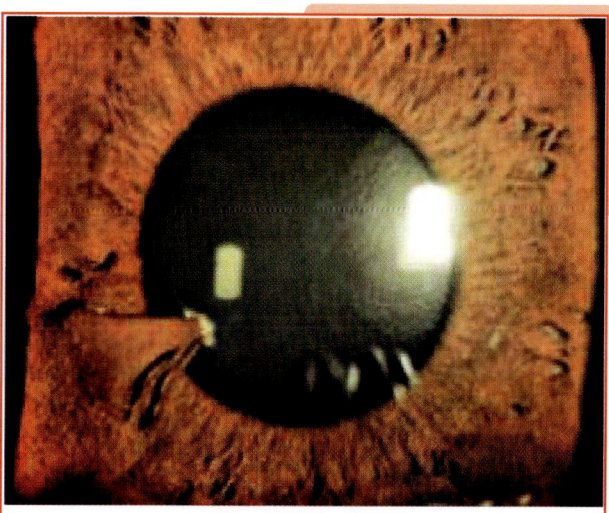

Fig. 5.11 : Anterior synechiae

7) *Lens :*

i) Pigment dispersal on anterior capsule.

ii) Exudates on lens.

iii) Complicated cataract :

Polychromatic lustre, bread crumb appearance.

8) *Vitreous & Retina :*

i) exudates, inflammatory cells.

ii) CME.

9) *IOP :*

➢ Normal

➢ Increased (in Secondary Glaucoma)

➢ Decreased (in Acute Iridocyclitis).

C) Complications :

1) Complicated cataract.

2) Secondary Glaucoma : can be early / late :

a) *Early glaucoma (hypertensive uveitis) :*

due to clogging of trabecular mesh-work of AC by inflammatory cells, exudates in active phase of disease.

b) *Late glaucoma : (post inflammatory)*

caused by seclusio pupillae/occlusio pupillae.

3) Cyclitic membrane

4) Choroiditis

5) Retina :

➢ CME

➢ Retinal scar

➢ Papillitis

➢ Macular scar, hole

➢ Exudative Retinal Detachment

➢ Epiretinal membrane

6) Papillitis (inflammation of optic disc)

7) Band keratopathy

8) Phthisis bulbi

9) Hyphaema

10) Hypopyon

11) Iris nodules

12) Posterior synechiae

13) Iris atrophy

14) Rubeosis iridis

15) Vitreous changes : Vitreous band leading to rhegmatogenous Retinal Detachment.

Phthisis bulbi : (Figs. 5.12 & 5.13)

✎ Final end stage of any form of chronic uveitis.

✎ Ciliary body is disorganised and so aqueous production is hampered.

✎ Eye becomes : soft, shrunken and eventually becomes soft atrophic globe (phthisis bulbi).

✎ Occurs in 3 stages :

1) Atrophic bulbi without shrinkage.

2) Atrophic bulbi with shrinkage.

3) Atrophic bulbi with disorganization.

✎ IOT is reduced, due to decrease aqueous formation.

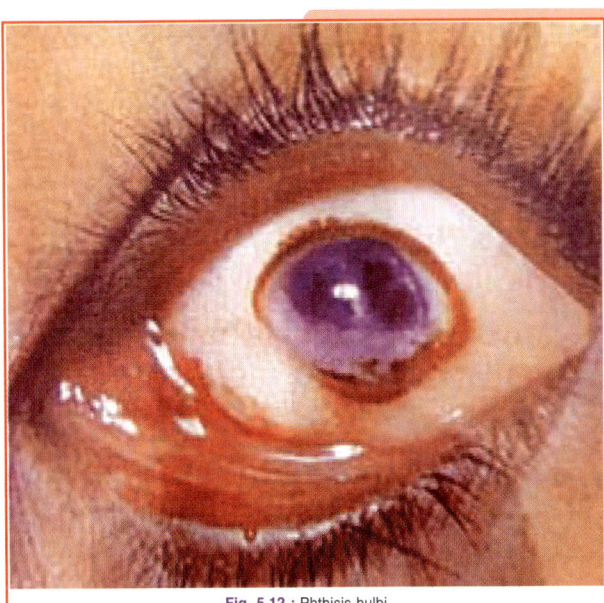

Fig. 5.12 : Phthisis bulbi

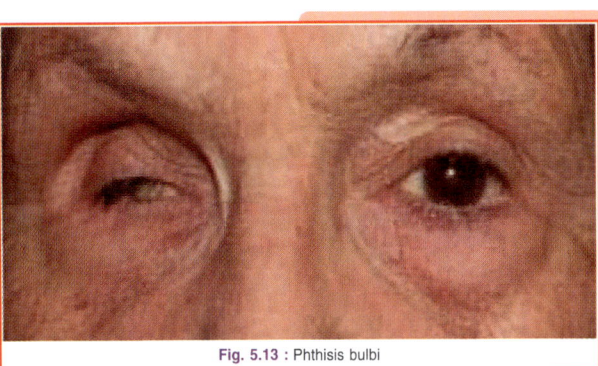

Fig. 5.13 : Phthisis bulbi

Histopathologically :

- Globe is small, shrunken with marked thickening of sclera.
- Disorganization, atrophy of intraocular contents.
- Retinal pigment epithelium undergo metaplasia leading to Intraocular ossification (calcification) in end stage.
- Calcification may also occur in Bowman's layer of cornea and lens.

D) Management :

Investigations :

1) *Hematological :*
   - TLC, DLC, ESR, Blood sugar, Blood uric acid.
   - Serological tests for syphilis, Toxoplasmosis.
   - Tests of ANA, CRP, Rh factor, LE cells.

2) *Urine :* for WBC, pus cells, RBC's.

3) *Stool :* Cysts, ova to rule out parasitic infections.

4) *Radiological :*
   - X-ray chest, paranasal sinuses, spine, sacroiliac joint.
   - CT scan, MRI.

5) *Skin tests.*

E) Treatment :

I) *Specific treatment of the cause.*

II) *Non-specific treatment :*

1) *Local :*

   Topical steroids are DOC.
   - Dexamethasone drops 4-6 times a day.
   - eye ointment at bed time.
   - Reduces inflammation.

   Mydriatics - cycloplegics (Atropine) are 2nd DOC. 2-3 times a day for 2-3 weeks
   - Mydricain (Atropine, Adrenaline, procaine).
   - Homatropine.
   - Tropicamide, cyclopentolate.
   - Relieves ciliary muscle spasm.
   - Prevents posterior synechiae formation.

   Broad spectrum antibiotic drops.

2) *Systemic :*

   Steroids (Prednisolone)

   NSAIDs (Aspirin)

   Immunosuppressants (cyclosporine, Methotrexate)

   Azithromycin, Tetracycline, Erythromycin

3) *General measures :*
   - Hot fomentation.
   - Dark goggles.

III) *Treatment of complications :*

1) Inflammatory Glaucoma → Timolol maleate

2) Post inflammatory Glaucoma → Laser Iridotomy

3) Complicated cataract → Lens extraction

4) Phthisis bulbi → when painful → Enucleation.

◻ **IRIS BOMBE**

◻ **KP's**

◻ **FESTOONED PUPIL**

◻ **SECLUSIO/OCCLUSIO PUPILLAE.**

discussed in Iridocyclitis

Chapter

6

Lacrimal Apparatus

Most Important (Must Read Topics)	Elective Topics
1) Epiphora, causes 2) Chronic Dacryocystitis 3) Acute Dacryocystitis 4) Congenital Dacryocystitis 5) Dacryocystorhinostomy	1) Dacryocystectomy

❑ EPIPHORA & IT's CAUSES : (Fig. 6.1)

⚮ Watering of eye is characterised by outflow of tears from conjunctival sac.

⚮ It may be due to :

1) Hyperlacrimation : excessive tears secretion.

2) Epiphora : obstruction to the outflow of normally secreted tears or due to lacrimal pump failure.

Epiphora causes :

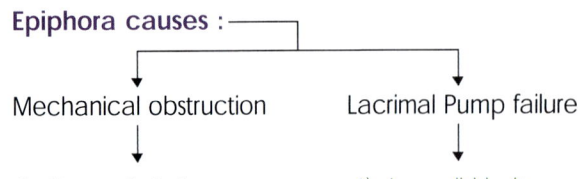

Mechanical obstruction

1) Congenital absence or occlusion of puncta
2) Congenital dacryocystitis
3) Chronic/Acute dacryocystitis
4) Canaliculitis
5) Canaliculi obstruction
6) Neoplasms of lacrimal sac

Lacrimal Pump failure

1) Lower lid laxity
2) Bell's palsy (weakness of orbicularis oculi)
3) Ectropion

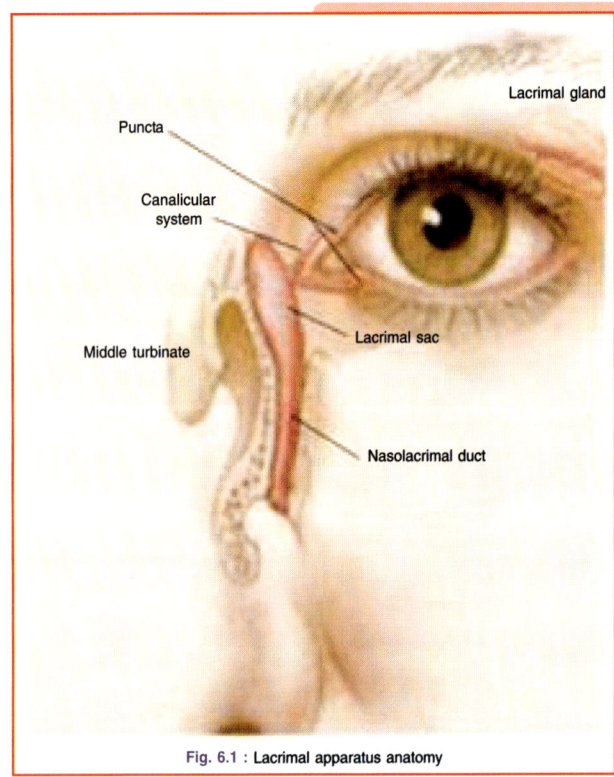

Fig. 6.1 : Lacrimal apparatus anatomy

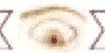

7) Nasal polyp

8) Tumors in inferior meatus.

Evaluation of Epiphora :

A) For mechanical obstruction :

1) ROPLAS (Regurgitation on pressure over lacrimal apparatus, sac).

2) Fluorescein dye test :
   - ➤ Normally, no dye is seen in conjunctival sac.
   - ➤ Prolonged retention in conjunctival sac indicates inadequate drainage.

3) Lacrimal Syringing :
   - ➤ Normal saline is pushed into the lacrimal sac from lower punctum with the syringe and lacrimal cannula.
   - ➤ Free passage into the nose rules out mechanical obstruction.

4) Jones dye test :
   - ➤ It is done in partial obstruction only, it has no value in total obstruction.

5) Dacryocystography

B) For lacrimal pump failure :

1) Dacryoscintigraphy

2) Radionucleotide dacryocystography
   └──▶ more sensitive

3) Fluorescein dye disappearance test.

◻ DACRYOCYSTITIS :

✠ It is inflammation of lacrimal sac at the inner corner of the eye.

✠ 2 types :

a) Congenital : low grade chronic inflammation

b) Acquired/adult : Acute or chronic

◻ CHRONIC DACRYOCYSTITIS : (Fig. 6.2)

✠ More common than Acute Dacryocystitis.

I) Etiology :

✎ Pre disposing factors :

1) Age : 4th to 6th decade of life.

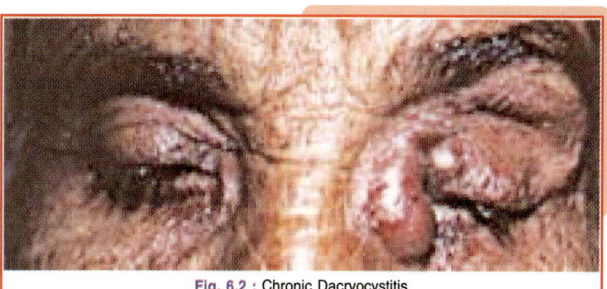
Fig. 6.2 : Chronic Dacryocystitis

2) Sex : in females 80%, due to the narrow lumen of bony canal.

3) Race : More common in whites than in Negroes.

4) Heredity.

5) Socioeconomic status : in low SE status.

6) Poor personal hygiene.

✎ Factors causing stasis of tears in lacrimal sac :

1) Anatomical factors :
   - ⇨ narrow bony canal
   - ⇨ partial canalization of membranous NLD.
   - ⇨ excessive membranous folds in NLD.

2) Foreign bodies in lacrimal sac.

3) Excessive lacrimation.

4) Inflammation due to conjunctivitis.

5) Obstruction of NLD by nasal diseases (polyp, hypertrophied inferior conchae, DNS, tumors, atrophic rhinitis).

✎ Source of infection :

from conjunctiva, nasal mucosa, paranasal sinuses.

✎ Causative organism :

Staphylococcus, streptococcus, pneumococcus, pseudomonas pyocyanea.

II) Clinical features :

4 stages :

1) Chronic catarrhal Dacryocystitis :

- ➤ Watering eye (epiphora) is the only symptom.
- ➤ Regurgitation : positive (clear fluid).

2) Lacrimal mucocele :

- ➢ Epiphora is associated with swelling below the inner canthus.

- ➢ *Encysted mucocele :* sometimes it is encysted due to continued chronic infection. Opening of both the canaliculi into the sac are blocked → large swelling with negative Regurgitation test (if mucocele is encysted).

- ➢ *Regurgitation :* positive (milky fluid).

3) Chronic suppurative dacryocystitis :

- ➢ mucocele becomes infected to form pyocele.

- ➢ Epiphora is associated with recurrent conjunctivitis, swelling at the inner canthus.

- ➢ Encysted pyocele : if the canaliculi are blocked.

- ➢ Regurgitation : positive (flank purulent fluid).

4) Chronic fibrotic sac :

- ➢ due to thickening of mucosa by low grade repeated infections for prolonged period.

- ➢ Persistent epiphora & discharge.

- ➢ Regurgitation : positive.

III) Complications :

1) Chronic conjunctivitis.

2) Ectropion of Lower lid.

3) Corneal ulceration.

4) Endophthalmitis

IV) Treatment :

1) Conservative :

- ➢ Massage

- ➢ Antibiotic drops

- ➢ Probing

- ➢ Lacrimal syringing

2) Balloon catheter dilatation

- ➢ also called Balloon dacryocystoplasty.

3) Dacryocystorhinostomy (DCR) :

- ➢ Surgery of choice

- ➢ Before surgery, pyocele should be controlled by topical antibiotics.

4) Dacryocystectomy (DCT) :

- ➢ It is done when DCR is contraindicated.

- ➢ DCT is done in :

  a) Too young (< 4 years) & too old (> 60 years).

  b) Shrunken & fibrosed sac.

  c) TB, Leprosy, Syphilis, Mycotic infections.

  d) Tumors of sac.

  e) Atrophic rhinitis.

  f) Unskilled surgeon : Good DCT is always better than bad DCR.

5) Conjunctivodacryocystorhinostomy (CDCR) : in blocked canaliculi.

◘ ACUTE DACRYOCYSTITIS :

- ⌀ Acute suppurative inflammation of lacrimal sac characterized by painful swelling in region of the sac.

- ⌀ Marked swelling, redness, tenderness over the lacrimal sac.

Etiology :

1) Acute exacerbation of chronic Dacryocystitis.

2) Acute peridacryocystitis from paranasal sinuses, bones, dental abscess, caries.

3) Causative organisms :

   Streptococcus, Pneumococcus, Staphylococcus.

Clinical features :

3 stages :

1) Cellulitis : (Fig. 6.3)

- ➘ Painful swelling in the lacrimal sac region.

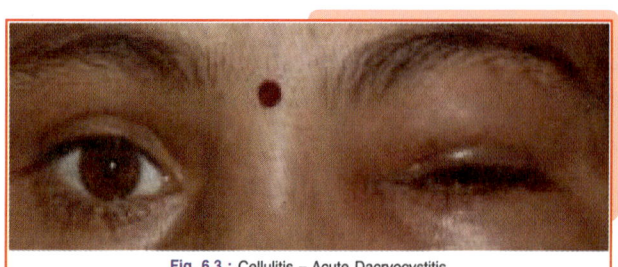

Fig. 6.3 : Cellulitis – Acute Dacryocystitis

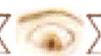

- Epiphora and presence of constitutional symptoms like fever, malaise.

- Swelling is red, hot, firm, tender.

2) Lacrimal abscess : (Fig. 6.4)

- Continued inflammation causes occlusion of canaliculi due to edema.

- Sac is filled with pus, sac distents, anterior wall ruptures forming a pericystic swelling.

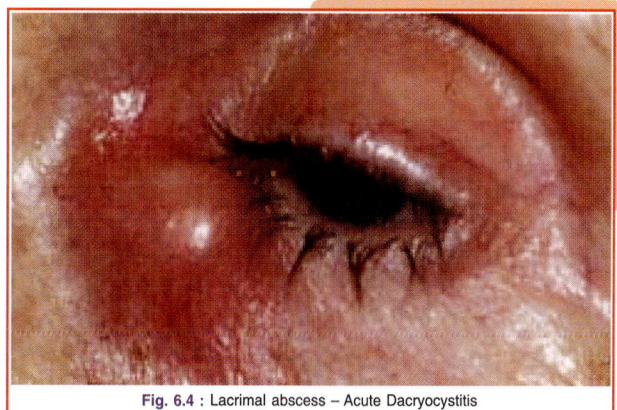

Fig. 6.4 : Lacrimal abscess – Acute Dacryocystitis

3) Fistula formation : (Fig. 6.5)

- when abscess is unattended, it discharges spontaneously leaving external fistula below the medial palpebral ligament.

- abscess open into the nasal cavity rarely → internal fistula.

Complications :

1) Acute conjunctivitis.
2) Corneal abrasion, ulcer.
3) Lid abscess.

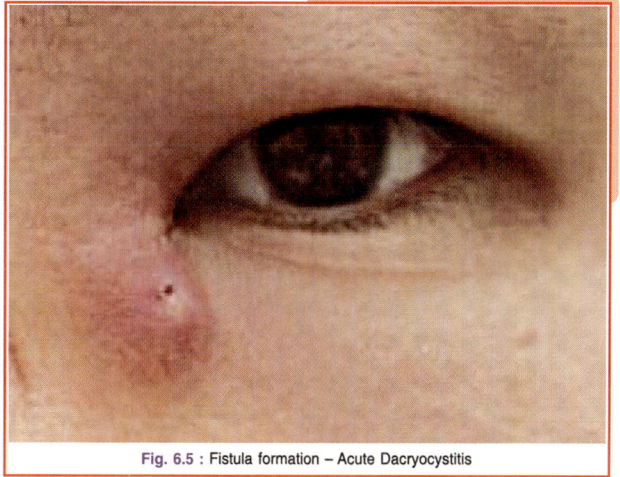

Fig. 6.5 : Fistula formation – Acute Dacryocystitis

4) Orbital cellulitis.
5) Osteomyelitis of lacrimal bone.
6) Facial cellulitis.
7) Cavernous sinus thrombosis.

Treatment :

1) Cellulitis :

- Systemic / Topical Antibiotics to control the infection.

- Systemic NSAIDs, steroids.

- Hot fomentation to relieve pain, swelling.

2) Lacrimal abscess :

- Above treatment as discussed.

- When pus starts pointing on the skin → It is drained with small incision, pus is squeezed out, dressing is done with betadine soaked gauze.

- Later depending upon the sac condition → DCT/DCR is done, otherwise Recurrence will occur.

3) External lacrimal fistula :

- Control the acute infection with systemic antibiotics then

- Fistulectomy along with DCT/DCR.

☐ CONGENITAL DACRYOCYSTITIS :

- Inflammation of the lacrimal sac in newborn infants.

- Also known as Dacryocystitis neonatorum. (Fig. 6.6)

Etiology :

1) Congenital blockage in NLD.

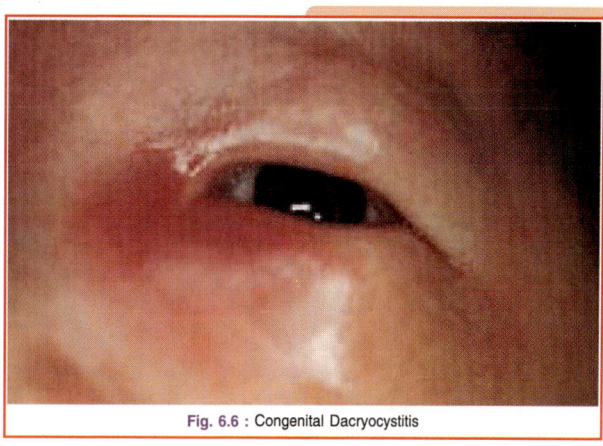

Fig. 6.6 : Congenital Dacryocystitis

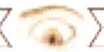

2) Membranous occlusion at lower end, near the Hasner valve - commonest cause.

3) Epithelial debris, membranous occlusion at upper end near the lacrimal sac, noncanalization, bony occlusion.

4) Common organisms :

Staphylococci, Streptococci, Pneumococci.

Clinical features :

1) Epiphora : after 7 days of birth, followed by mucopurulent discharge.

2) Swelling on the sac.

3) Regurgitation is positive.

Complications :

1) Conjunctivitis.

2) Acute/chronic Dacryocystitis

3) Lacrimal abscess/fistula.

Treatment :

1) Massage over the lacrimal sac with topical antibiotics : 4 times a day followed by instillation of antibiotic drops.

   - cures obstruction in 90% Infants.

   - spontaneous recanalization of obstructed NLD can occur upto 9 months.

2) Lacrimal syringing :

   - with normal saline and antibiotic solution if condition is not cured upto 3 months.

3) Probing of NLD with Bowman's probe :

   - if it is not cured upto 6-12 months.

4) Balloon catheter dilatation :

   - when repeated probing is failure.

5) Intubation with silicone tube :

   - if probing, balloon catheter dilatation are failure.

6) Dacryocystorhinostomy (DCR) :

   - when intubation also fails.

   - Conservative management by massaging, topical antibiotics & intermittent lacrimal syringing should be continued till 4 years of age, then the DCR is performed.

☐ DACRYOCYSTORHINOSTOMY :

⚗ It is a surgical procedure to restore the flow of tears into the nose from the lacrimal sac when the nasolacrimal duct does not function.

⚗ 3 Types :

1) Conventional External DCR.

2) Endonasal (Surgical or laser) DCR.

3) Endocanalicular laser DCR.

I) Conventional external DCR :

Indications :

1) Primary acquired Nasolacrimal duct obstruction.

2) Secondary acquired Nasolacrimal duct obstruction (due to trauma, nasal surgery etc.)

3) Functional obstruction of outflow, due to lacrimal pump weakness or after facial nerve palsy.

4) Congenital nasolacrimal duct obstruction, after failed probing, intubation.

5) History of Dacryocystitis.

Steps of Surgery :

1) General Anaesthesia is given.

2) Curved skin incision along medial to medial canthus.

3) Exposure of medial palpebral ligament (MPL) by blunt dissection to expose anterior lacrimal crest.

4) Separation of periosteum from anterior lacrimal crest.

5) Dissection of lacrimal sac with blunt dissector and is reflected laterally.

6) Exposure of nasal mucosa.

7) Probe is introduced into the sac through lower canaliculus and sac is incised vertically.

8) Fashioning of nasal mucosa flaps by converting them into H shape.

9) Suturing of the flaps by 6-0 vicryl.

10) Suturing of medial palpebral ligament to periosteum, suturing of orbicularis muscle with 6-0 vicryl.

11) Skin is closed with 6-0 silk.

📖 ***Success rate is over 90%.***

II) Endonasal (Surgical or Laser) DCR :

This is preferred over conventional external DCR because of certain disadvantages of external approach.

Indications :

1) Failure of conservative treatment.
2) Chronic Dacryocystitis.
3) Failure of conventional external DCR.

Steps of Surgery :

1) Preparation of nasal mucosa with nasal decongestants drops, local anaesthetics before the operation.
2) Infiltration of conjunctival sac with 2% lignocaine.
3) Identification of sac area with nasal endoscope and further injection of lignocaine.
4) Creation of opening in the nasal mucosa, bones forming lacrimal fossa, and posteromedial wall of the sac by cutting the tissues or by Holmium YAG laser.
5) Stenting of Rhinostomy opening :
   ⇨ Silicon tubes are passed through the upper and lower puncta, pulled out through ostium and tied within the nose.
6) Nasal packing and dressing is done.
7) Post operative care (decongestants, antibiotics, steroids for 4 weeks) and after 24 hours nasal packs are removed.
8) Removal of Sialistic lacrimal stents after 8-12 weeks of surgery.

📖 ***Success rate is about 85%.***

Endonasal DCR	Conventional External DCR
Advantages	**Disadvantages**
1) No external scar	1) Cutaneous scar present.
2) Relatively blood less surgery	2) Relatively more bleeding.
3) Better visualization of nose	3) —
4) Less chances of injury to ethmoidal vessels & cribriform plate	4) Potential injury to medial canthus structures.
5) Less time required (15-30 mins)	5) More time required (upto 60 mins)
6) No postoperative morbidity	6) Significant post-op. morbidity.

Endonasal DCR	Conventional External DCR
Disadvantages	**Advantages**
1) Less success rate (70-90%)	1) More success rate (95%).
2) Requires skilled ophthalmologist and/or rhinologist	2) Easily performed by Ophthalmologists
3) Expensive	3) Cheap
4) Requires familiarity with endoscopic anatomy	4) Not required

III) Endocanalicular Laser DCR :

Steps of Surgery :

1) Local anaesthesia is given.
2) Identification of sac area.
3) Creation of opening in nasal mucosa, bones forming lacrimal fossa and posteromedial wall of sac by Holmium YAG or KTP laser.
4) Laser probe is passed through canaliculus upto the medial wall of sac.

📖 ***Success rate is only 70%.***

🔲 **DACRYOCYSTECTOMY (DCT) :**

☞ It is complete surgical extirpation of lacrimal sac.

Indications :

1) When DCR is contraindicated.
2) In too young (< 4 years) & too old (> 60 years).
3) Shrunken and fibrosed sac.
4) TB, Leprosy, Syphilis, Mycotic infections.
5) Tumors of sac.
6) Atrophic Rhinitis.
7) Unskilled surgeon : Good DCT is always better than bad DCR.

Steps of surgery :

(1-5) Steps of External DCR.
6) Removal of Lacrimal Sac by blunt dissection.
7) Curettage of bony NLD to remove the infected parts of membranous NLD.
8) Closure with 6-0 silk.

Chapter

7

Retina

Most Important (Must Read Topics)	Elective Topics
1) Diabetic Retinopathy 2) Retinal Detachment 3) Hypertensive Retinopathy 4) Retinopathy in Toxaemia of pregnancy 5) Differential Diagnosis of White pupillary reflex (Leukocoria) 6) Retinoblastoma	1) Macular Function tests 2) Retinal Hemorrhage

◻ DIABETIC RETINOPATHY : (DR)

✔ Diabetic Retinopathy is damage to the retina caused by complications of Diabetes Mellitus, which can eventually lead to blindness.

✔ Risk of DR is higher in patients with Type I DM (Insulin dependent) which is juvenile onset and almost all Type I DM patients develops DR in 15 years.

✔ And as type II DM (maturity onset) is more common, it contributes to significant portion of DR.

I. Etiopathogenesis :

Risk factors :

1) Duration of the disease : most important risk factor.

   It is duration of the disease after onset of puberty which acts as risk factor.

2) Age of onset of diabetes :
   ➤ Risk of Retinopathy in children with onset of diabetes at 2 years is negligible for first 10 years.
   ➤ After onset of puberty, age of onset is not a risk factor.

3) Poor glycemic control.

4) *Sex :* more in females.

5) Heredity.

6) *Pregnancy :* accelerate changes of DR.

7) *Hypertension :* accelerate changes of DR.

8) *Others :* Smoking, Obesity, Hyperlipidemia, Anemia.

Pathogenesis :

✎ DR including macular edema is Microangiopathy affecting Retinal

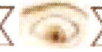

venules, capillaries, pre capillary arterioles.

- Chronic Hyperglycemia is important factor leading to microvasculature complications of DM (Diabetic Retinopathy, Neuropathy, Nephropathy)

- Excessive Glucose is reduced by aldose reductase to sorbitol.

- Accumulation of sorbitol & advanced glycosylated products results in :

  a) Activation of protein kinase C.

  b) Oxidative stress

  c) Increase production of growth factors.

     i)   VEGF-A

     ii) TGF-B

     iii) PDGF

     iv) EGF

     v)   IGF

- These results in endothelial metabolic dysfunction and cause microangiopathy & manifestations of DR. **(Fig. 7.1)**

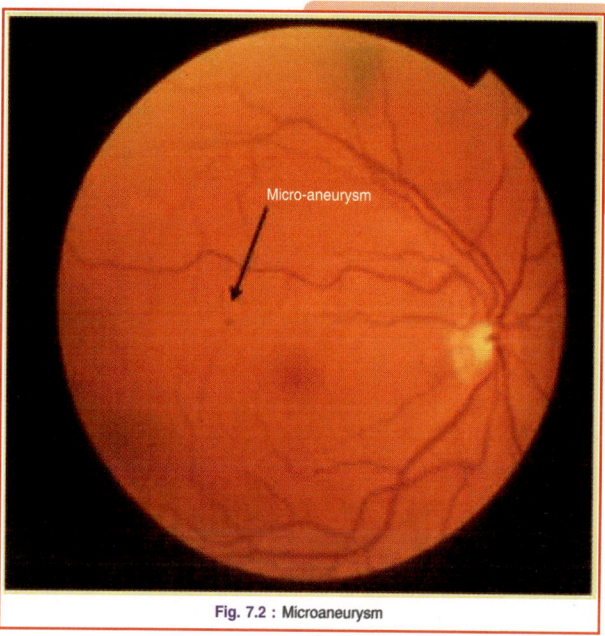

Fig. 7.2 : Microaneurysm

Retinopathy (advanced NPDR).

1) *Microaneurysms :* **(Fig. 7.2)**

   Earliest ophthalmoscopically detectable change, involves inner nuclear layer.

2) *Venous abnormalities :*

   ❑ Venous beading, looping, dilation.

3) Retinal edema at macular area.

4) Hard exudates, and in advanced NPDR : Soft exudates (cotton wool spots) **(Fig. 7.3)**

5) Retinal hemorrhage : **(Fig. 7.4)**

   both deep (dot blot) and

   superficial (flame shaped).

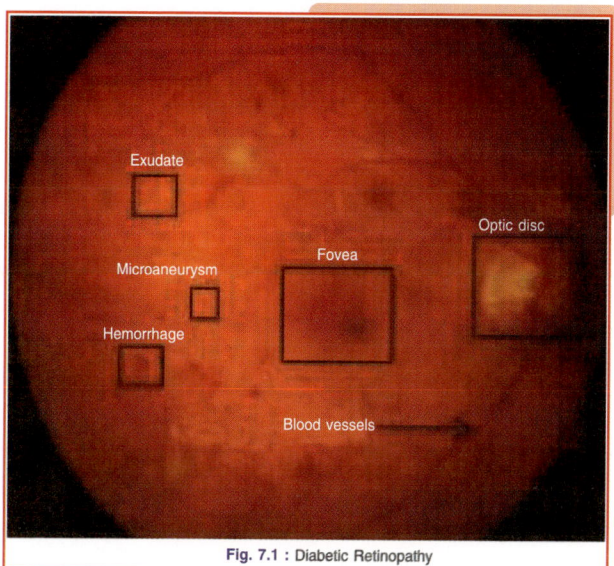

Fig. 7.1 : Diabetic Retinopathy

II. Classification/Manifestations of DR :

A) Non proliferative DR (NPDR) :

- It may be mild, moderate, severe, very severe.

- Earliest stage of DR.

- It includes Background Retinopathy (early NPDR), Pre proliferative

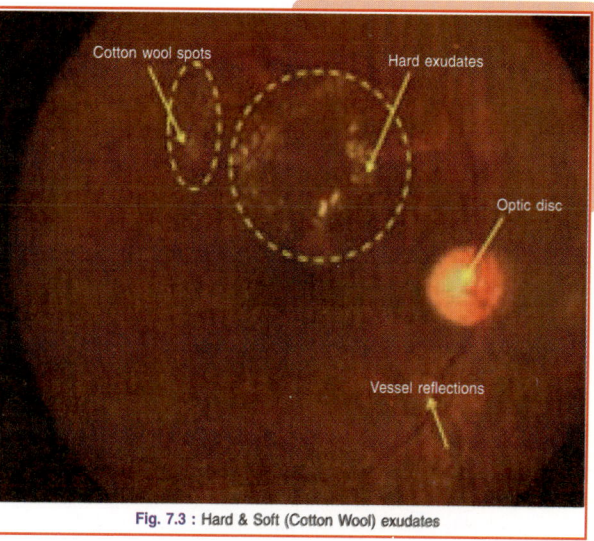

Fig. 7.3 : Hard & Soft (Cotton Wool) exudates

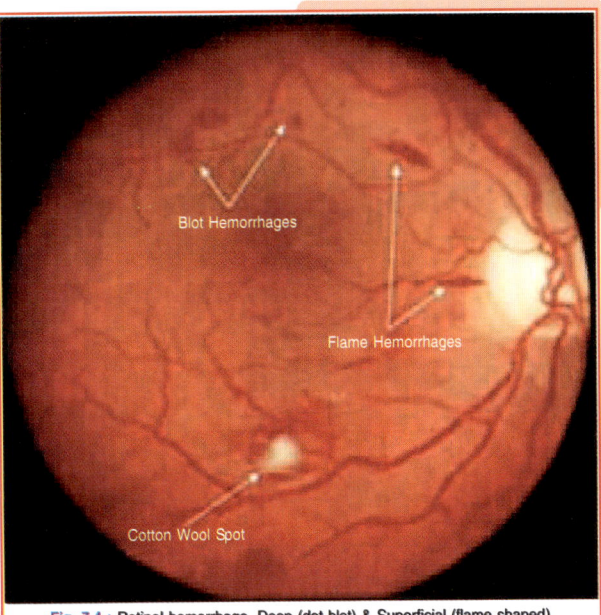

Fig. 7.4 : Retinal hemorrhage, Deep (dot blot) & Superficial (flame shaped)

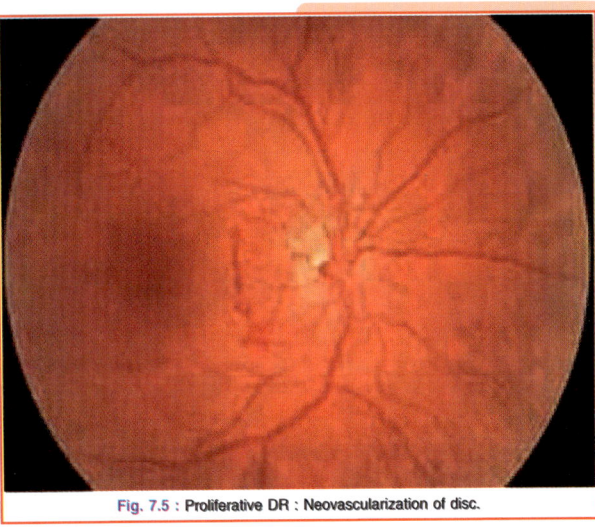

Fig. 7.5 : Proliferative DR : Neovascularization of disc.

B) Proliferative DR : (Fig. 7.5)

Hallmark of Proliferative DR is 'Neovascularization'.

↓

i) within one disc diameter of optic disc, is referred to as Neovascularization of Disc. (NVD)

ii) farther than one disc diameter of optic disc, is referred to as Neovascularization elsewhere (NVE).

Complications :

i) Vitreous hemorrhage.

ii) Fibrovascular proliferation

iii) Tractional Retinal Detachment.

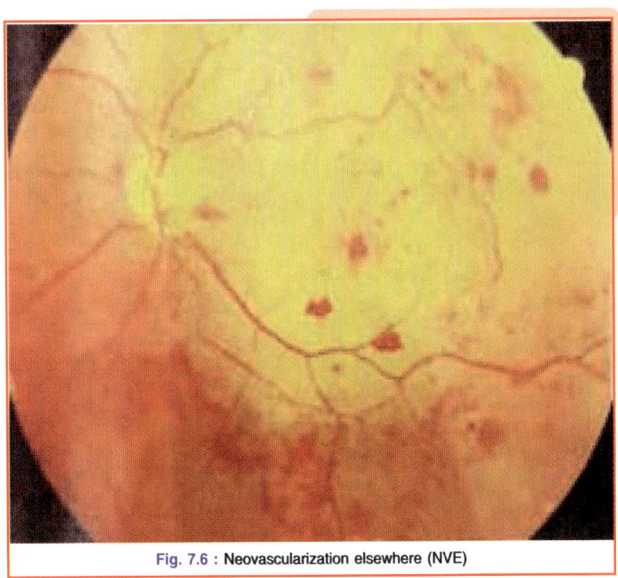

Fig. 7.6 : Neovascularization elsewhere (NVE)

C) Diabetic Maculopathy : (Fig. 7.7)

➢ may be associated with NPDR or PDR.

➢ Macular edema occurs due to increased permeability of Retinal capillaries.

➢ Macular edema is termed as clinically significant macular edema (CSME) if one of the following three criterias are present : (Fig. 7.8)

i) Thickening of retina at or within 500 micron of centre of fovea.

ii) Hard exudate at or within 500 micron of centre of fovea associated with retinal thickening.

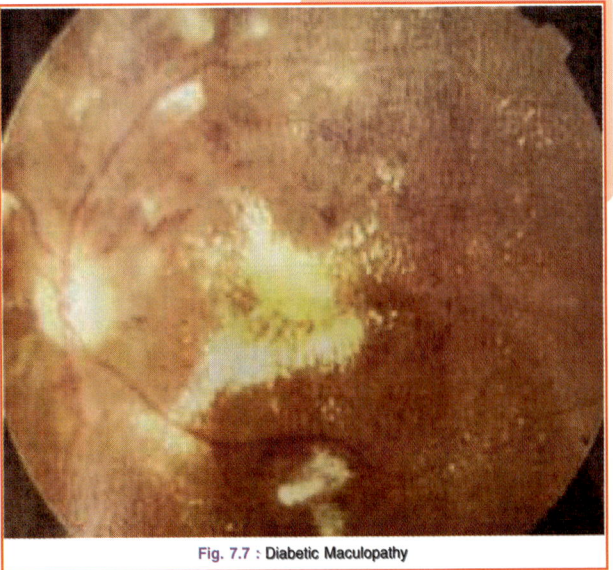

Fig. 7.7 : Diabetic Maculopathy

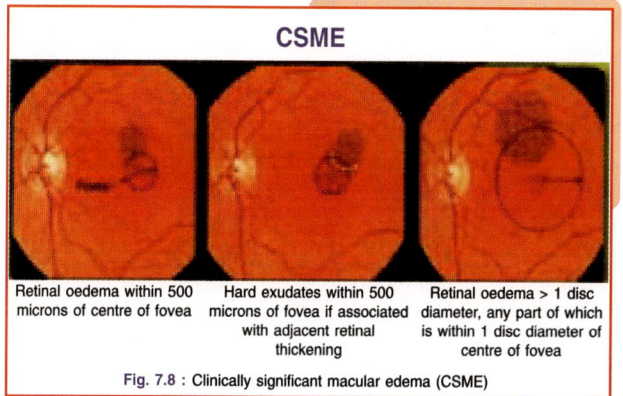

CSME

Retinal oedema within 500 microns of centre of fovea | Hard exudates within 500 microns of fovea if associated with adjacent retinal thickening | Retinal oedema > 1 disc diameter, any part of which is within 1 disc diameter of centre of fovea

Fig. 7.8 : Clinically significant macular edema (CSME)

iii) Development of zone of retinal thickening which is one disc diameter or larger, at least a part of which is within one disc diameter of foveal centre.

D) Advanced Diabetic Eye disease :

➢ End stage of uncontrolled PDR.

➢ *Complications* :

   i) Persistent vitreous hemorrhage.

   ii) Neovascular Glaucoma (Rubeosis Iridis).

   iii) Tractional Retinal Detachment.

III) Management :

A) Screening.

B) Investigations.

C) Treatment.

A) Screening :

Periodic fundus examination :

i) First examination, 5 years after the diagnosis of Type I DM and at the time of diagnosis in Type II DM.

ii) Every year till there is no DR or mild NPDR.

iii) Every 6 months in moderate NPDR.

iv) Every 3 months in severe NPDR.

v) Every 2 months in PDR.

B) Investigations :

1) Urine examination.

2) Blood sugar.

3) 24 hour urinary protein

4) Retinal function tests

5) Lipid profile

6) Hemogram

7) HbA1c

8) Fundus fluorescein angiography

9) Optical coherence tomography (OCT)

C) Treatment :

1) Strict Glycemic control and control of associated hypertension.

2) *Pharmacological* :

   a) Protein kinase Inhibitors.

   b) Anti VEGF drugs :

      Bevacizumab ⎱ intravitreal
      Ranibizumab ⎰

   c) Antioxidants

   d) Vit. E

   e) Intravitreal steroids (Triamcinolone)

3) *Photocoagulation* : Mainstay for the treatment of Diabetic Retinopathy, Maculopathy.

   ⇨ done by using laser (Krypton or diode argon)

     a) for Proliferative DR :

       Panretinal photocoagulation.

     b) for CSME :

       Focal laser and grid pattern photocoagulatiion.

4) *Surgery* :

   for advanced PDR and complications. 'Pars plana vitrectomy' is treatment of choice.

   a) Advanced PDR with vitreous hemorrhage :

      Vitrectomy with removal of opaque vitreous gel and endophotocoagulation.

   b) Advanced PDR with extensive fibrovascular epiretinal membrane :

      Vitrectomy with removal of mebrane and endophoto-coagulation.

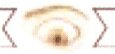

c) Advanced PDR with Tractional Retinal Detachment

Vitrectomy with reattachment of detached retina and endophotocoagulation.

RETINAL DETACHMENT :

- It is separation of neurosensory epithelium of retina from pigmented epithelium, because there is a potential space between these two layers where fluid can accumulate and cause separation.
- Divided into 3 types :

A) Rhegmatogenous Retinal Detachment.

B) Tractional Retinal Detachment.

C) Exudative Retinal Detachment.

A) Rhegmatogenous / Primary Retinal Detachment (Figs. 7.9 & 7.10)

➢ Most common type.

➢ Due to Retinal break/tear/hole which allows liquid vitreous to seep into subretinal space and separates sensory retina from pigmentory epithelium.

Etiology :

Pre disposing factors :

1) Myopia

2) Previous intraocular surgery : (Aphakia/Pseudophakia)

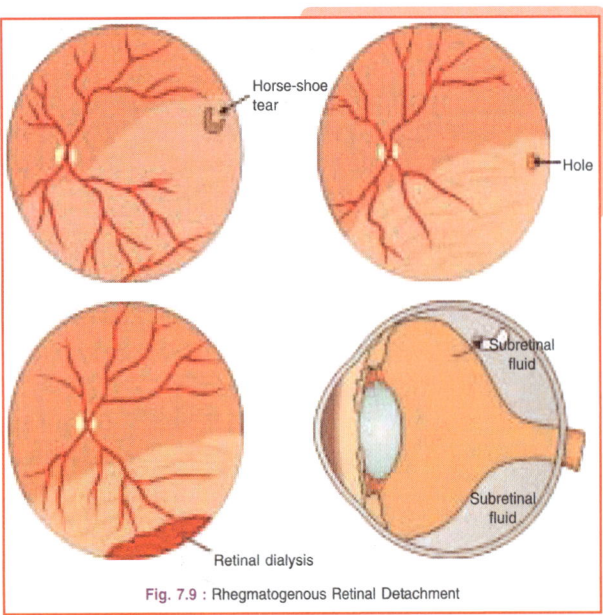

Fig. 7.9 : Rhegmatogenous Retinal Detachment

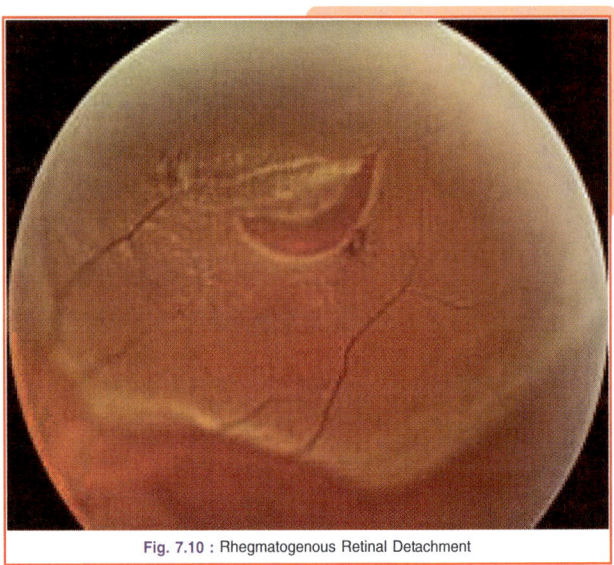

Fig. 7.10 : Rhegmatogenous Retinal Detachment

3) Trauma.

4) Retinal degeneration :
⇨ Lattice, Snail track degeneration.
⇨ Senile or degenerative retinoschisis.

5) Age : 40-60 years.

6) Sex : More in males.

Clinical features :

1) Photopsia (flashes of light).

2) Sudden onset of floaters i.e. dark spots infront of the eye (muscae volitantes) (Fig. 7.11)

3) Visual field defects corresponding to the area of detachment. (often there is peripheral loss in field of vision).

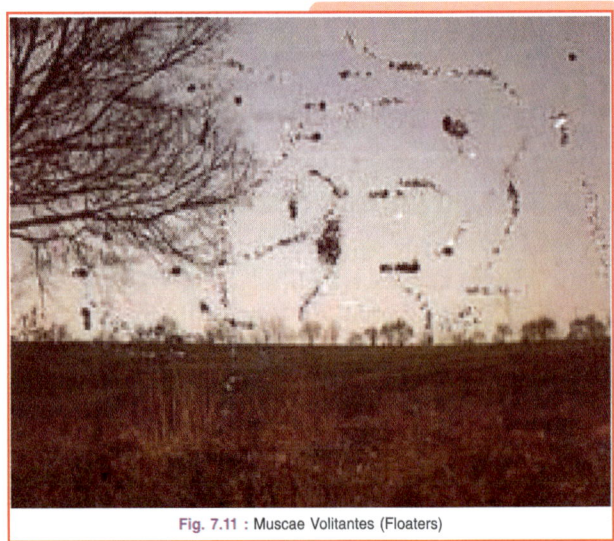

Fig. 7.11 : Muscae Volitantes (Floaters)

4) Sudden appearance of dark cloud, 'curtain' or 'veil' obscuring field of vision. **(Fig. 7.12)**

5) Sudden painless loss of vision.

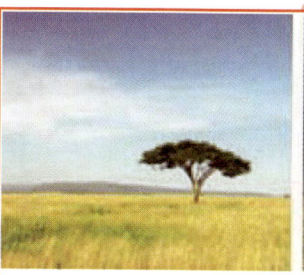
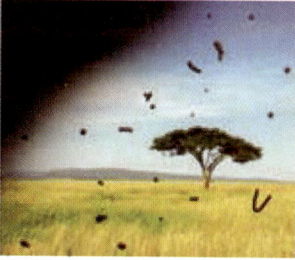

Fig. 7.12 : Curtain / Veil obscuring field of vision

Signs :

1) Ophthalmoscopy :

   ⇨ RD is best examined by Indirect Ophthalmoscopy using scleral indentation.

   ⇨ Freshly detached retina gives 'Grey Reflex' instead of normal pink reflex.

   ⇨ Retinal breaks are seen in the periphery (upper temporal quadrant commonly).

   ⇨ Vitreous shows pigment in anterior vitreous 'Tobacco dusting or Shaffer sign'. In absence of prior ocular surgery, it is pathognomic of Rhegmatogenous Detachment. **(Fig. 7.13)**

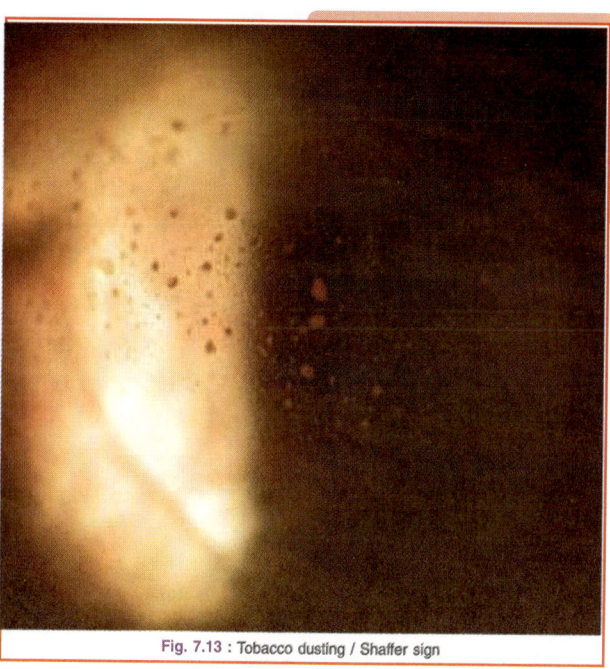

Fig. 7.13 : Tobacco dusting / Shaffer sign

2) *Perimetry* :
   Visual field defect corresponding to area of detached Retina (Scotomas).

3) Goldmann three mirror fundus lens & indirect slit lamp biomicroscopy by high power lens (+ 90 D or + 78 D), Central fundus examination by 55D, Hruby lens for macular detachment.

4) *ERG :* Subnormal or Absent.

5) *B scan USG :* done in presence of dense cataract to find the detachment.

6) *Plane mirror :* Altered red reflex in pupillary area.

7) Marcus Gunn pupil in extensive RD.

B) Tractional Retinal Detachment :

Due to the pulling on Retina from fibrovascular band in vitreous cavity *i.e.* vitreoretinal band. **(Figs. 7.14 & 7.15)**

Etiology :

1) Proliferative Diabetic Retinopathy.

2) Retinopathy of Prematurity.

3) Eale's disease.

4) Penetrating injury to the eye.

5) Post hemorrhagic retinitis proliferans.

6) Sickle cell Retinopathy.

7) Plastic cyclitis.

8) CRVO

9) Toxocariasis.

Clinical features :

1) Asymptomatic (no photopsia or floaters) unless macula is involved.

2) Presence of vitreoretinal bands.

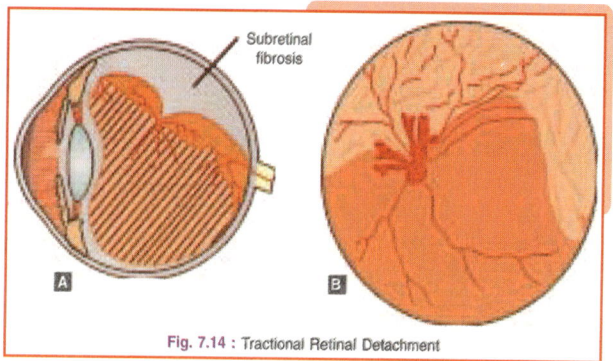

Fig. 7.14 : Tractional Retinal Detachment

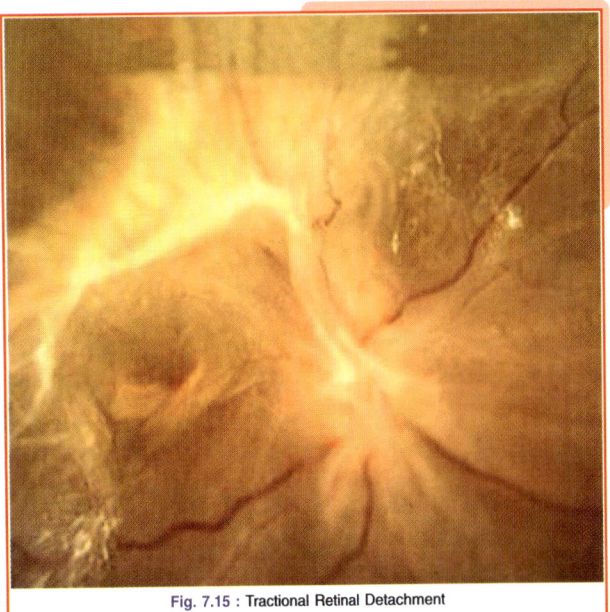

Fig. 7.15 : Tractional Retinal Detachment

3) Retinal breaks.

4) Highest elevation of Retina at the site of vitreoretinal traction.

C) Exudative or solid Retinal Detachment :

Occurs due to retina being pushed away by accumulation of fluid or neoplasm beneath the retina following vascular or inflammatory lesions. **(Figs. 7.16 & 7.17)**

Etiology :

Systemic Diseases :

➤ Toxaemia of Pregnancy.

➤ Renal Hypertension.

➤ Blood dyscrasias & PAN.

Ocular diseases :

1) Inflammation :

   ⇨ Harada's disease

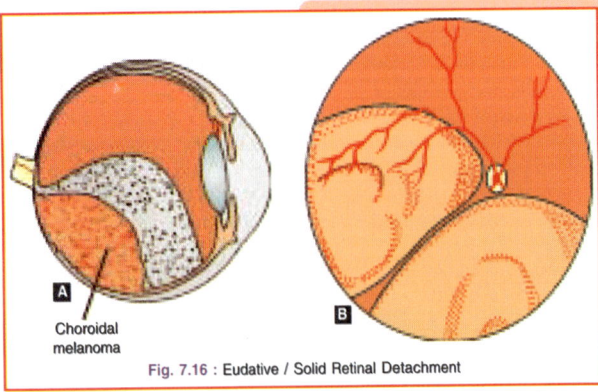

A
Choroidal melanoma
B

Fig. 7.16 : Eudative / Solid Retinal Detachment

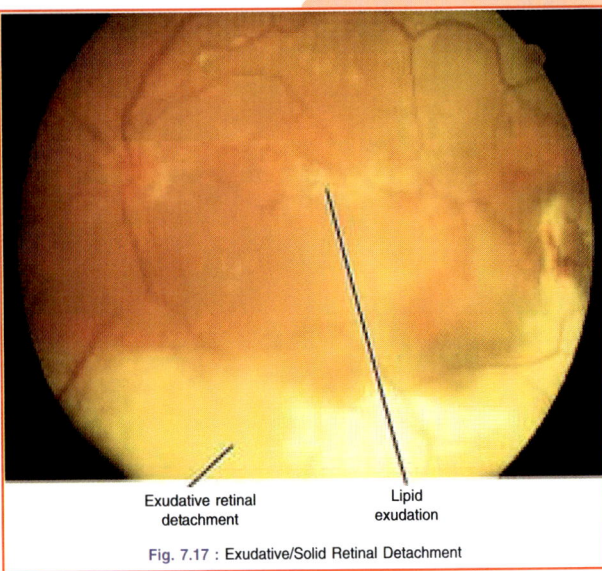

Exudative retinal detachment   Lipid exudation

Fig. 7.17 : Exudative/Solid Retinal Detachment

   ⇨ Posterior scleritis

   ⇨ Sympathetic ophthalmitis.

   ⇨ Orbital cellulitis.

2) Vascular diseases :

   ⇨ Central serous Retinopathy.

   ⇨ Exudative Retinopathy of Coats.

3) Neoplasms :

   ⇨ Retinoblastoma (exophytic type).

   ⇨ Malignant melanoma of choroid.

   ⇨ Metastatic tumor of choroid, hemangioma.

4) Sudden hypotony :

   ⇨ Perforation of the globe.

   ⇨ Intraocular operations.

5) Choroidal neovascularization.

6) Uveal effusion syndrome.

7) Congenital :

   ⇨ Nanophthalmos.

   ⇨ Coloboma.

   ⇨ Familial exudative vitreo-retinopathy.

Clinical features :

1) Occasional floaters but no photopsia.

2) Sudden painless loss of vision.

3) Smooth & convex detachment.

4) Shifting fluid characterised by

changing position of detached area : Hallmark of exudative Retinal Detachment.

Treatment of Retinal Detachment :

A) *Rhegmatogenous :*

1) Sealing the retinal breaks & tears :

   ❑ finding the retinal tears (holes) and sealing them by laser photocoagulation, diathermy, cryoapplication.

2) Drainage of SRF :

   ❑ allows apposition between sensory and retinal pigment epithelium.

3) Maintenance of Chorioretinal apposition by 'scleral buckling, external plombage, encirclage.

4) Pneumatic Retinopexy (gas injection into the vitreous).

5) Pars plana vitrectomy, endolaser photocoagulation, internal tamponade.

B) *Tractional :*

⇨ Treatment of causative factor.

⇨ Reducing the vitreous traction.

⇨ Pars plana vitrectomy, internal tamponade with gas or silicon oil.

C) *Exudative :*

⇨ Treatment of the cause.

⇨ Enucleation in presence of intraocular tumor.

▢ HYPERTENSIVE RETINOPATHY :

✦ Fundus changes occuring in patients suffering from systemic hypertension is Hypertensive Retinopathy. **(Fig. 7.18)**

Clinical Types :

1) Chronic Hypertensive Retinopathy.

2) Acute / Malignant Hypertensive Retinopathy.

1) Chronic Hypertensive Retinopathy :

Fundus changes occuring are :

a) Generalised (diffuse) arteriolar attenuation.

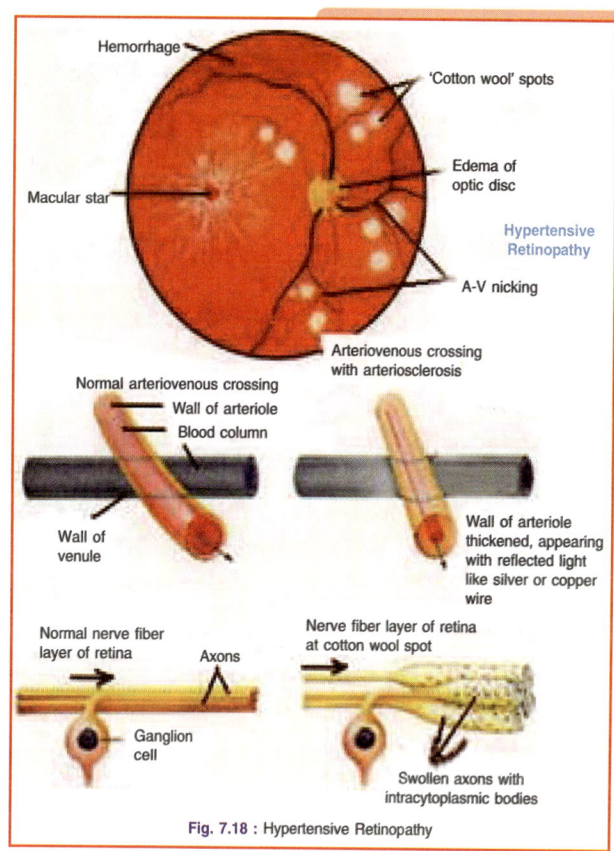
Fig. 7.18 : Hypertensive Retinopathy

b) Focal arteriolar narrowing / attenuation **(Fig. 7.19)**

   ↳ Earliest sign.

c) Arteriovenous crossing (nicking) changes:

   i) Right angle deflection at AV crossing

      ↳ 'Salu's sign'. **(Fig. 7.20)**

   ii) Banking of veins distal to AV crossing

      ↳ 'Bonnet sign'. **(Fig. 7.21)**

   iii) Tapering of veins on either side of crossing

      ↳ 'Gunn sign'. **(Fig. 7.22)**

d) Arteriolar reflex changes : **(Fig. 7.23)**

   Broadening of arteriolar light reflex 'Scheie classification' :

   Grade 0 → Normal (bright, thin)

   Grade 1 → Broadening of light reflex (diffuse, less bright).

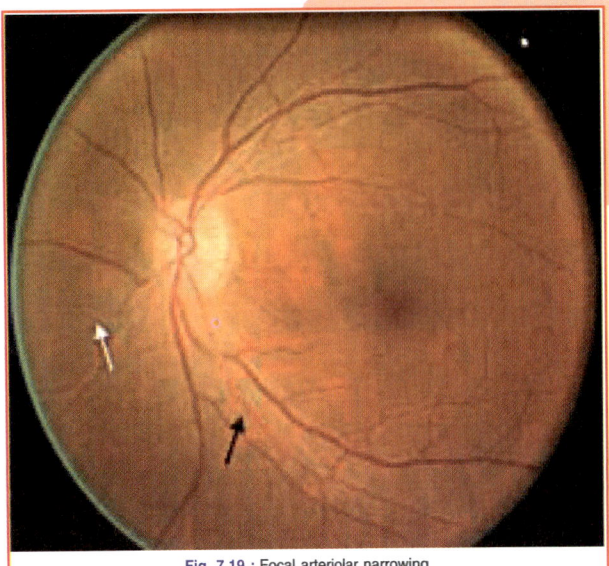

Fig. 7.19 : Focal arteriolar narrowing

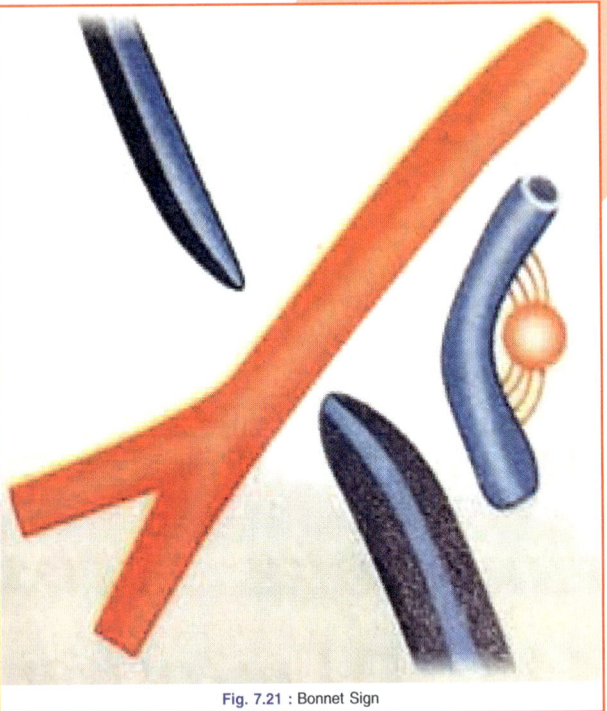

Fig. 7.21 : Bonnet Sign

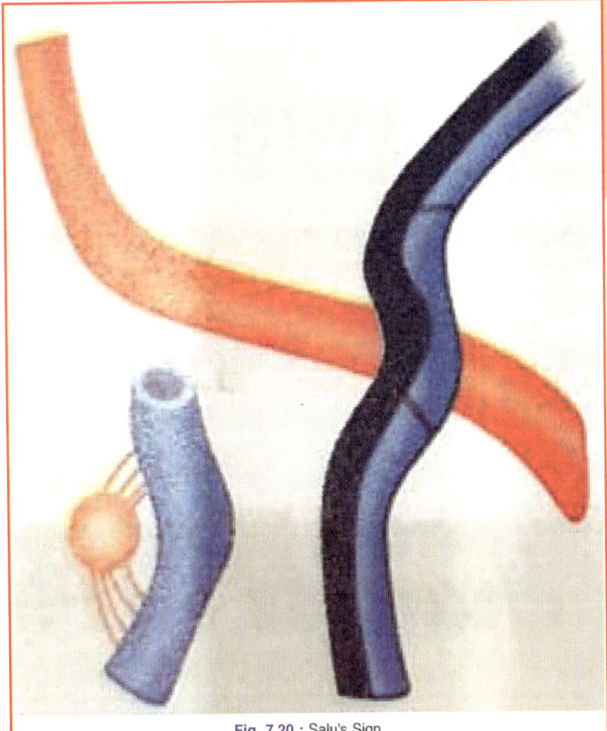

Fig. 7.20 : Salu's Sign

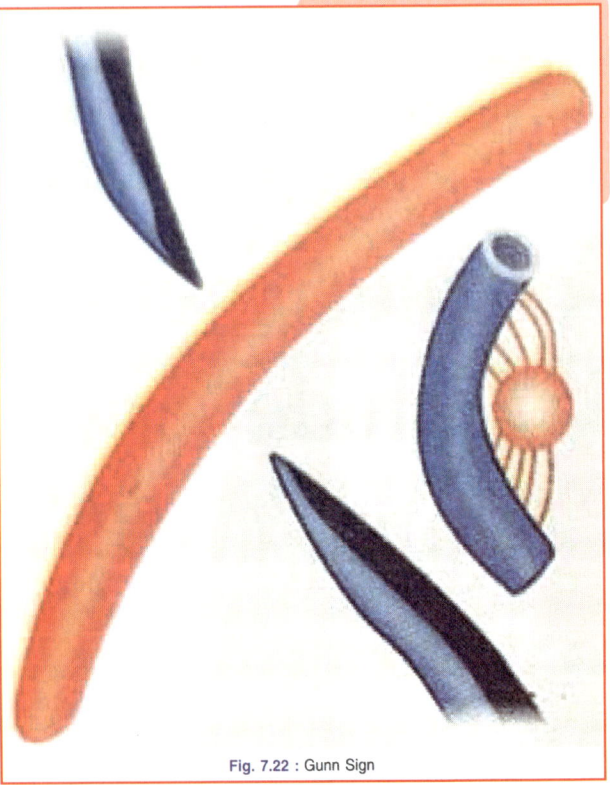

Fig. 7.22 : Gunn Sign

Grade 2 → Copper wire starts appearing.

Grade 3 → Copper wire appearance (reddish brown)

Grade 4 → Silver wire appearance (opaque white)

e) Superficial Retinal hemorrhages

'Flame shaped hemorrhages'.

f) Hard exudates

'Macular fan, Macular star'.

g) Soft exudates

'Cotton wool patches'.

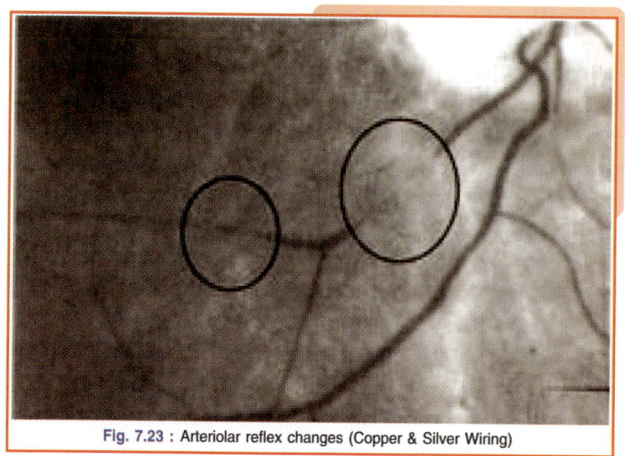

Fig. 7.23 : Arteriolar reflex changes (Copper & Silver Wiring)

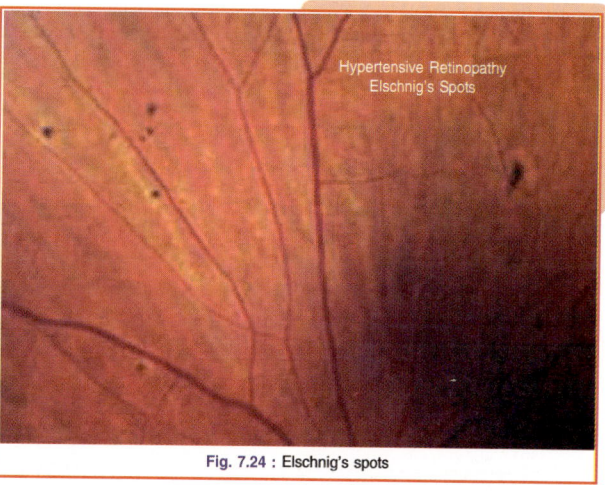

Fig. 7.24 : Elschnig's spots

2) Malignant Hypertensive Retinopathy : (Acute)

Fundus picture characterized by :

a) Acute hypertensive Retinopathy :
  - ➢ marked arteriolar narrowing
  - ➢ superior retinal hemorrhage
  - ➢ microaneurysms
  - ➢ Cotton wool spots
  - ➢ FIPTs (focal intraretinal periarteriolar transudates)

b) Acute hypertensive choroidopathy :
  - ➢ Acute focal retinal pigment epitheliopathy.
  - ➢ Elschnig's spots (focal small black dots). **(Fig. 7.24)**
  - ➢ Siegrist streaks (linear pigments along the choroid). **(Fig. 7.25)**
  - ➢ Serous neurosensory Retinal Detachment.

c) Acute hypertensive Optic Neuropathy :
  - ➢ Disc edema, hemorrhages.
  - ➢ Disc pallor.

Staging of Hypertensive Retinopathy :

I) Keith-Wagner - Barker Classification :

  Grade I : Mild to moderate arteriolar attenuation

  Grade II : Moderate to marked arteriolar attenuation, Salu's sign.

  Grade III : Bonnet's sign
  Gunn sign
  Flame shaped hemorrhages.

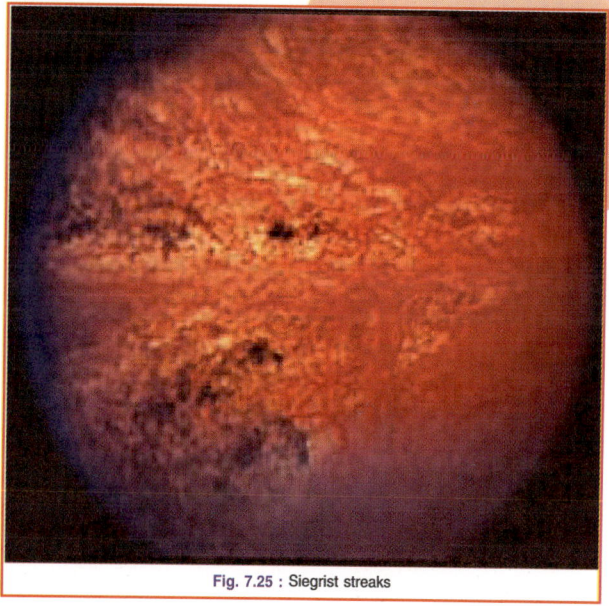

Fig. 7.25 : Siegrist streaks

  Cotton wool spots
  Hard exudates

  Grade IV : Grade III plus silver wiring, Papilloedema, macular star.

II) Scheie Classification :

  ✍ mentioned above

III) Wong & McIntosh Classification :

  1) Mild Retinopathy
  2) Moderate Retinopathy
  3) Accelerated Retinopathy

Management :

1) Mid Hypertensive Retinopathy :
   Blood pressure control.

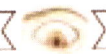

2) Moderate Hypertensive Retinopathy :

BP control + Assessment of Risk factors + Risk Reduction therapy.

3) Accelerated Hyertensive Retinopathy :

☞ Stepwise BP control (as sudden BP reduction reduce optic nerve head perfusion & may cause stroke) & Hypertensive Treatment.

❏ RETINOPATHY IN TOXAEMIA OF PREGNANCY/RETINOPATHY IN PREGNANCY INDUCED HYPERTENSION :

✍ PIH was previously known as 'Toxaemia of pregnancy'.

✍ Characterized by :

a) Raised BP

b) Proteinuria

c) Generalised edema.

✍ Retinal changes occur when BP rises above 160/100 mm Hg.

✍ Changes are marked at 200/130 mmHg.

Clinical features :

1) Narrowing of nasal arterioles, followed by generalised narrowing → Earliest change.

2) Superficial hemorrhages, cotton wool spots.

3) Retinal edema, exudates, macular star.

4) Exudative Retinal Detachment.

Management :

Changes are reversible and disappear after delivery.

1) *Pre organic state :*

If patient responds well to conservative treatment, Pregnancy is continued under close observation.

2) *Hypoxic Retinopathy :*

(Cotton wool spots, Retinal edema, Hemorrhage). Termination of pregnancy otherwise permanent visual loss or even loss of life (both mother & foetus) may occur.

❏ DIFFERENTIAL DIAGNOSIS OF WHITE PUPILLARY REFLEX : (Leukocoria)

✍ Also known as 'Pseudoglioma'.

I) **Hereditary :**

1) Norrie's disease.

2) Congenital Retinoschisis.

3) Dominant exudative vitreoretinopathy.

II) **Developmental :**

1) PHPV (Persistent hyperplastic primary vitreous).

2) Congenital Cataract.

3) Coloboma.

4) Congenital corneal opacity.

5) Myelinated nerve fibres.

6) Morning glory syndrome.

7) Congenital Retinal fold.

III) **Inflammatory :**

1) Congenital CMV Retinitis.

2) HSV Retinitis.

3) Toxoplasmosis.

4) Toxocariasis.

5) Uveoretinitis.

6) Endophthalmitis.

7) Orbital cellulitis.

IV) **Tumors :**

1) Retinal Astrocytic Hamartoma.

2) Glioneuroma.

3) Lymphoma, Leukemia, Hemangioma.

V) **Miscellaneous :**

1) Coat's Disease.

2) Retinopathy of Prematurity. (Retrolental fibroplasia).

❏ RETINOBLASTOMA :

✍ Common malignant tumor arising from neurosensory retina in one or both the eyes.

✍ Most common intraocular tumor in children.

✍ Confined to infancy and very young children (1-2 years of age).

✍ No sex predisposition.

✍ *Unilateral :* 70-75% cases.

✍ *Bilateral* : 25-30% cases.

(Figs. 7.26 & 7.27)

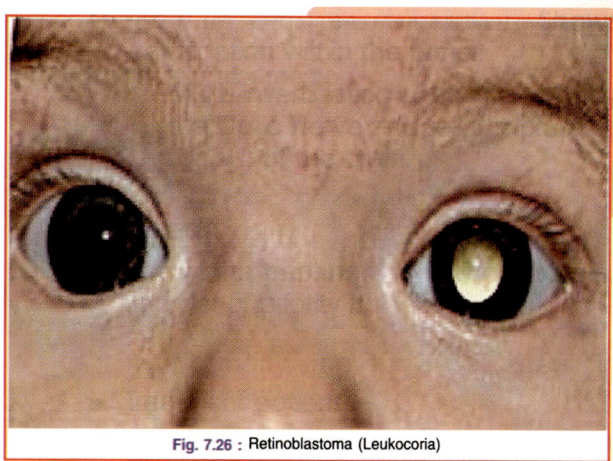

Fig. 7.26 : Retinoblastoma (Leukocoria)

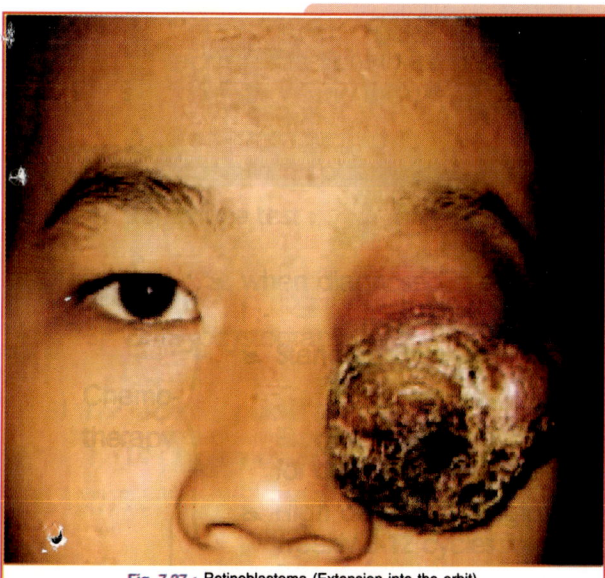

Fig. 7.27 : Retinoblastoma (Extension into the orbit)

I) Etiology :

- Retinoblastoma (RB) gene is located on 13q14 (14 band on long arm of Chr 13). which is tumor suppressor gene.

- Retinoblastoma develops when both the alleles of RB gene are inactivated/altered.

- Typical *e.g.* of Knudson's two hit hypothesis.

- In hereditary Retinoblastoma first genetic change (first hit) in RB gene is inherited from affected parent, second hit occurs in postnatal life and both alleles are lost : (40%)

- In non hereditary Retinoblastoma, both mutations (hits 1st & 2nd) occur postnataly. (60%)

II) Pathology :

1) Tumor arises from small round cells with large nuclei *i.e.*

   'small round blue cell tumor'.

2) *Microscopic features :* **(Fig. 7.28)**

   a) Flexner-Wintersteiner Rosettes (specific for Rb).

   b) Homer-Wright Rosettes.

   c) Pseudorosettes.

   d) Fleurettes formation.

   e) Necrosis & calcification.

III) Clinical features : ☺ RETINOBLAS₂CC :

1) **L**eukocoria (**A**maurotic cat's eye reflex) :

   ➤ most commonest manifestation.

   ➤ caused by the reflection of light from white intraocular tumor whichs gives white glow in the pupil (Leukocoria).

2) **S**trabismus, squint (Convergent)

   ➤ 2nd commonest manifestation

3) **S**econdary Glaucoma.

4) **C**orneal **C**louding due to ↑ IOP.

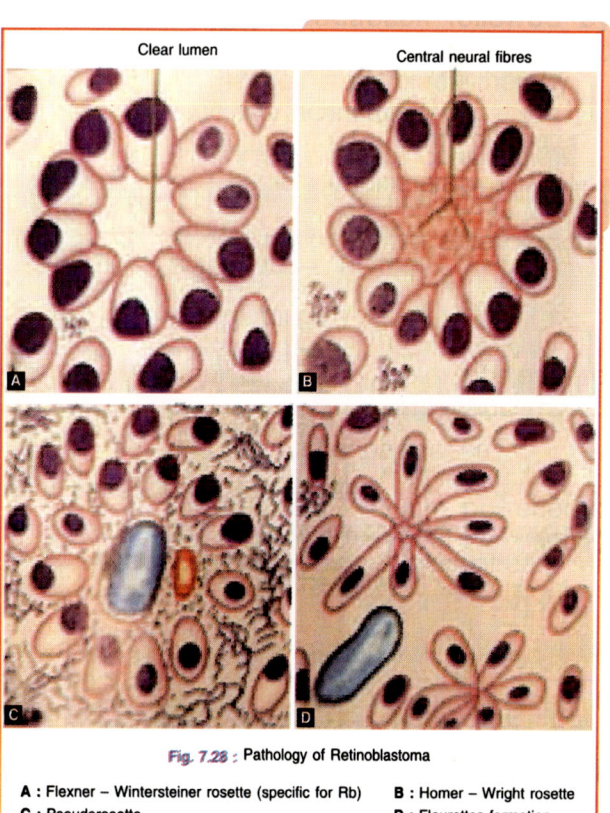

Fig. 7.28 : Pathology of Retinoblastoma

A : Flexner – Wintersteiner rosette (specific for Rb)   B : Homer – Wright rosette
C : Pseudorosette   D : Fleurettes formation

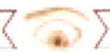

5) **R**ed eye.

6) **E**xcessive **T**ears

7) **I**ris discoloration (**N**eovascularization of iris).

8) **O**rbital cellulitis.

9) **B**uphthalmos & Proptosis.

10) **P**ainful Red eye associated with Pseudohypopyon or Hyphaema.

Spread occurs by :

1) Direct extension by the continuity of optic nerve and brain. Therefore, after enucleation, optic nerve is always examined to *see* the invasion into the optic nerve.

2) Lymphatic spread to preauricular lymph nodes.

3) Metastasis by blood stream to cranial/other bones.

On basis of ophthalmoscopy, 3 types of Retinoblastoma : **(Fig. 7.29)**

a) Endophytic : grows inwards into the retina, vitreous cavity, cottage cheese appearance on calcification.

b) Exophytic : grows outwards, separates the retina from choroid.

c) Diffuse infiltrating tumors.

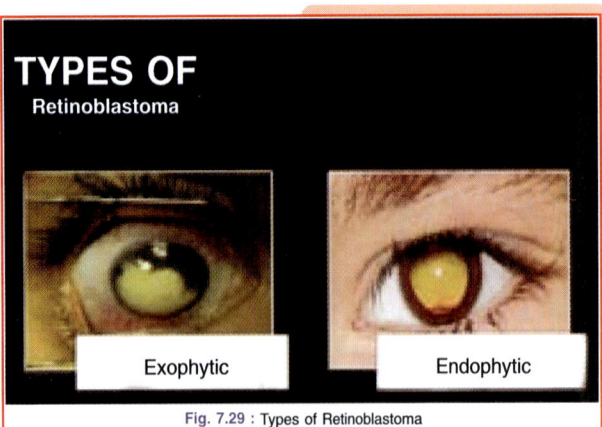

TYPES OF
Retinoblastoma

Exophytic   Endophytic

Fig. 7.29 : Types of Retinoblastoma

IV) Differentiating features of Retinoblastoma from Pseudoglioma :

1) IOP ↑ in Retinoblastoma (↓ in pseudoglioma).

2) Calcification in intraocular mass occurs in Retinoblastoma, not in leucocoria.

3) Enlargement of optic foramen with calcified mass is seen in Retinoblastoma, not in pseudoglioma.

V) Classification of Retinoblastoma :

1) Reese - Ellsworth classification
   ➤ for prognostic significance.

2) ICRB (International classification of Retinoblastoma).
   ➤ to decide the treatment modality.

i) Group A (very low risk)
   ➤ small tumor < 3 mm in greatest dimension.
   ➤ confined to the Retina.
   ➤ located > 3 mm from fovea & > 1.5 mm from optic disc.

ii) Group B (low risk)
   ➤ large tumor > 3 mm in dimension.
   ➤ located < 3 mm from fovea & < 1.5 mm from optic disc.

iii) Group C (moderate risk)
   ➤ focal seeds characterised by subretinal, vitreous seeds ≤ 3 mm from Retinoblastoma.

iv) Group D (high risk) :
   ➤ diffuse seeds characterized by subretinal, vitreous seeds > 3 mm from Retinoblastoma.

v) Group E (very high risk) :
   Retinoblastoma with tumor touching the lens, neovascular glaucoma, diffuse infiltrating tumor, orbital cellulitis, invasion of optic nerve, choroid, sclera, orbit, anterior chamber or phthisis bulbi.

VI) Management :
Investigations :

1) LDH is increased in aqueous humor.

2) Direct/Indirect Ophthalmoscopy :
   ➤ done under the anaesthesia.
   ➤ whitish mass that fills the vitreous chamber is seen.

3) ↑ IOP on tonometry.

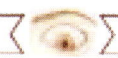

4) Plain X ray/USG/CT/MRI : Shows calcification within the tumor.

> MRI is investigation of choice to study the Optic Nerve and sellar/suprasellar regions of the brain.

Treatment :

✎ Aim of the treatment in Retinoblastoma, in order of priority is to save :

Life > eye > sight > cosmetic.

✎ Treatment options :

Standard	Newer
1) Enucleation	1) Subtenon chemotherapy
2) Radiotherapy	2) Ophthalmic artery infusion therapy
3) Chemotherapy	3) High dose chemotherapy with stem cell rescue
4) Cryotherapy	
5) Thermotherapy by diode laser or laser photocoagulation.	

A) Conservative tumor destruction therapy :

Chemo-therapy
- ✎ when diagnosed in early stage I :-
- ✎ Standard dose CVE Regimen Carboplatin, Vincristine, Etoposide, 3 weekly 6 cycles for group A, B, C patients.
- ✎ High dose CVE Regimen, 3 weekly 6-12 cycles for group D patients

✎ Focal therapy : depending upon the location, size of tumor.
- i) Cryotherapy
- ii) Thermotherapy
- iii) Laser photocoagulation
- iv) Plaque Radiotherapy
- v) External beam Radiotherapy

✎ If above modalities are not available

→ Enucleation.

B) Enucleation : when
i) Tumor involves half of the retina.
ii) Optic nerve is involved.

iii) Glaucoma is present.
iv) Anterior chamber is involved.

Eyeball is enucleated with maximum length of the optic nerve. If the optic nerve shows invasion, post operative treatment is given :
i) External beam Radiotherapy
ii) Chemotherapy (CVE with Cyclosporin)

C) Palliative therapy :

For : ✎ Rb with orbital extension.
    ✎ Rb with intracranial extension
    ✎ Rb with distant metastasis.

done with : chemotherapy (CVE),
    surgical debulking,
    external beam Radiotherapy.

D) Treatment according to stages :

1) Tumor is small (involve less than half of the globe) & no optic nerve involvement : Local tumor destructive procedures. Now, SALT (sequential aggressive therapy) *i.e.* multimodal therapy is given :

> Large tumor (> 12 mm diameter) :
⇨ Chemoreduction followed by destruction by cryotherapy, thermotherapy, brachytherapy.

> Medium tumor (< 12 mm diameter)
⇨ Chemo + Radiotherapy

> Small tumor (< 4.5 mm, anterior to the equator)
⇨ cryotherapy

> Small tumor (< 4.5 mm, posterior to the equator) (near the macula)
⇨ Laser photocoagulation

> Small tumor (< 4.5 mm, posterior to the equator) (away from the macula)
⇨ Thermotherapy

Bilateral Retinoblastoma :

Chemotherapy is the first line of treatment. If vision cannot be preserved in both the eyes, enucleation of eye with more advanced tumor & chemoreduction with local destruction of eye with less advanced tumor.

☐ MACULAR FUNCTION TESTS (MFT) :

These are the tests which are used for :

1) Diagnosis and follow-up of macular diseases.

2) Evaluating potential macular functions in eyes with opaque media such as cataract and dense vitreous hemorrhage.

Classification of MFT :

I) MFT with clear Media :

1) Visual acuity.

2) Slit lamp Biomicroscopy.

3) Contrast sensitivity.

4) Photostress test.

5) Color vision.

6) Amsler grid test.

7) Microperimetry.

8) Fundus Fluorescein Angiography (FFA)

9) Optical Coherence Tomography (OCT).

II) MFT with opaque media :

Simple Tests	Other Tests
1) Two light discrimination test	1) Laser Interferometry
2) Maddox Rod test	2) Potential acuity meter test
3) Entoptic visualization	3) Blue field entoptoscopy
4) Color perception	4) Flying corpuscle test

III) Objective tests for Retina Evaluation :

1) Ultrasonic evaluation of posterior segment.

2) ERG (Electroretinogram).

3) EOG (Electroculogram)

4) VER (Visually evoked response)

Few Important Types :

1) Two light discrimination test :

   ✎ Opaque disc is perforated with two pin-holes which are 2 inches apart and kept about 2 feet away from the eye.

   ✎ Light is held behind the two pin holes and patient looks through the pin hole.

   ✎ If two lights are perceived, it indicates normal macular function.

2) Maddox Rod test :

   ✎ Patient looks at distant bright light through Maddox Rod.

   ✎ Accurate perception of red line indicates the normal function of macula.

3) Color perception :

   ✎ Indicates some macular funtion is present and optic nerve is relatively normal.

4) Entoptic visualisation :

   ✎ A point source of light is rubbed against the closed eyelids.

   ✎ If the patient perceives the retinal vascular pattern in black outline, it is favourable indication of retinal function.

   ✎ Being subjective in nature, so importance of negative test can be considered if the patient can perceive the pattern with the opposite eye.

☐ RETINAL HEMORRHAGE :

   ⚡ It is a disorder of the eye in which bleeding occurs into the light sensitive tissue on the back wall of the eye.

Cause :

1) High altitude climbing.

2) Hypertension.

3) Diabetes mellitus.

4) Retinal vein occlusion.

5) Shaken baby syndrome.

6) Severe blows to the head.

Diagnosed by an Ophthalmoscope or by Fundus fluorescein angiography.

Classification :

1) Superficial Hemorrhage (flame/splinter shaped) in the superficial nerve fibre layer.

2) Deep hemorrhage : (dot blot)

   in the deeper retinal layers.

3) Retrohyaloid (subhyaloid) hemorrhage : **(Fig. 7.30)**

   ✎ boat shaped or scaphoid.

   ✎ located anterior (internal) to the retina within retrohyaloid space.

   (hyaloid is another name for vitreous humor).

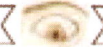

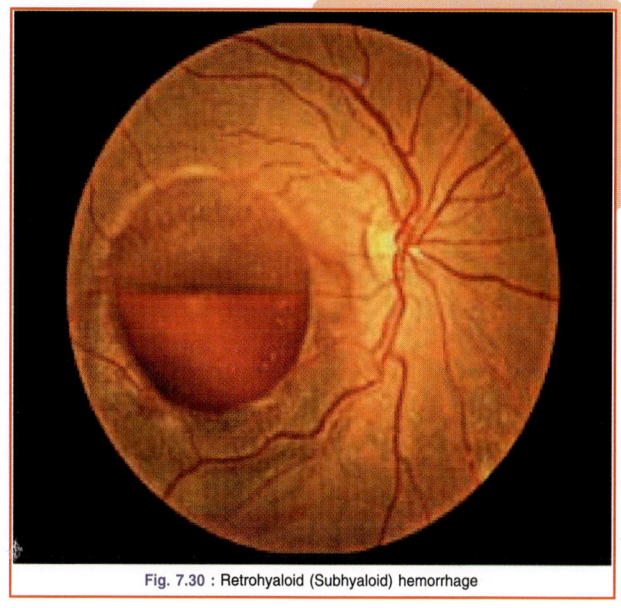

Fig. 7.30 : Retrohyaloid (Subhyaloid) hemorrhage

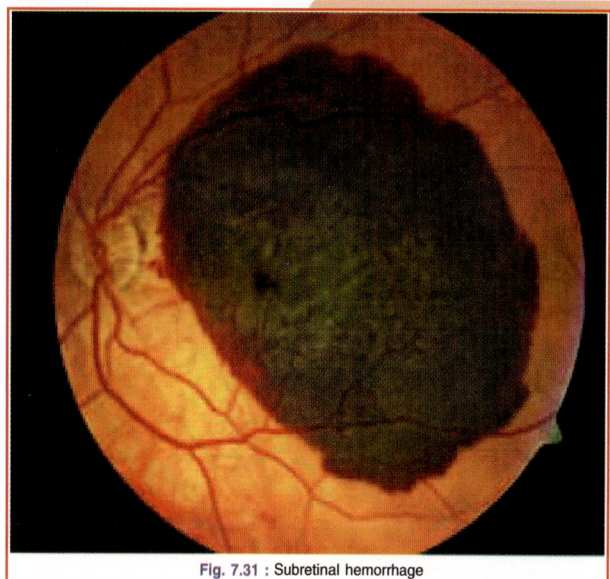

Fig. 7.31 : Subretinal hemorrhage

4) Subretinal hemorrhage : **(Fig. 7.31)**

    located deep (external) to the retina.

5) Vitreous hemorrhage. **(Fig. 7.32)**

Treatment :

1) Laser endophotocoagulation to seal off damaged blood vessels.

2) Anti VEGF drugs (Bevacizumab, Avastin) in retinal hemorrhage due to diabetes.

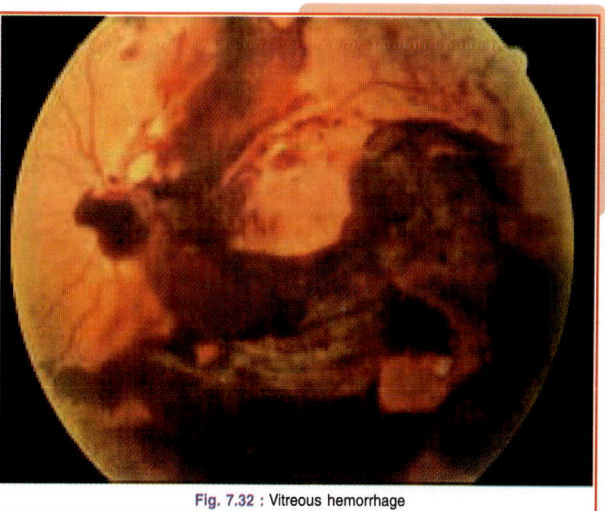

Fig. 7.32 : Vitreous hemorrhage

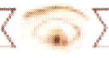

Chapter

8

Neuro-Ophthalmology

Most Important (Must Read Topics)	Elective Topics
1) Optic Neuritis	1) Optic Atrophy
2) Papilloedema	2) Papilloedema Vs Papillitis Vs Pseudopapillitis
3) Marcus Gunn Pupil	

❏ OPTIC NEURITIS : (Fig. 8.1)

Optic neuritis is inflammatory and demyelinating disorder of Optic Nerve.

A) Etiology :

1) Idiopathic.

2) Hereditary Optic Neuritis (Leber's disease).

3) Demyelinating disorders :

   are most common cause of Optic neuritis :

   ➢ Multiple sclerosis

   ➢ Neuromyelitis optica (Devic's disease)

   ➢ Encephalitis of Schilder.

   ➢ Krabbe's galactocerebroside dystrophy

   ➢ Pelizaeus Merzbacher disease

4) Infections :

   ➢ Cat scratch fever

   ➢ Syphilis

   ➢ Lyme's disease

   ➢ TB

   ➢ Cryptococcal meningitis in AIDS

5) Viral infections :

   ➢ Measles

   ➢ Mumps

   ➢ Chickenpox

   ➢ Whooping cough, Glandular fever

6) Autoimmune disorders :

   ➢ SLE, PAN, Wegener's granulomatosis

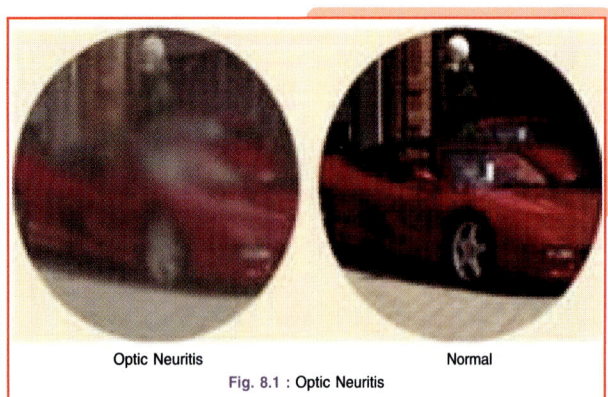

Optic Neuritis   Normal

Fig. 8.1 : Optic Neuritis

7) Toxic optic Neuritis :

> Chloroquine, Isoniazid, Ethambutol, Digoxin, Methyl alcohol etc.

8) Metabolic / Nutritional deficiency :

> B_1, B_2, B_6, B_{12}, folic acid deficiency, Diabetes.

B) Types : <u>3 types</u> (Fig. 8.2)

1) Papillitis	: Involvement of Optic Nerve, Disc.
2) Neuroretinitis	: Involvement of Optic disc + surrounding retina
3) Retrobulbar neuritis	: Involvement of Optic nerve behind the eyeball.

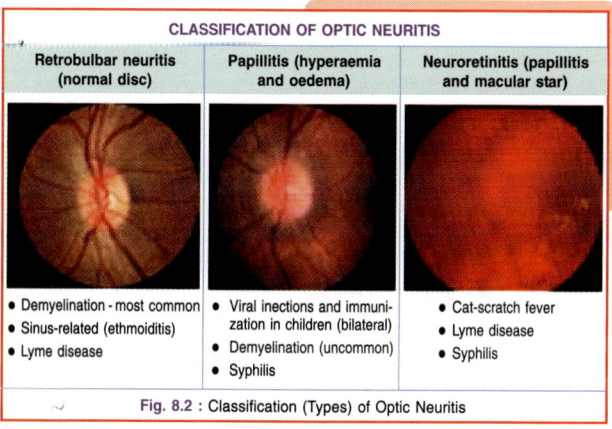

CLASSIFICATION OF OPTIC NEURITIS

Retrobulbar neuritis (normal disc)	Papillitis (hyperaemia and oedema)	Neuroretinitis (papillitis and macular star)
• Demyelination - most common • Sinus-related (ethmoiditis) • Lyme disease	• Viral inections and immunization in children (bilateral) • Demyelination (uncommon) • Syphilis	• Cat-scratch fever • Lyme disease • Syphilis

Fig. 8.2 : Classification (Types) of Optic Neuritis

C) Clinical features :

Symptoms :

1) Monocular sudden progressive profound visual loss → Hallmark.

2) Dark adaptation is lowered.

3) Visual obscuration in bright light.

4) Impairment of color vision.

5) Movement phosphenes and sound induced phosphenes **(Fig. 8.3)**

6) *Uhthoff's symptom :*

Episodic transient obscuration of vision on exertion and exposure to heat, which recovers on resting and on moving away from heat.

7) *Pulfrich phenomena :*

Impairment in depth perception.

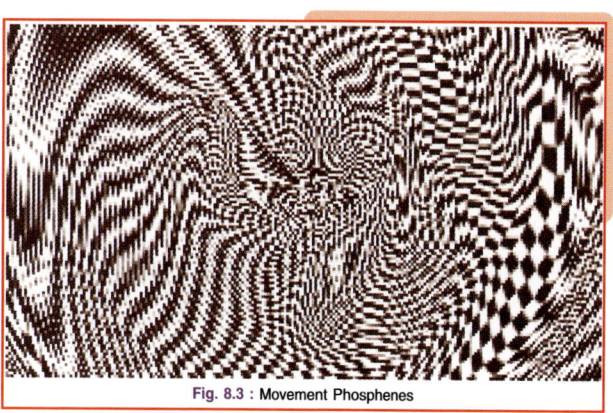

Fig. 8.3 : Movement Phosphenes

8) *Pain :*

Behind the eyeball, particularly in Retrobulbar neuritis which is aggravated by ocular movements in upward & downward direction.

Signs :

1) Visual acuity is reduced.

2) Color vision is impaired (Red desaturation)

3) *Visual field changes :*

central/centrocaecal scotoma. **(Figs. 8.4 & 8.5)**

4) *RAPD (Relative Afferent Pupillary Defect)* **(Fig. 8.6)**

Marcus Gunn pupil, detected by swinging flash light test.

5) *Ophthalmoscopy :*

i) <u>Papillitis</u> : Hyperaemia of disc and blurring of margins.

⇨ Obliteration of physiological cup.

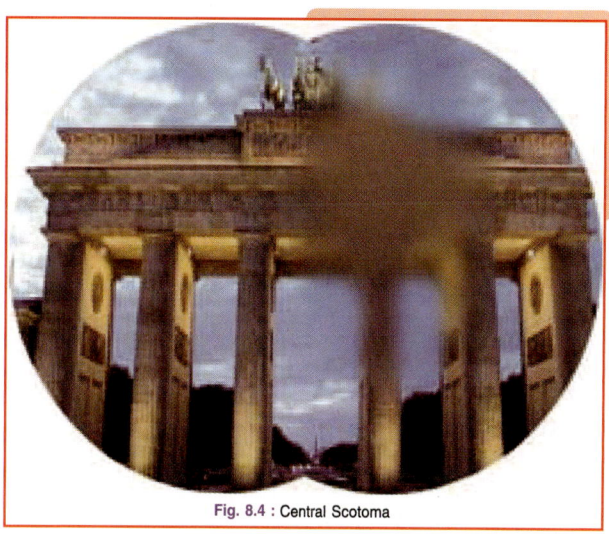

Fig. 8.4 : Central Scotoma

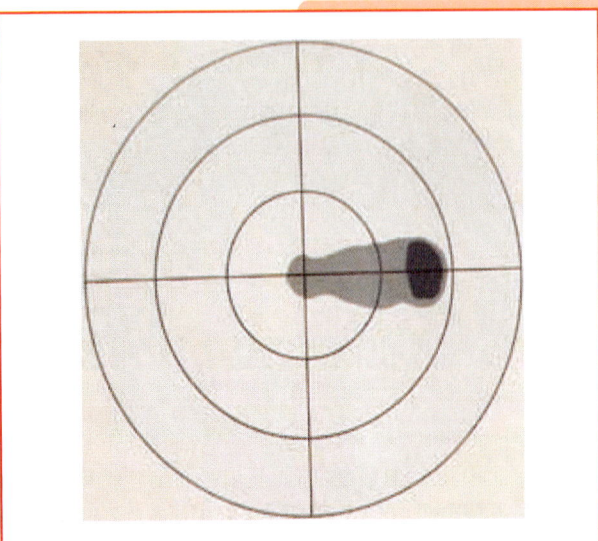

Fig. 8.5 : Central Scotoma

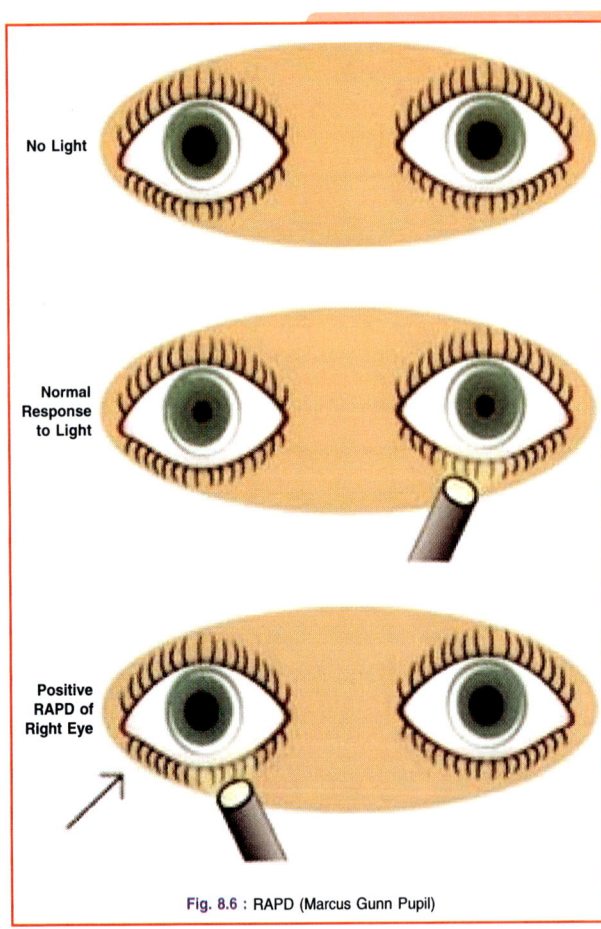

No Light

Normal
Response
to Light

Positive
RAPD of
Right Eye

Fig. 8.6 : RAPD (Marcus Gunn Pupil)

⇨ Retinal veins are congested, tortuous.

⇨ Splinter hemorrhages, fine exduates are seen.

⇨ Inflammatory cells in the vitreous.

ii) <u>Neuroretinitis</u> : Macular star formation

6) Contrast sensitivity is impaired.

7) *VER* : Reduced amplitude & delay in transmission time.

8) Fundus fluorescein angiography : mild to moderate leak.

D) Treatment :

1) Treatment of the cause.

2) Corticosteroid Therapy :

   ➢ Oral prednisolone is contraindicated in acute Optic Neuritis.

   ➢ iv methylprednisolone (if brain shows lesions supportive of multiple sclerosis on MRI) 1 gm daily for 3 days followed by oral prednisolone 1 mg/kg/day for 11 days, then taper prednisolone over 4 days.

   ➢ iv dexamethasone is also effective.

3) Interferon therapy :

   to reduce recurrence in patients of multiple sclerosis.

▢ PAPILLOEDEMA :

⚐ It is non-inflammatory edema of Optic disc caused by increased Intracranial Tension (ICT).

⚐ Edema of the disc can also be caused by other causes (other than ↑ ICT) so the term Disc edema or Disc swelling is then used to include all types of edema of optic disc (by inflammation, uveitis, orbital tumors, vascular causes) **(Fig. 8.7)**

A) Causes of Disc Oedema :

1) Inflammation (papillitis, neuroretinitis, uveitis).

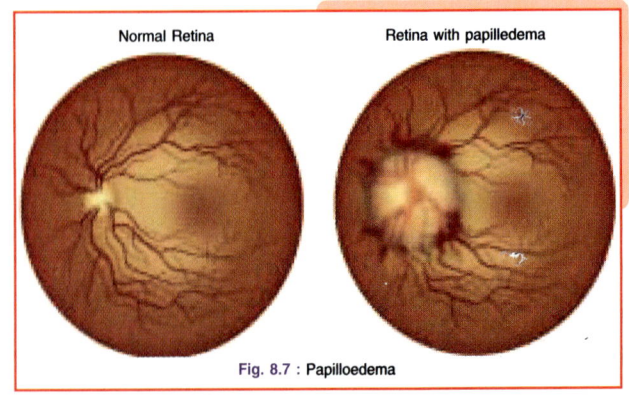

Normal Retina　　　　　Retina with papilledema

Fig. 8.7 : Papilloedema

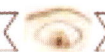

2) Orbital causes : (tumors, cellulitis).

3) Vascular causes : (CRVO, diabetic papillopathy, uremia).

4) Ocular Hypotony.

5) Infiltrative conditions (leukemias, lymphomas).

B) Pathogenesis :

✍ Principal pathophysiology is due to blockage of axoplasmic transport. (Hayreh's theory)

✍ ↑ CSF pressure → Axoplasmic stasis in the Optic disc

↓

Swelling of the optic disc. (without signs of inflammation)

✍ ↑ ICT may be due to :

1) Congenital – Aqueductal stenosis,

Craniosynostosis

2) Intra cranial space occupying lesion (SOL).

3) Intracranial infections.

4) Intracranial hemorrhages.

5) Obstruction to CSF absorption.

6) Tumors of spinal cord.

7) Idiopathic Intracranial Hypertension.

8) Diffuse cerebral edema.

9) Cerebral Venous Sinus Thrombosis.

10) Systemic conditions (Malignant Hypertension, PIH etc.).

C) Clinical features :

✍ *General :*

due to ↑ ICT - (Headache, Nausea, Projectile vomiting, Diplopia)

✍ *Ocular :*

1) Initially vision is normal.

2) Visual symptoms occur in Advanced severe papilloedema :

⇨ Transient visual obscurations (Amaurosis fugax) lasting less than 30 seconds in which vision turns grey or black, like veil has fallen over the eyes.

⇨ Affect both the eyes, as papilloedema is bilateral.

⇨ Enlargement of the blind spot & progressive contraction of visual field.

↓

'Gradual painless progressive loss of vision'.

⇨ Eventually, complete blindness sets in.

✍ *Ophthalmoscopic features :*

1) Blurring (obscuration) of disc margin (First sign) starts at upper and lower nasal margins.

⇨ Temporal margin is last to involve.

2) Venous engorgement, congestion.

3) Loss of venous pulsations even on applying pressure on the globe.

4) Gradual obliteration of physiological cup.

5) Hyperaemia of the disc.

6) Disc is elevated (mushroom, dome shaped) so vessels bends sharply over the margin. **(Figs. 8.8 & 8.9)**

⇨ There is difference of 2-6 D between the vessels at top and those on retina, So, Definitive parallax is obtained on Indirect Ophthalmoscopy.

7) Cotton wool spots (soft exudates), Hard exudates (macular fan, star).

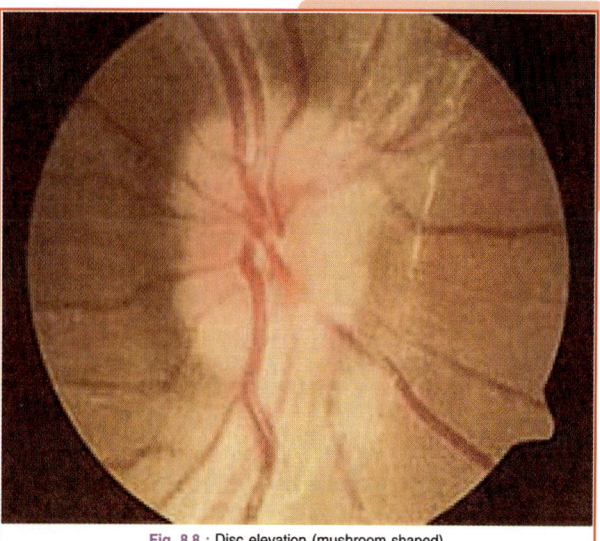

Fig. 8.8 : Disc elevation (mushroom shaped)

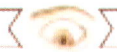

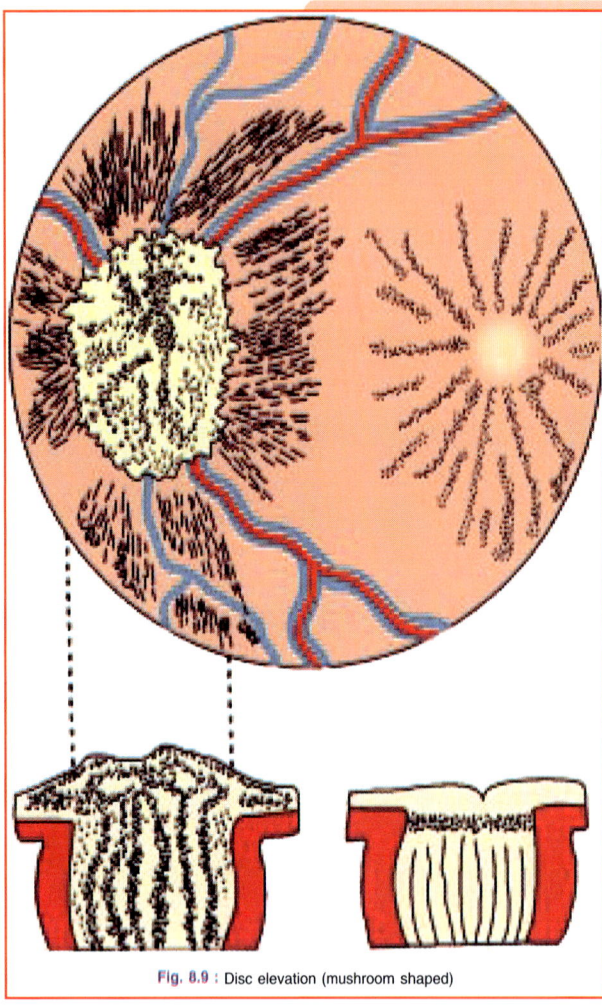

Fig. 8.9 : Disc elevation (mushroom shaped)

8) Flame shaped (superficial) & Punctate (Deep) hemorrhages.

9) *Paton's Line* : Radial Retinal lines cascading from the optic disc. **(Fig. 8.10)**

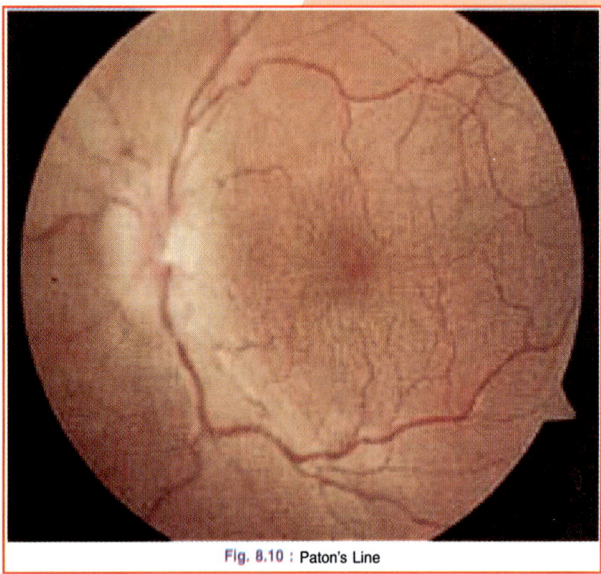

Fig. 8.10 : Paton's Line

10) In long standing (Vintage papilloedema) :

⇨ Disc is markedly elevated with 'Champagne cork appearance' **(Fig. 8.11)**.

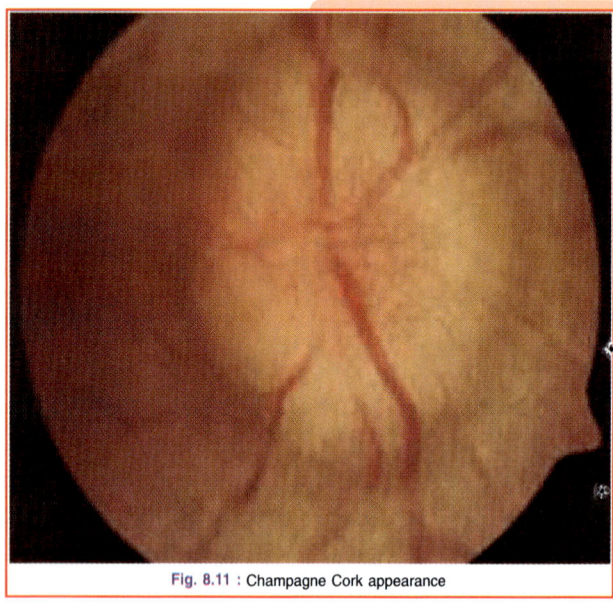

Fig. 8.11 : Champagne Cork appearance

⇨ Corpora amylacea (crystalline deposits on the optic disc) can be seen.

⇨ Postneuritic Optic Atrophy.

D) Facts about papilloedema :

1) Visual symptoms occur only in 25%. So, loss of vision is not a common feature.

2) Central vision is not impaired until late.

3) No afferent pupillary defect, except late.

4) Pseudopapilloedema (pseudopapillitis) is elevation of disc similar to papilloedema in conditions such as :

 a) Optic disc drusen (stony nodule) **(Fig. 8.12)**.

 b) Hypermetropia.

 c) Persistent hyaloid tissue.

Unilateral vs Bilateral Papilloedema :

ᔕ Disc swelling is usually unilateral.

ᔕ Papilloedema (due to ↑ ICT) is Bilateral.

ᔕ But ↑ ICT and unilateral swelling may occur in few conditions (unilateral papilloedema) :

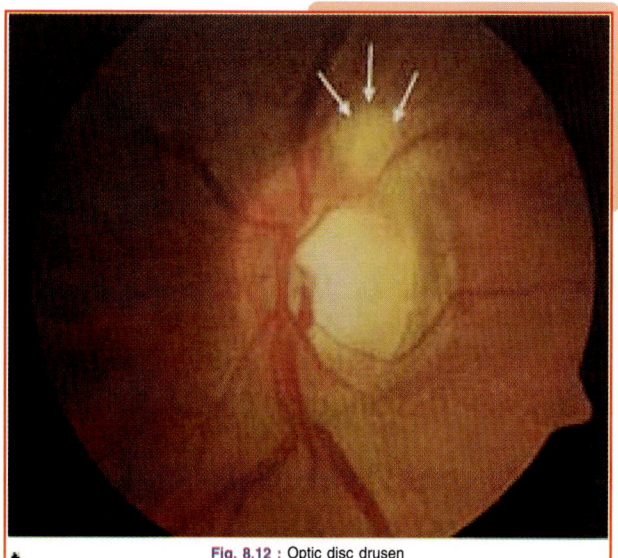

Fig. 8.12 : Optic disc drusen

1) <u>Foster-Kennedy syndrome</u> :

due to frontal lobe, olfactory tumors → Pressure optic atrophy on the side of lesion & papilloedema on the other side (due to ↑ ICT).

2) <u>Pseudo Foster Kennedy Syndrome</u> :

Unilateral papilloedema associated with ↑ ICT (due to any cause) and pre-existing optic atrophy on other side (due to any cause).

E) Treatment :

Immediate Hospitalization

↓

CT, MRI with Gadolinium enhancement.

↓

Treatment of the cause & cerebral decompression.

☐ OPTIC ATROPHY :

- Optic Atrophy refers to the optic nerve shrinkage, from any cause which produces degeneration of axons in the anterior visual system *i.e.* from retinal ganglionic cells to lateral geniculate body.

- *Ophthalmoscopic classification :*

Based on ophthalmoscopic appearance :

1) Primary (simple) optic atrophy.

2) Consecutive optic atrophy.

3) Secondary optic atrophy.

4) Glaucomatous optic atrophy.

5) Post neuritic optic atrophy (Type of Secondary)

6) Vascular (Ischaemic) optic atrophy.

7) Toxic optic atrophy.

- *Pathological classification :*

1) *Ascending or autograde optic atrophy (Wallerian degeneration)*

➢ damage to the ganglion cells or nerve fibre layer due to diseases of retina or Optic disc.

➢ ascends from eyeball towards the geniculate body.

➢ consecutive atrophy is a type of ascending atrophy.

2) *Descending or retrograde optic atrophy :*

➢ Proceeds from the region of Optic tract, chiasma, retrobulbar portion of the Optic nerve towards the Optic disc.

➢ Primary atrophy is a type of descending atrophy.

3) *Cavernous (Schnable's) optic atrophy :*

➢ Here, mucoid degeneration of glia occurs.

➢ Seen in chronic simple glaucoma, methyl alcohol poisoning, high myopia.

Etiology :

1) *Primary (simple) optic atrophy :*

a) Trauma to the optic nerve or chiasma : most common cause.

b) Tumor compressing optic nerve or chiasma.

c) Multiple sclerosis.

d) Retrobulbar neuritis.

e) Leber's hereditary neuritis.

f) Toxic amblyopia.

g) Tabes dorsalis due to syphilis.

h) Hydrocephalus.

i) Vitamin B deficiency.

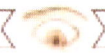

2) *Consecutive optic atrophy :*

✎ destruction of ganglionic cells secondary to degenerative, inflammatory lesions of the choroid or retina.

  a) Retinitis pigmentosa ⎫
                     ⎬ Common cause
  b) CRAO ⎭

  c) Diffuse chorioretinitis

  d) Glaucoma

  e) Pathological myopia.

3) *Secondary optic atrophy :*

✎ occurs after disc edema, so also called post papilledematous optic atrophy :

  a) Papilledema

  b) Optic neuritis (papillitis)

  c) Neuroretinitis.

  d) Ischaemic optic neuropathy

4) *Glaucomatous optic atrophy :*

✎ due to long standing raised IOP :

  a) Chronic open angle Glaucoma.

  b) Closed angle Glaucoma.

5) *Post neuritic optic atrophy (type of secondary) :*

✎ due to long standing :

  a) papilledema.

  b) papillitis.

6) *Vascular (Ischaemic) optic atrophy :*

  a) Giant cell arteritis

  b) Severe hemorrhage

  c) Severe anemia

7) *Toxic optic atrophy :*

✎ due to chronic retrobulbar neuritis secondary to toxic amblyopia :

  a) Tobacco

  b) Ethyl, methyl alcohol

  c) Quinine

  d) Chloroquine

  e) Lead

Clinical features :

1) *Loss of vision :*

  Sudden / Gradual → depends upon the cause

  Partial / Total   → depends upon the degree of atrophy

2) Semidilated, fixed pupil.

  Swinging flash light test shows Marcus Gunn pupil (RAPD)

3) Visual field loss (concentric contraction of visual field).

4) *Ophthalmoscopic appearance :*

  i) <u>Primary (simple) optic atrophy</u> : **(Fig. 8.13)**

    ➢ Greyish white or chalky white colour of the optic disc with clear margin.

    ➢ Surrounding retina and retinal vessels are normal.

    ➢ Shallow, saucer shaped atrophic cupping of the optic disc.

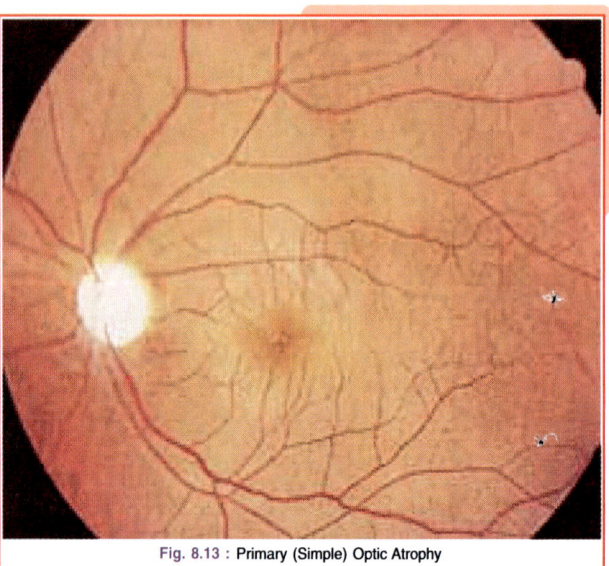

Fig. 8.13 : Primary (Simple) Optic Atrophy

  ii) <u>Consecutive optic atrophy</u> : **(Fig. 8.14)**

    ➢ Yellow-waxy colour of optic disc.

    ➢ Retinal vessels are attenuated.

  iii) <u>Secondary optic atrophy</u> : **(Fig. 8.15)**

    ➢ Disappearance of vascularity of the disc which causes increase in pallor of the disc.

    ➢ Attenuation of arteries.

    ➢ Surrounding retina shows hyaline bodies/drusen.

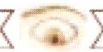

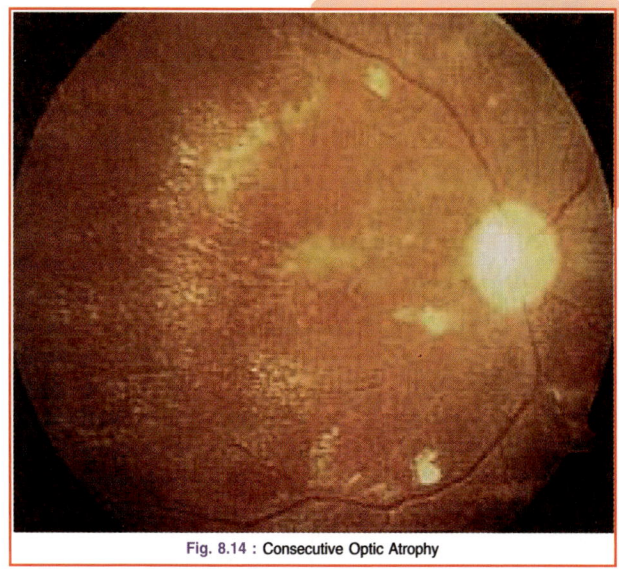

Fig. 8.14 : Consecutive Optic Atrophy

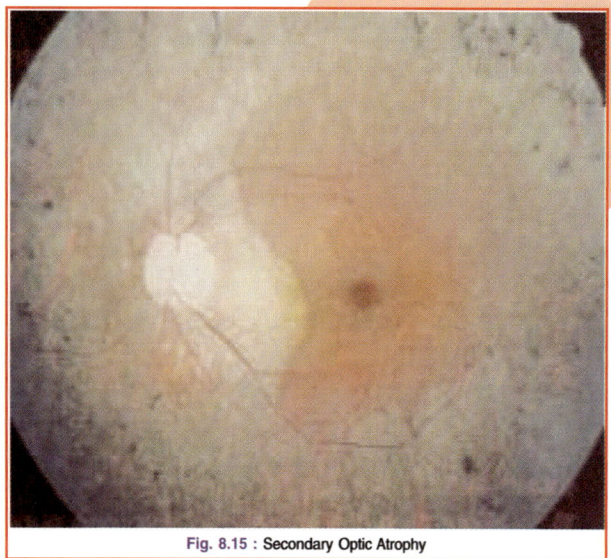

Fig. 8.15 : Secondary Optic Atrophy

iv) <u>Glaucomatous optic atrophy</u> :

➤ Deep and wide cupping of the optic disc.

➤ Nasal shift of blood vessels.

v) <u>Post neuritic optic atrophy</u> (type of secondary) :

➤ Dirty white colour of the optic disc.

➤ Perivascular sheathing is present.

vi) <u>Vascular (Ischaemic) optic atrophy</u> :

➤ Disc is pale (pallor of the disc).

➤ Obliteration of Retinal vessels.

Treatment :

1) Treatment of the underlying cause in cases of partial optic atrophy.

✎ No treatment is effective if complete optic atrophy sets in.

☐ PAPILLOEDEMA vs PAPILLITIS vs PSEUDOPAPILLITIS :

Feature	Papilloedema	Papillitis	Pseudopapillitis
1) Laterality	Bilateral	Unilateral	Unilateral or Bilateral
2) Visual Acuity	Transient attacks of blurred vision, later vision decreases	Sudden onset, marked loss of vision	Defective vision, depends upon degree of Refractive error
3) Pain, Tenderness	Absent	Present with ocular movements	Abent
Fundus examination :			
4) Media	Clear	Posterior vitreous haze	Clear
5) Disc color	Red & Juicy	Hyperaemic	Reddish
6) Disc margins	Blurred	Blurred	Not well defined
7) Disc swelling	2-6 D	< 3 D	Depends on the degree of hypermetropia.
8) Peripapillary edema	Present	Present	Absent
9) Venous engorgement	More marked	Less marked	Absent
10) Retinal hemorrhage	Marked	Absent	Absent
11) Retinal exudates	More marked	Less marked	Absent
12) Macula	Macular star	Macular fan	Absent
13) Visual field	Enlarged blind spot	Central scotoma	No defect
14) FFA	Vertical oval pool of the dye due to leakage	Minimal leakage	No leakage

☐ MARCUS GUNN PUPIL :

☞ It is paradoxical response of pupil to the light in presence of RAPD (Relative afferent pupillary defect).

☞ It is earliest indication of optic nerve disease even in the presence of normal visual acuity in the affected eye.

Causes :

1) Incomplete optic nerve lesions.
2) Severe retinal diseases.

Test :

Tested by swinging flash light test :

1) A bright flash of light is shone onto one pupil and constriction is noted.

2) Then, flashlight is quickly moved to the contralateral pupil and response is noted.

3) This swinging to and fro of flashlight is repeated several times and pupillary response is observed.

4) Normally, both the pupil constrict equally and the pupil to which light is transferred remains tightly constricted.

5) In presence of RAPD in one eye, the affected pupil will dilate when the flash of light is moved from normal eye to the abnormal eye.

This response is called as RAPD or 'Marcus Gunn Pupil'.

Chapter

9

Ocular Motility

Most Important (Must Read Topics)	Elective Topics
1) Squint, Classification	1) Diplopia
2) Concomitant Squint (Esotropia)	2) Heterophoria
3) Paralytic squint	3) Tropia Vs Phoria
4) Paralytic vs Concomitant squint	

☐ SQUINT (STRABISMUS) & CLASSIFICATION:

☞ Normally, visual axis of two eyes are parallel to each other in 'primary position of gaze' and this alignment is mantained in all the positions of gaze.

☞ 'Misalignment of visual axes of two eyes is called squint or strabismus'.

(Fig. 9.1)

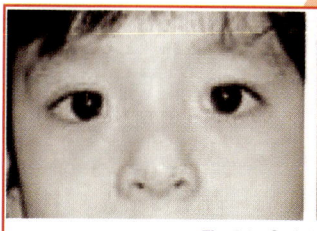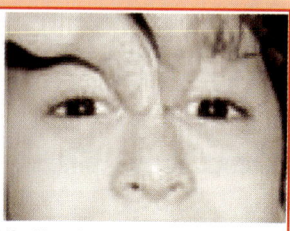
Fig. 9.1 : Squint (Strabismus)

```
                    Squint
      ┌───────────────┼───────────────┐
 Apparent/          Latent          Manifest
Pseudostrabismus  (Heterophoria)  (Heterotropia)
                      └───────┬───────┘
                   Concomitant   Incomitant squint/
                     squint       Paralytic squint
                        │
(Convergent ←  1) Esotropia (deviation of eyeball
   squint)             inwards)
```

(Divergent   ← 2) Exotropia (deviation of eyeball
squint)   outwards)

                 3) Hypertropia (upwards)

                 4) Hypotropia (downwards)

☐ CONCOMITANT SQUINT (ESOTROPIA) : (Fig. 9.2)

Eyes are not in alignment and degree of misalignment remains constant in all the directions of gaze and there is no limitation of ocular movements. It can be :

1) Esotropia   3) Hypertropia

2) Exotropia   4) Hypotropia

STRABISMUS

Normal

Esotropia-eye turns inward

Exotropia-eye turns outward

Hypertropia-eye turns upward

Hypotropia-eye turns downward

Fig. 9.2 : Concomitant Squint (Strabismus) types.

Esotropia (convergent squint) :

☞ Inward deviation of eye.

☞ Most common type in children.

☞ It can be unilateral or alternating.

a) Unilateral :

Same eye always deviates inwards, and the other takes fixation.

b) Alternating :

either of eye deviates inwards, and other takes fixation alternately.

A) Clinico-etiological types :

1) Infantile (Congenital) esotropia

2) Accommodative esotropia

3) Acquired non accommodative esotropia

4) Sensory esotropia

5) Consecutive esotropia

1) Infantile esotropia :

➤ occurs at 1-2 months of age.

➤ angle of deviation is constant (> 30^0).

➤ Binocular vision does not develop (both eyes are fixing simultaneously).

➤ There is alternate fixation in primary gaze.

➤ Cross fixation in lateral gaze.

➤ Amblyopia (in 25-40% cases)

➤ Inferior oblique overaction & DVD (dissociated vertical deviation) is present.

➤ There is latent horizontal nystagmus.

Treatment :

a) Amblyopia treatment by covering the normal eye before surgery.

b) Recession of both medial recti.

c) Surgery to be done at 6 month - 2 years of age (preferably before age of 1 year).

2) Accommodative Esotropia :

➤ due to the overaction of convergence associated with accommodation reflex.

➤ occurs at 2-3 years of age.

➤ most common type in children :

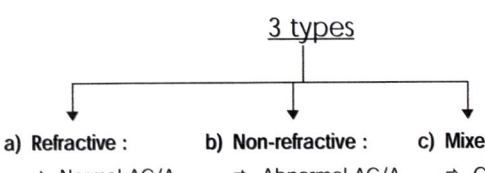

3 types

a) Refractive :	b) Non-refractive :	c) Mixed :
⇨ Normal AC/A ratio (Acc. convergence/ Accommodation	⇨ Abnormal AC/A ratio	⇨ Combination of hypermetropia & high AC/A ratio
⇨ In hypermetrops	⇨ occurs in patient with no refractive errors	⇨ Rx : correction of hypermetropia with + 3 DS lens.
⇨ Rx : spectacle use	⇨ Rx : Bifocal glasses with + 3 DS for near vision.	
	Miotics as they reduce AC/A ratio	

3) Acquired non accommodative esotropia :

➤ Includes : i) essential acquired or late onset esotropia

      ii) Acute concomitant esotropia.

      iii) Cyclic esotropia.

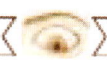

iv) Nystagmus blockage syndrome

v) Esotropia in myopia/ microtropia.

➤ Essential acquired or late onset esotropia is common. <u>3 types</u> :

a) Basic type.

b) Convergence excess type.

c) Divergence insufficiency type.

➤ *Treatment :*

i) Amblyopia correction before surgery.

ii) Correction of associated refractive error.

iii) Surgery.

4) *Sensory Esotropia :* due to monocular lesions in childhood (cataract, aphakia, Retinoblastoma)

5) *Consecutive Esotropia :* due to surgical over correction of Exotropia.

▢ INCOMITANT SQUINT (Paralytic Squint) :

✍ Type of heterotropia, in which amount of deviation varies in different direction of gaze and there is limitation of ocular movements.

✍ <u>3 types</u> :

1) Paralytic squint (common).

2) Restrictive squint

3) 'A' & 'V' pattern heterotropias.

Paralytic squint :

Due to complete / incomplete paralysis of one or more extraocular muscles.

A) Etiology :

Lesions may be neurogenic, myogenic, or at level of NMJ.

1) *Neurogenic :*

Meningitis, Cranial nerve palsy, Neoplastic / Vascular lesions, Trauma, Toxic, Demyelinating lesions.

2) *Myogenic :*

Myopathies (chronic progressive ophthalmoplegia), Bilateral ptosis, diplopia, trauma, Inflammation.

3) *NMJ :*

Myasthenia Gravis.

B) *Clinical Features :*

Symptoms :

1) Diplopia (Main symptom) and is more marked in the direction of action of paralysed muscle.

➤ It is more when patient looks downwards & right.

2) <u>Confusion</u> :

➤ due to the formation of image of two different objects on corresponding points of two retinae.

3) <u>Nausea, Vertigo. Vomiting</u> :

➤ due to diplopia.

4) Ocular deviation

5) Loss of stereopsis

Signs :

1) Secondary Deviation is more than Primary Deviation : (Fig. 9.3)

➤ Primary deviation is deviation in the affected eye and is away from the action of paralysed muscle.

➤ Secondary deviation is deviation in the normal eye under cover, when patient is made to fix with squinting eye.

2) Restriction of Ocular movements :

in the direction of action of paralysed muscle.

3) Compensatory Head Posture :

➤ Patient with paralytic squint move their head in such a way that eye

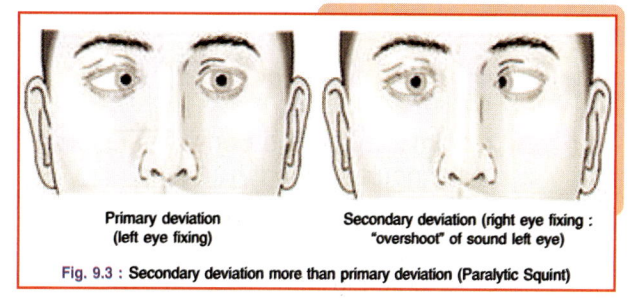

Primary deviation (left eye fixing)

Secondary deviation (right eye fixing : "overshoot" of sound left eye)

Fig. 9.3 : Secondary deviation more than primary deviation (Paralytic Squint)

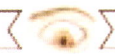
occupy position in orbit where angle of squint is minimal and thus can avoid diplopia, confusion.

➢ Head is turned towards the action of paralysed muscle.

4) **False projection / orientation :**

➢ due to increased innervational impulse to the paralysed muscle.

5) **No amblyopia and Visual Acuity is normal,** as paralytic squint develops in adults when visual acuity has already developed.

C) Management :

Investigations :

1) Diplopia charting.

2) Hess screen Test.

3) **FDT (Forced Duction Test)**

➢ To differentiate between incomitant squint due to paralysis of extraocular muscle and due to mechanical restriction of ocular movements.

➢ FDT is +ve if it is due to mechanical obstruction.

4) Field of binocular fixation.

Treatment :

1) Treatment of the cause of paralysis of extraocular muscle.

2) Treatment of Diplopia :

Occluder use on affected eye.

3) Conservative measure :

Wait and watch for 6 months for self improvement. Vit. B complex, steroids are given.

4) Chemodenervation of contralateral muscle with Botulinum toxin in recovery period.

5) Orthoptic exercises.

6) Surgery : if Recovery doesn't occur in 6 months.

➢ Aim is to provide comfortable field of binocular vision (fixation).

➢ Strengthening of paralysed muscle by Resection and/or weakening of overacting muscle by Recession.

❑ PARALYTIC (Incomitant) vs NON PARALYTIC (Concomitant) SQUINT :

Features	Paralytic	Non paralytic
1) Onset	Sudden	Slow
2) Diplopia	Present	Absent
3) Ocular movements	Limited in direction of action of the paralyzed muscle	Full Range
4) False Projection	Present (+ve)	Absent (–ve)
5) Head Posture	Depends upon the muscle paralysed, present	Normal
6) Nausea, Vertigo	Present	Absent
7) Secondary deviation	more than primary deviation	Equal to primary deviation
8) Pathological sequelae in muscles.	Present	Absent

❑ DIPLOPIA (Double Vision) : (Fig. 9.4)

✍ It is simultaneous perception of two images of a single object.

✍ It may be binocular or uniocular.

Binocular Diplopia :

✍ It is due to misalignment of the two eyes relative to each other.

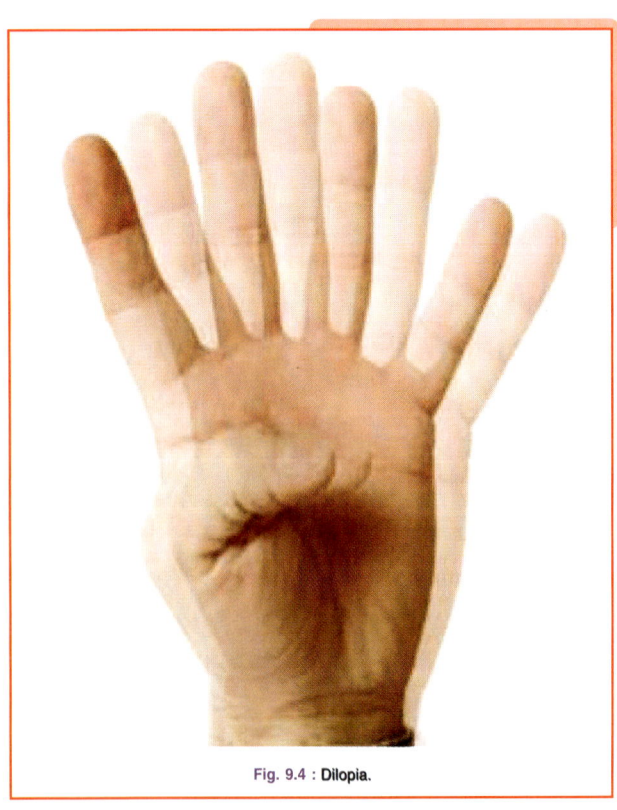

Fig. 9.4 : Dilopia.

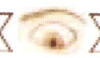

⚘ Image of single object is formed on dissimilar points of two retinae.

⚘ **Causes :**

1) Paralytic squint is the most commonest cause of binocular diplopia.

2) Displacement of eyeball (fracture of orbit, space occupying lesion in orbit).

3) Mechanical restriction of ocular movements (pterygium, symblepharon, Thyroid ophthalmopathy).

4) Anisometropia.

5) Deviation of ray of light in one eye. (by decentred spectacles)

Types of Binocular Diplopia :

1) *Uncrossed (Harmonious) Diplopia :*

   ⧫ false image is formed on same side as the deviation of eye.

   ⧫ Occurs in convergent squint (Esotropia), lateral rectus palsy.

2) *Crossed (Non-harmonious) Diplopia :*

   ⧫ false image is formed on opposite side of the deviation of eye.

   ⧫ Occurs in Divergent squint (Exotropia), medial rectus palsy.

Uniocular Diplopia :

⚘ Double vision arising in single eye (even if the other eye is closed).

⚘ **Causes :**

1) Subluxated clear lens.

2) Subluxated intraocular lens.

3) Double pupil due to congenital anomaly, large peripheral Iridectomy, Iridodialysis.

4) Incipient cataract (usually polyopia)

5) Keratoconus.

Treatment :

1) Treatment of the cause.

2) Occluding the affected eye for temporary relief.

❑ HETEROPHORIA/PHORIA/LATENT SQUINT :

⚘ As the name, latent squint remains latent (does not manifest) due to fusion.

⚘ It is a condition in which tendency of the eyes to deviate is kept latent by fusion.

⚘ Eyes have tendency to squint when one of the eye is covered thus abolishing the fusion.

⚘ Orthophoria is perfect alignment of two eyes even after the removal of influence of fusion, this is only theoretical.

⚘ Physiological Heterophoria is small amount of Heterophoria which is universal.

(Fig. 9.5)

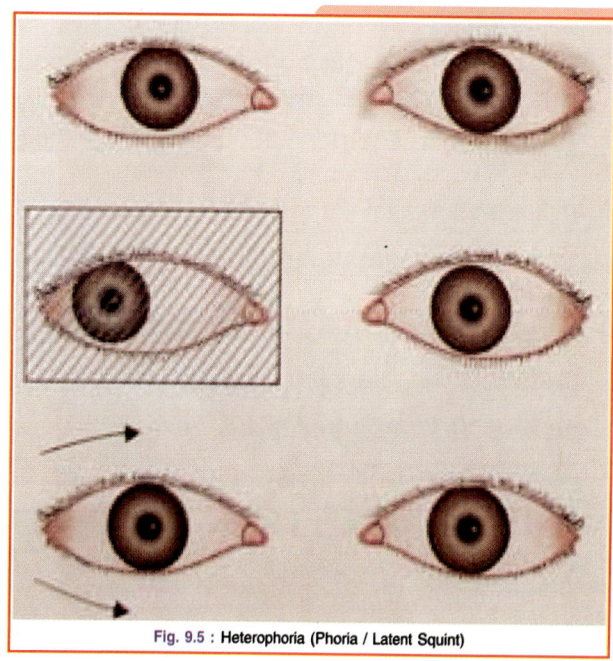

Fig. 9.5 : Heterophoria (Phoria / Latent Squint)

Types :

1) Esophoria :

   ⧫ tendency for deviation of eyeball inwards (converge).

2) Exophoria :

   ⧫ tendency for deviation of eyeball outwards (diverge).

3) Hyperphoria :

   ⧫ tendency for deviation of eyeball upwards.

4) Cyclophoria :

   ⧫ torsional deviation of eye :

   a) *Incyclophoria :*

   Upper pole of cornea rotates nasally.

   b) *Excyclophoria :*

   Upper pole of cornea rotates temporally.

5) <u>Anisophoria</u> :

    ⤷ deviation of eyeball varies with the direction of gaze.

Etiology :

1) Increased requirement of accommodation and convergence as in Hypermetropia, causes Esophoria.

2) Decreased requirement of accommodation and convergence as in Myopia, causes Exophoria.

3) Occupation requiring too much close work such as goldsmith, watchmakers.

4) Advancing age, general poor health, fatigue.

Clinical features :

1) Eyeache, headache after prolonged near work.

2) Photophobia.

3) Difficulty in changing the focus.

4) Blurring, crowding of words while reading.

5) Intermittent diplopia.

6) Intermittent squint.

Diagnosis :

1) Vision testing and Refraction testing.

2) Cover-Uncover test.

3) Prism cover test

4) Maddox Rod test

5) Maddox wing test

6) Measurement of convergence, accommodation, fusional reserve.

Treatment :

1) Correction of Refractive error.

2) Orthoptic exercises by use of synoptophore, pencil exercise.

3) Use of prism in spectacles.

4) Surgical treatment :

    Resection or Recession of the muscle.

5) General improvement of health, nutrition.

☐ TROPIA vs PHORIA :

Tropia	Phoria
1) Misalignment of two eyes when patient is looking with binocular vision.	1) Misalignment of two eyes appears only when binocular viewing is broken.
2) Occurs when two eyes are looking at same subject.	2) Occurs when two eyes are no longer looking at same subject.
3) Manifest deviation.	3) Latent deviation.
4) Unmasked i.e. always visible.	4) Can be unmasked by covering either of the eye.
5) Diagnosed by Unilateral cover test	5) Diagosed by Alternating cover test.
6) Tropia is "Always Present".	6) Phoria is "Present some of the time" as when patient is tired, misalignment of eyes starts appearing.

Chapter

10

Sclera

Most Important (Must Read Topics)	Elective Topics
1) Staphyloma 2) Episcleritis 3) Scleritis	

▢ STAPHYLOMA :

☞ It is an abnormal protrusion of uveal tissue through a weak and thin portion of cornea or sclera.

☞ It is lined :

Internally → by Uveal Tissue

Externally → by Weak cornea or sclera

☞ Types : **(Fig. 10.1)**

1) *Anterior staphyloma :* **(Fig. 10.2)**

   ➢ Protrusion & adhesion of iris to ectatic cornea.

   ➢ *Commonest cause :* Corneal ulcer. It perforates and heals with the formation of pseudocornea.

2) *Intercalary staphyloma :* **(Fig. 10.3)**

   ➢ occurs at limbus.

   ➢ lined by iris and anterior portion of ciliary body.

   ➢ Causes : Injury to the limbus,

      ⇨ marginal corneal ulcer,

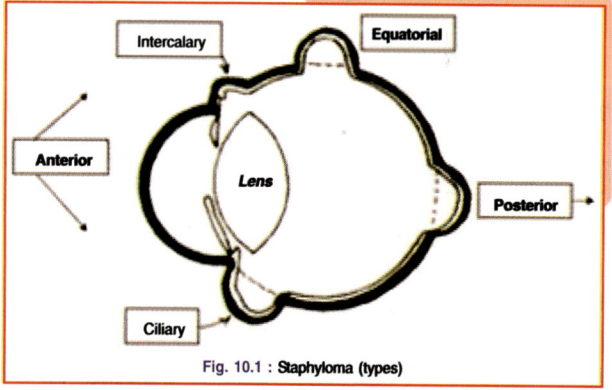

Fig. 10.1 : Staphyloma (types)

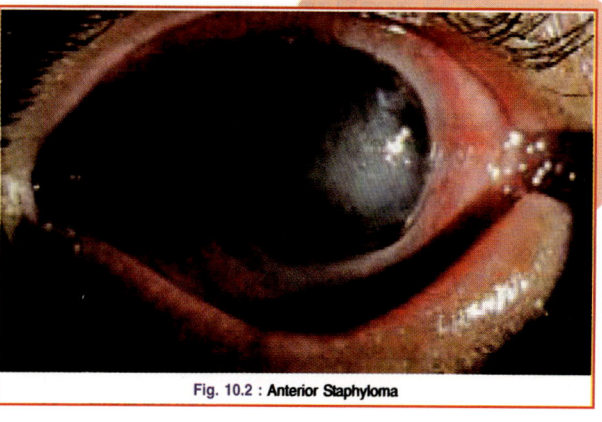

Fig. 10.2 : Anterior Staphyloma

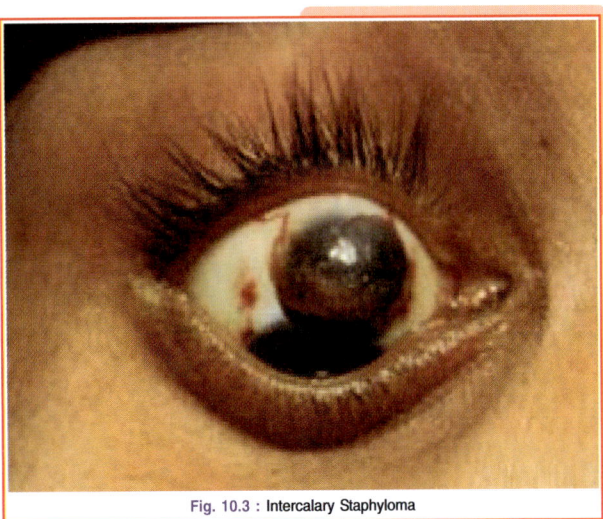

Fig. 10.3 : Intercalary Staphyloma

⇨ complicated cataract surgery,

⇨ secondary angle closure glaucoma,

⇨ Anterior scleritis,

⇨ Scleromalacia perforans.

➤ Defective vision occurs

➤ Treatment : staphylectomy + Heavy dose oral steroids.

3) Ciliary staphyloma : (Fig. 10.4)

➤ affects ciliary zone (8 mm behind the limbus)

➤ *Causes* : Injury, Scleritis, Absolute Glaucoma,

Developmental Glaucoma.

4) Equatorial staphyloma :

➤ at equatorial region of the eye.

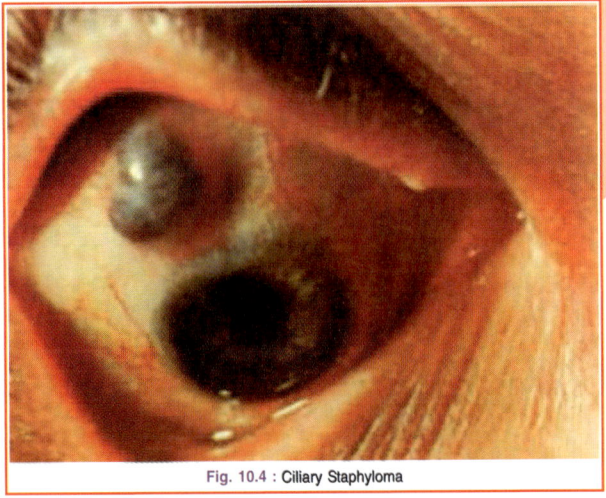

Fig. 10.4 : Ciliary Staphyloma

➤ *Causes* : Scleritis, Pathological myopia,

Chronic uncontrolled glaucoma.

5) Posterior staphyloma : (Fig. 10.5)

➤ at the posterior pole lined by choroid behind the equator.

➤ *Causes* : Degenerative high axial myopia,

posterior scleritis, injuries.

➤ Area is excavated with retinal vessels dipping in it (just like marked cupping of optic disc in Glaucoma)

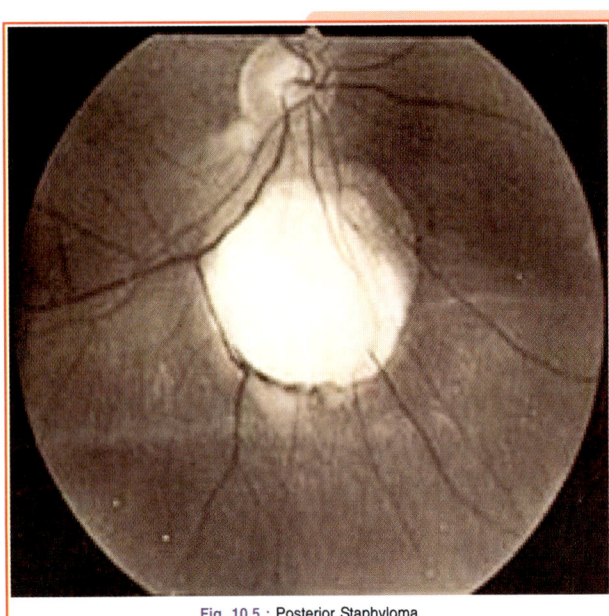

Fig. 10.5 : Posterior Staphyloma

Treatment :

1) No effective treatment.

2) Enucleation in cases of extreme disfigurement.

3) Posterior staphyloma :

Reinforcement surgery by fascia lata or

Silicon band in cases of high myopia.

4) Evisceration in bleeding anterior staphyloma.

☐ EPISCLERITIS :

✒ It is benign recurrent inflammation of the subconjunctival and episcleral tissue, involving the overlying Tenon's capsule but not the underlying sclera.

Etiology :

1) Idiopathic.

2) Hypersensitivity Reaction to endogenous tubercular, streptococcal toxins.

3) Infections (Herpes zoster, syphilis, Lyme disease, Tuberculosis).

4) Systemic diseases (RA, Gout, Psoriasis, collagen disease).

Pathology :

Lymphocytic infiltration of subconjunctival, episcleral tissue.

Types :

1) Simple diffuse episcleritis.

2) Nodular episcleritis.

Clinical features :

Symptoms :

1) Redness.

2) Gritty, burning, foreign body sensation.

3) Photophobia, lacrimation.

Signs :

1) *Simple diffuse episcleritis :* **(Fig. 10.6)**

 ➤ Sectorial diffuse inflammation of episclera.

 ➤ Episcleral vessels are large, engorged, run in radial direction below the conjunctiva.

2) *Nodular episcleritis :* **(Fig. 10.7)**

 ➤ Pink purple flat nodule, 2-3 mm away from the limbus.

 ➤ firm, non tender, can be moved freely from the sclera and overlying conjunctiva.

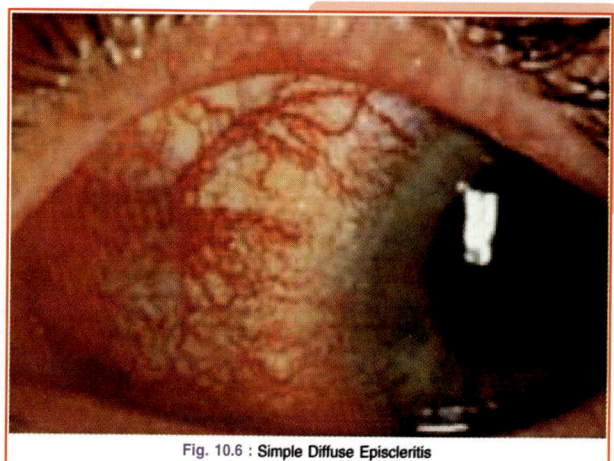
Fig. 10.6 : Simple Diffuse Episcleritis

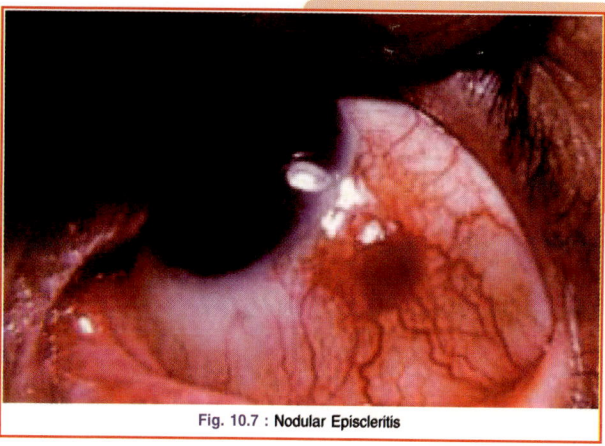
Fig. 10.7 : Nodular Episcleritis

Treatment :

1) *Local :*

 a) Cold compress.

 b) Topical NSAIDs (ketorolac)

 c) Topical steroids eyedrops (Fluorometholone)

 d) Topical artificial tears (methyl cellulose).

2) *Systemic :*

 a) NSAIDs (flurbiprofen)

 b) Analgesics to relieve the pain.

❑ SCLERITIS :

 ⚘ Inflammation of sclera proper.

 ⚘ Characterized by cellular infiltration, collagen destruction and vascular remodelling.

 ⚘ Usually bilateral, more frequently in women.

Etiology :

Associated with connective tissue diseases in 50% cases.

1) Rheumatoid arthritis is the most common cause. Other autoimmune collagen disorders like PAN, SLE, Ankylosing spondylitis, Wegener's granulomatosis, dermatomyositis, Reiter's syndrome, Gout, Polychondritis.

2) Metabolic disorders – Thyrotoxicosis.

3) Infections (Herpes zoster ophthalmicus, Staphylococcus, Streptococcus)

4) Granulomatous diseases (TB, Leprosy, Syphilis).

5) SIS (Surgery induced scleritis).

6) Miscellaneous (Vogt-Koyanagi-Harada Syndrome, Behcet's disease).

7) Idiopathic.

Pathology :

Dense lymphocytic infiltration of the sclera.

Classification :

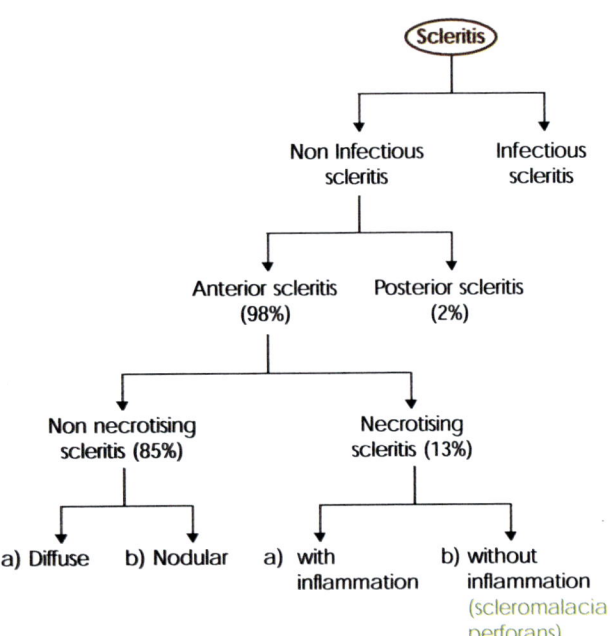

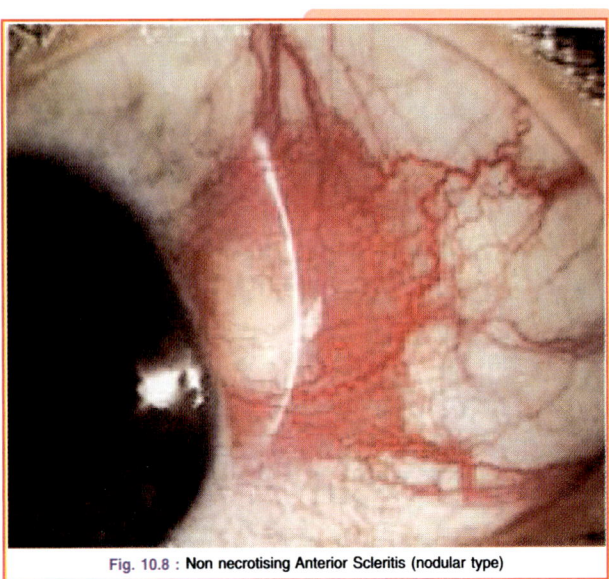

Fig. 10.8 : Non necrotising Anterior Scleritis (nodular type)

3) <u>Necrotising Anterior Scleritis (with inflammation)</u> : **(Fig. 10.9)**

➤ intense localised inflammation, with areas of infarction due to vasculitis.

➤ Sclera becomes transparent, ectatic and uvea shines through it.

Clinical features :

Symptoms :

1) Moderate to severe, deep boring pain which radiates to jaw and temple, wakes the patient early in the morning.

2) Redness.

3) Photophobia, Lacrimation.

4) Diminution of vision.

Signs :

A) *Non infectious :*

1) <u>Non necrotising Anterior Scleritis (diffuse type)</u>

➤ widespread inflammation.

➤ involved area is raised, salmon pink to purple in colour.

2) <u>Non-necrotising Anterior scleritis (nodular type)</u> : **(Fig. 10.8)**

➤ one or two hard, purplish, elevated, immovable scleral nodules near the limbus.

➤ When arranged in ring around the limbus it is known as 'annular scleritis'.

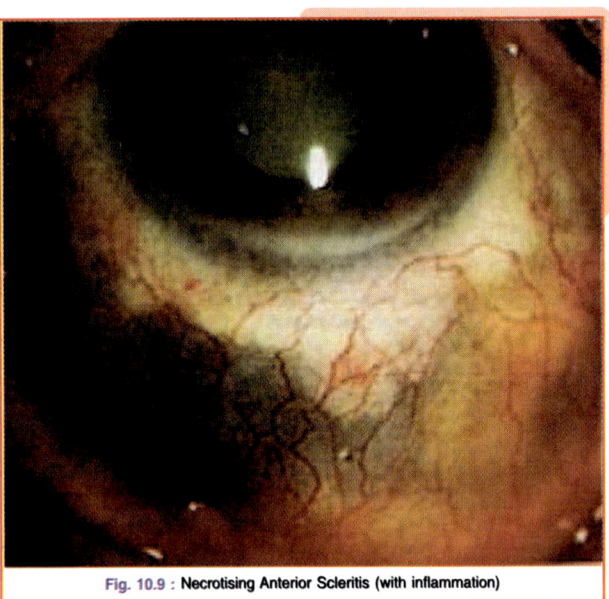

Fig. 10.9 : Necrotising Anterior Scleritis (with inflammation)

4) <u>Necrotising Anterior Scleritis (without inflammation)</u> : (Scleromalacia Perforans) **(Fig. 10.10)**

➤ in elderly females suffering from RA.

➤ yellowish patch of melting sclera.

➤ sclera is dead white in color and punched out through which uvea shines.

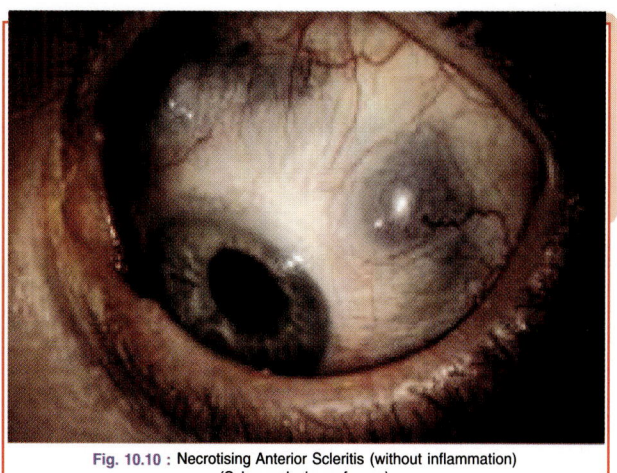

Fig. 10.10 : Necrotising Anterior Scleritis (without inflammation)
(Scleromalacia perforans)

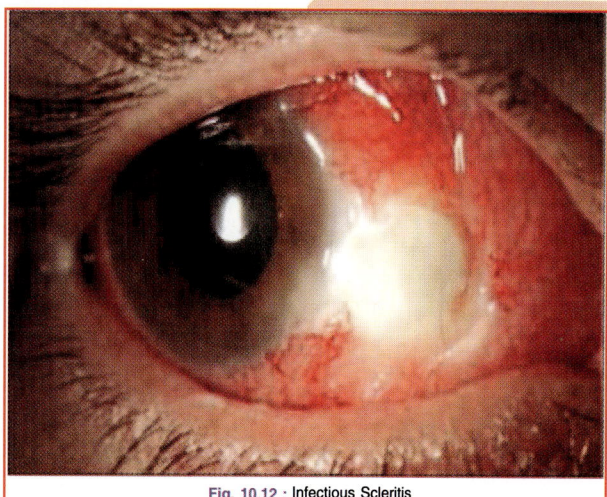

Fig. 10.12 : Infectious Scleritis

B) *Posterior scleritis :* **(Fig. 10.11)**

- ✎ Inflammation behind the equator.

- ✎ Macular edema, Exudative retinal detachment, proptosis, limitation of ocular movements occurs.

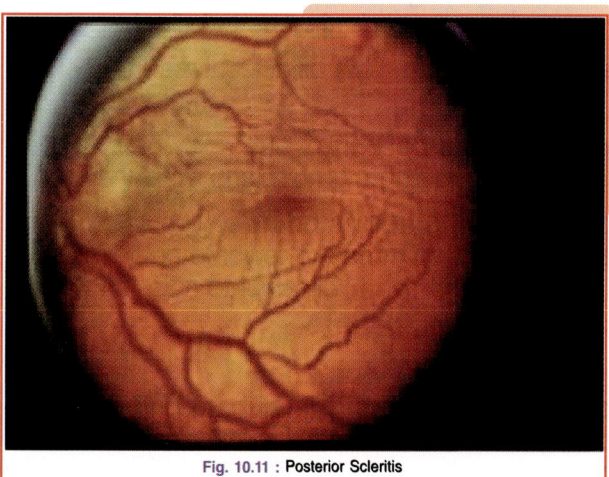

Fig. 10.11 : Posterior Scleritis

C) *Infectious scleritis :* **(Fig. 10.12)**

- ✎ purulent exudates are seen.

- ✎ fistulae formation, painful nodules, conjunctival, scleral ulcers are seen.

Complications :

⚐ Common in necrotising scleritis :

1) Complicated cataract.
2) Secondary Glaucoma.
3) Retinal Detachment **(rarely)**
4) Sclerosing keratitis.
5) Keratolysis.
6) Uveitis
7) Macular edema.

Management :

Investigations :

1) TLC, DLC, ESR.
2) Serum complement [C3], ANA, Rheumatoid factor, LE cells.
3) VDRL, FTA-ABS for syphilis.
4) Serum uric acid for Gout.
5) Urine test.
6) Mantoux test
7) X-ray chest, sacroiliac joint.
8) FFA for vasculitis.

Treatment :

1) Medical :

➤ First line of defence.

a) Local steroids eyedrops (fluorometholone).

b) Systemic steroids :
⇒ at high doses in starting and then is tapered gradually.

c) Analgesics, anti inflammatory drugs :
⇒ to relieve pain, inflammation.

d) Cytotoxic Immunosuppressants (cyclophosphamide, Methotrexate)

e) Antibiotics for infectious scleritis.

2) Surgical :

a) Reinforcement : for scleral thinning and perforation by donor sclera, cornea.

b) Lamellar keratoplasty : for extreme marginal corneal ulceration or keratolysis.

Chapter

11

Eyelids

Most Important (Must Read Topics)	Elective Topics
1) Chalazion	1) Ptosis
2) Hordeolum Externum (Stye)	2) Symblepharon
3) Stye vs. Chalazion vs Hordeolum Internum	3) Trichiasis
4) Entropion	
5) Ectropion	
6) Ulcerative Blepharitis	

❑ CHALAZION (Meibomian/Tarsal Cyst) :

☞ It is chronic non-infective lipogranulomatous inflammation of sebaceous glands called Meibomian glands. (non suppurative) **(Fig. 11.1)**

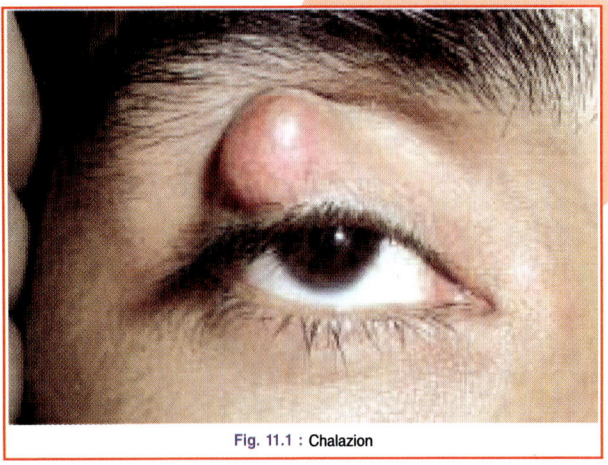

Fig. 11.1 : Chalazion

Etiology :

☞ *Predisposing factors :*

1) *Age :* more common in children, young adults.

2) Habitual rubbing of the eyes.

3) *Metabolic factors :* excessive alcohol, carbohydrates.

4) Trachoma, Blepharitis.

☞ *Pathogenesis :*

Obstruction of Meibomian gland duct by low grade infection that causes proliferation of Meibomian gland duct epithelium and infiltration of wall of ducts, which eventually gets blocked.

Low grade infection

↓

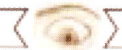

Proliferation, infiltration of the wall of ducts of Meibomian

↓

Duct is blocked

↓

Retention of sebum in gland, causing enlargement

↓

Extravasation of lipids

↓

Non infective lipogranulomatous inflammation of blocked Meibomian gland and surrounding tissue.

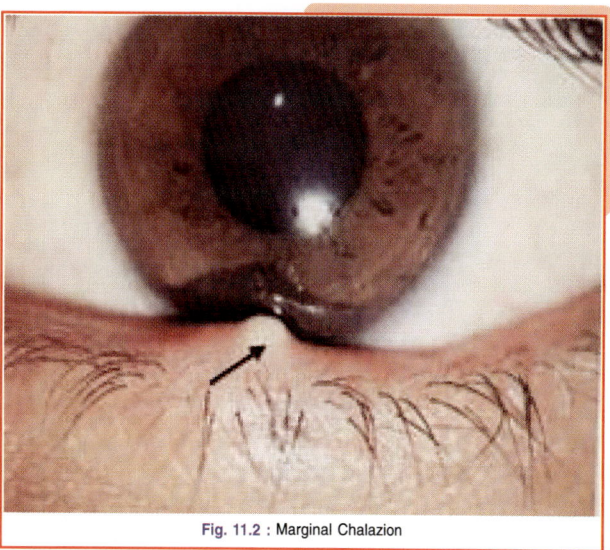

Fig. 11.2 : Marginal Chalazion

Clinical features :

Symptoms :

1) Painless, non tender swelling in eyelid which gradually increases in size.

2) Mild heaviness in lid (with moderately large chalazion).

3) Blurred vision due to induced astigmatism by very large chalazion pressing on the cornea.

4) Watering (epiphora) sometimes due to eversion of lower punctum caused by large chalazion of lower lid.

Signs :

1) Swelling (nodule) is present away from the lid margin which is firm, non tender. Upper lid is involved more commonly than lower lid because of the fact that upper lid contains more Meibomian gland than the lower lid.

2) If swelling (nodule) is present at the lid margin → Marginal Chalazion. **(Fig. 11.2)**

3) Reddish purple area where chalazion points is seen on palpebral conjunctiva after eversion of lid.

Clinical course & complications :

1) Complete spontaneous resolution is rare.

2) Slowly size increases and eventually becomes large.

3) Secondary infection leading to Hordeolum internum.

4) Calcification may occur, rarely.

5) Malignant change to Meibomian gland adenocarcinoma.

6) Recurrence occurs in seborrhoeic dermatitis, acne rosacea, malignant change.

Treatment :

1) *Conservative :*

for soft, small & recent Chalazion

↳ Hot fomentation, Topical antibiotic drops,

Oral antiinflammatory drugs.

2) Intralesional injection of long acting steroid (Triamcinolone)

3) Drainage by Transconjunctival Incision & curettage.

4) Diathermy for marginal Chalazion.

5) Oral Tetracycline in recurrent Chalazion.

❑ HORDEOLUM EXTERNUM (Stye) :

✍ It is acute suppurative inflammation of lash follicle and its gland of Zeis or Moll. **(Figs. 11.3 & 11.4)**

Etiology :

✍ Pre disposing factors

Same as Chalazion

✍ Causative organisms

Staphylococcus aureus

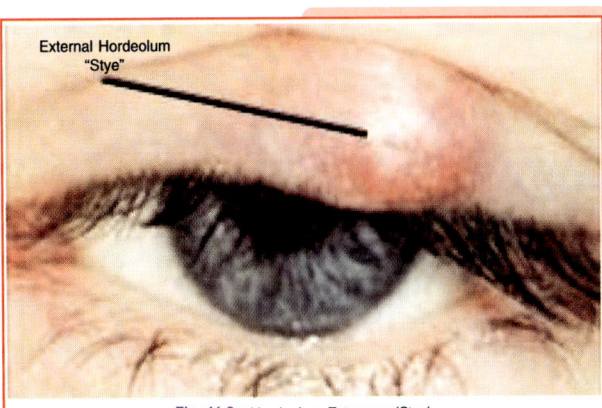

Fig. 11.3 : Hordeolum Externum (Stye)

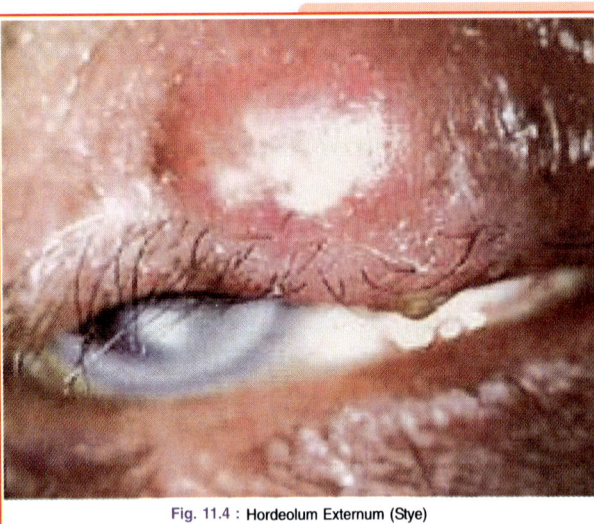

Fig. 11.4 : Hordeolum Externum (Stye)

Clinical features :

Symptoms :

1) Pain.
2) Swelling of the lid.
3) Mild watering.
4) Photophobia.

Signs :

1) *Stage of cellulitis :*
   - localized firm, red, tender lid swelling at lid margin with edema.
   - usually single, may be multiple
2) *Stage of abscess formation :*
   Visual pus point on the lid margin.

Treatment :

1) Hot compress 2-3 times a day (in cellulitis stage)

2) Evacuation of pus (in abscess stage).
3) Surgical incision for large abscess.
4) Antibiotic eye drops (3-4 times a day), eye ointment at bed time.
5) Systemic NSAIDs, analgesics to relieve pain, edema.
6) Systemic antibiotics.
7) In Recurrent stye, find & treat the cause.

FEATURE	STYE	CHALAZION	HORDEOLUM INTERNUM
1) Onset	Acute	Chronic	Acute (also called Acute Chalazion)
2) Gland	Zeis/Moll	Meibomian	Meibomian
3) Type of inflammation	Suppurative	Lipogranulo-matous	Suppurative
4) Symptoms	Acute pain, swelling	Painless, swelling	Severe pain
5) Signs	Hard, tender, swelling near the lid margin	Hard, non-tender swelling away from lid margin	Yellow point seen on lid everting.
6) Treatment	Hot compress, Antibiotics, Lash Removal	Drainage by I&C, Intralesional steroid, Diathermy, Antibiotics	Incision & Drainage, Antibiotics, Analgesics.

ENTROPION : (Fig. 11.5)

- It is inward rolling and rotation of lid margin towards the globe.

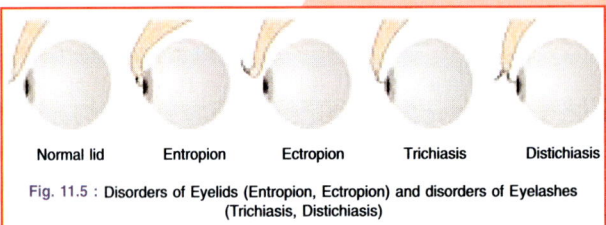

Fig. 11.5 : Disorders of Eyelids (Entropion, Ectropion) and disorders of Eyelashes (Trichiasis, Distichiasis)

- **Etiological types :**
  A) Congenital
  B) Cicatrical
  C) Spastic
  D) Senile (Involutional)

- *A) Congenital entropion :* **(Fig. 11.6)**
  ➤ Rare, present since birth.
  ➤ more commonly in lower eyelid.
  ➤ due to improper development of lower lid retractors.

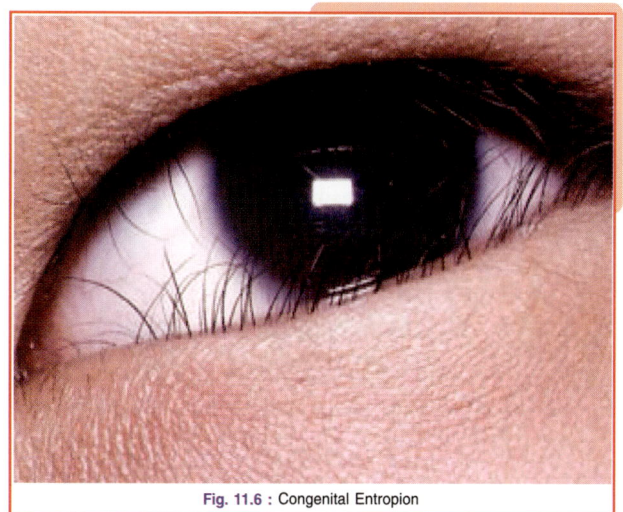

Fig. 11.6 : Congenital Entropion

➢ *Management :*

Plastic Reconstruction (Hotz Procedure)

B) *Cicatrical entropion :* (Fig. 11.7)

➢ more commonly in upper eyelid.

➢ due to Trachoma, burns, pemphigus, Steven Johnson Syndrome.

➢ *Management :*

1) Modified Burrow's operation.

2) Joesche Arlt's operation.

3) Modified Ketessey operation.

4) Resection of skin, muscle, tarsus.

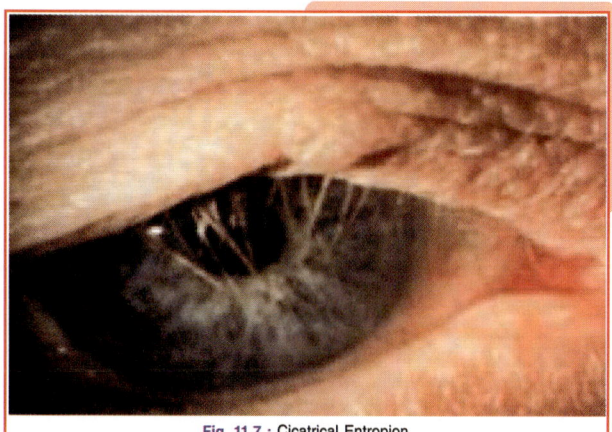

Fig. 11.7 : Cicatrical Entropion

C) *Spastic entropion :*

➢ due to orbicularis oculi spasm.

➢ *Management :*

1) Treat the cause of spasm.

2) Injection of Botulinum toxin

D) *Senile (Involutional) Entropion :* (Fig. 11.8)

➢ most commonly in lower lid.

➢ in elderly.

➢ due to horizontal laxity of lid caused by orbicularis weakening.

➢ *Management :*

1) Jones, Reech, Wobig operation (plication or tuckling of inferior lid retractors)

2) Modified Wheeler's operation.

3) Weiss operation.

4) Bick's procedure

5) Quickert procedure

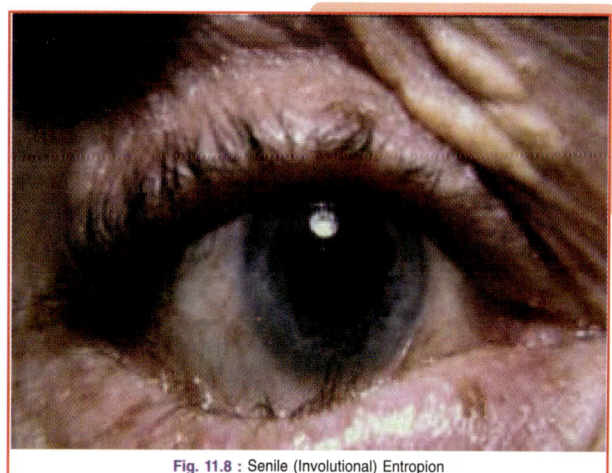

Fig. 11.8 : Senile (Involutional) Entropion

ECTROPION :

⚘ It is outward rolling or turning of lid margin away from the globe.

⚘ **Etiological types :**

A) Congenital Ectropion.

B) Cicatrical Ectropion.

C) Paralytic Ectropion.

D) Involutional (Senile) Ectropion

E) Mechanical Ectropion.

A) *Congenital Ectropion :* (Fig. 11.9)

➢ Rare, present since birth.

➢ Occur in both upper & lower lid.

➢ due to Down Syndrome, blepharophimosis syndrome, congenital shortage of skin.

➢ *Management :*

Mild ectropion   → No treatment

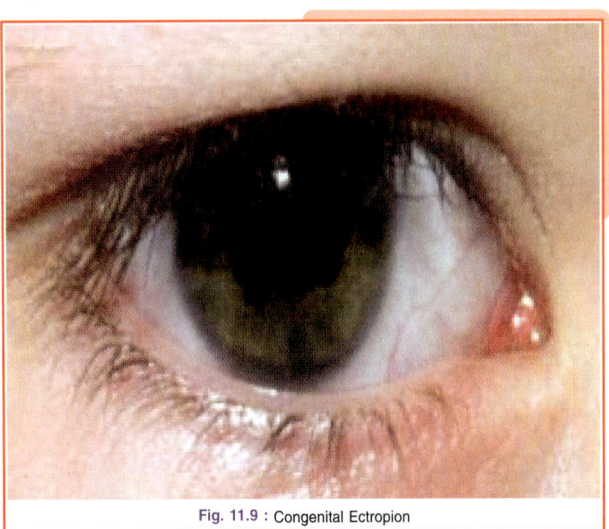
Fig. 11.9 : Congenital Ectropion

<u>Moderate/Severe</u> → ⇨ Horizontal lid
<u>Ectropion</u>   tightening

⇨ full thickness
skin graft

B) Cicatrical Ectropion : (Fig. 11.10)

➢ can involve both the lids.

➢ due to the scarring of skin by thermal, chemical burns, lacerating injuries, skin ulcers.

➢ *Management :*

1) V-Y operation.

2) Z plasty (Elsching's operation)

3) excision of scar tissue and full thickness skin graft.

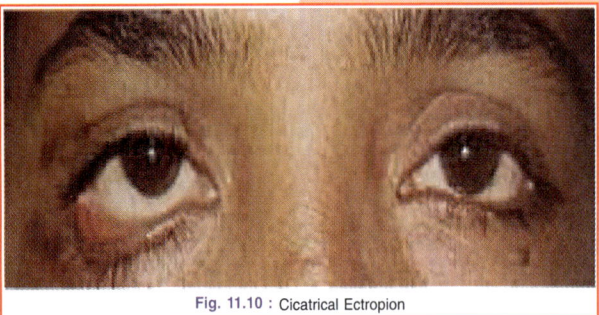
Fig. 11.10 : Cicatrical Ectropion

C) Paralytic Ectropion :

➢ occurs in lower lid.

➢ due to VIIth nerve paralysis (Bell's palsy, head injury, middle ear infection, operation on parotid).

➢ *Management :*

1) Resolve within 6 month if it is due to Bell's palsy → Temporary measures are taken.

2) Non resolving → Permanent surgical measures are needed.

3) <u>Temporary measures</u> :

❑ topical lubricants

❑ suture tarsorrhaphy

4) <u>Permanent measures</u> :

❑ Horizontal lid tightening

❑ Palpebral sling operation.

D) Involutional (Senile) Ectropion : (Fig. 11.11)

➢ commonest form.

➢ affects the lower lid only.

➢ due to : ⇨ horizontal laxity of lid,

⇨ medial/lateral canthal tendon laxity,

⇨ disinsertion of lower lid retractors.

➢ *Management :*

1) Medial conjunctivoplasty.

2) Byron Smith's modified Kuhnt-Szymanowski operation.

3) Horizontal lid shortening.

4) Lateral tarsal strip technique.

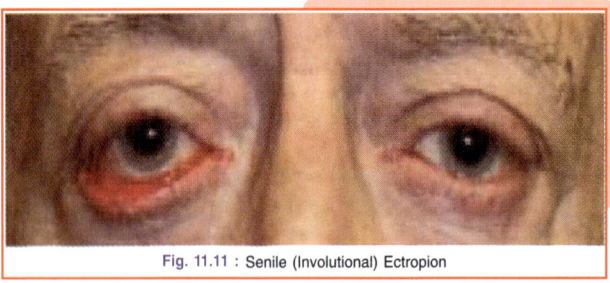
Fig. 11.11 : Senile (Involutional) Ectropion

E) Mechanical Ectropion :

➢ involve lower lid.

➢ due to the pulling down of lower lid as in tumors or pushing out and down as in proptosis and chemosis of conjunctiva.

➢ *Management :*

Treat the underlying mechanical force causing ectropion.

Clinical features :

Symptoms :

1) Epiphora (main symptom)
   in lower lid ectropion.

2) Irritation, discomfort, photophobia is due to associated chronic conjunctivitis.

Signs :

1) lid margin is outrolled.

   <u>Grade I</u> : Only punctum everted.

   <u>Grade II</u> : Lid margin everted & palpebral conjunctiva is visible.

   <u>Grade III</u> : fornix is visible

2) Signs of etiological conditions
   (scars, VIIth nerve palsy)

3) In involutional ectropion :
   Horizontal lid laxity,
   Medial/lateral canthal tendon laxity.

Complications :

1) Dryness, thickening of conjunctiva, exposure keratitis.

2) Eczema, dermatitis of lower lid skin due to epiphora.

☐ PTOSIS/BLEPHAROPTOSIS : (Fig. 11.12)

- ✆ It is abnormal drooping of the upper eyelid.
- ✆ Normally upper eyelid covers upper 1/6th of the cornea (2 mm).
- ✆ In ptosis it covers more than 2 mm.
- ✆ It occurs when muscles that raise the eyelid (Levator palpebrae superioris and Muller's muscle) are not strong enough to do so properly.

Etiological – Clinical Types :

A) *Congenital myogenesis ptosis :* **(Fig. 11.13)**

   ➘ most common type, bilateral.

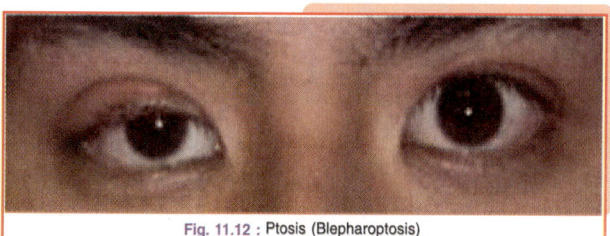

Fig. 11.12 : Ptosis (Blepharoptosis)

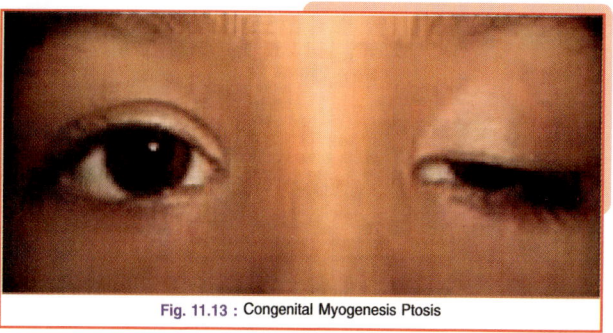

Fig. 11.13 : Congenital Myogenesis Ptosis

➘ associated with maldevelopment or congenital weakness of levator palpebrae superioris.

Characteristic features :

1) Drooping of one or both the lids at birth (may be mild, moderate, severe).

2) Diminished or absent lid crease.

3) Lid lag on downgaze (ptotic lid is higher than the normal) due to tethering effect of abnormal muscle.

   In acquired ptosis : Ptotic lid is lower than the normal in downgaze also.

➘ It may occur in following forms :

1) Simple congenital ptosis
   no other anomaly is present.

2) Congenital ptosis with superior rectus weakness.

3) Blepharophimosis syndrome : ☺ BCET
   a) Blepharophimosis.
   b) Congenital ptosis.
   c) Epicanthus inversus.
   d) Telecanthus.

4) Congenital synkinetic ptosis : (Marcus Gunn jaw winking ptosis) **(Fig. 11.14)**
   ⇨ Retraction of the ptotic lid with jaw movement like chewing.

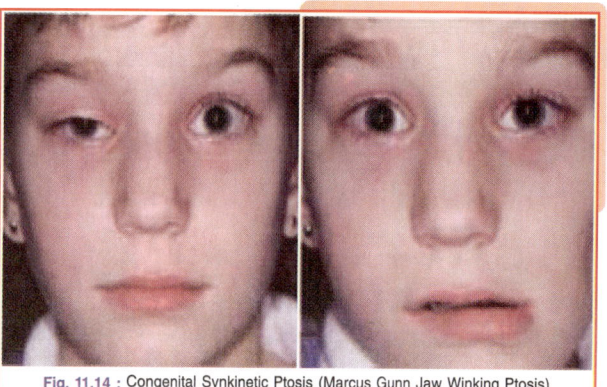

Fig. 11.14 : Congenital Synkinetic Ptosis (Marcus Gunn Jaw Winking Ptosis)

(*i.e.* with stimulation of ipsilateral pterygoid muscle there is spasm of levator palpebrae).

⇨ Due to trigemino-oculomotor synkinesis (V[th] and VIIIth cranial nerve) *i.e.* two or more muscles innervated independently by these two cranial nerves have simultaneous or co-ordinated movement.

B) Acquired Ptosis :

Depending upon the cause it may be :

1) Neurogenic : due to :

a) Third nerve palsy.

b) Horner's syndrome (Triad of mild ptosis, miosis, Anhydrosis).

c) Ophthalmoplegic migraine.

d) Multiple sclerosis.

e) Sympathetic nerve lesion supplying Muller's muscle.

2) Myogenic : **(Fig. 11.15)**

➤ Acquired defect of LPS muscle as seen in myasthenia gravis, thyrotoxicosis, Lambert-eaton myasthenia syndrome, dystrophia myotonica, ocular myopathy.

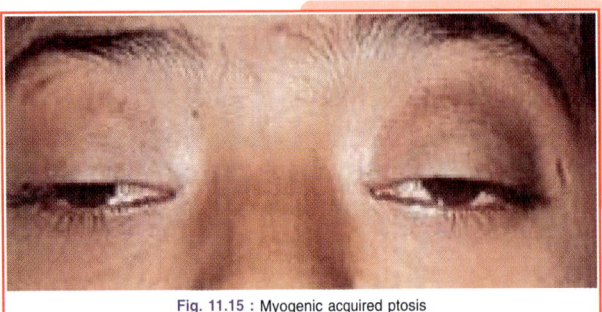
Fig. 11.15 : Myogenic acquired ptosis

3) Mechanical :

➤ due to the excessive weight on upper lid as in lid tumors, multiple chalazion, lid edema.

➤ also due to scarring (cicatrical ptosis) in patients with ocular pemphigoid and trachoma.

4) Aponeurotic ptosis :

➤ due to the defect of levator aponeurosis in presence of normal functioning muscle .

➤ as in involutional (senile) ptosis, post operative ptosis.

C) Pseudoptosis : (Simulated ptosis)

✎ due to the lack of support of upper lid as in microphthalmos, phthisis bulbi, enophthalmos, empty socket.

Clinical features :

Symptoms :

1) No symptoms, if pupil is not covered with the lid.

2) Visual disturbances, if pupil is covered with the lid.

3) Cosmetic disfigurement is the most common symptom.

4) Compensatory changes such as wrinkling of forehead skin, elevation of eyebrow.

Signs :

1) Margin of upper lid covers more than 2 mm of cornea.

2) Palpebral fissure is narrower than the normal.

3) No skin folds in the skin of upper lid.

4) On attempt to elevate upper lid, there is elevation of eyebrow and wrinkling of skin of forehead due to hyperaction of frontalis.

5) Head is lifted backwards so as to draw the lid upwards beyond the pupillary area.

Investigations :

1) History (Age, family history, Trauma, surgery).

2) **Examination :**

a) Exclude Pseudoptosis.

b) Observe if unilateral / bilateral, jaw winking phenomena, Bell's phenomena.

3) **Measurement of ptosis :**

a) In unilateral ptosis, difference between the vertical height of palpebral fissures of two sides indicates degree of ptosis.

b) In bilateral ptosis, it is determined by measuring amount of cornea covered by the upper eyelid and substracting 2 mm. Depending upon its amount, ptosis is graded as :

Mild ptosis   : 2 mm

Moderate ptosis : 3 mm

Severe ptosis   : 4 mm

4) **MRD (Margin reflex distance)** : (Fig. 11.16)
  ➤ Distance between the upper lid margin and corneal light reflex.
  ➤ Normal is 4-5 mm.

5) Levator function assessment.

6) Special investigations :
  a) Tensilon test
  b) Phenylephrine test.
  c) Neurological investigations for neurogenic ptosis.

7) Photographic record for comparison.

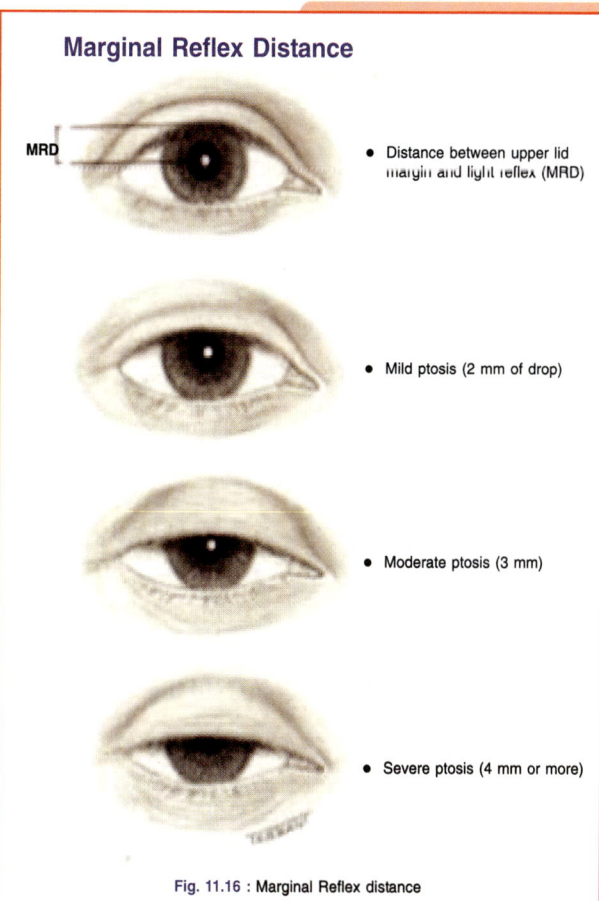

Marginal Reflex Distance

MRD

- Distance between upper lid margin and light reflex (MRD)

- Mild ptosis (2 mm of drop)

- Moderate ptosis (3 mm)

- Severe ptosis (4 mm or more)

Fig. 11.16 : Marginal Reflex distance

Treatment :
✍ Surgical correction is needed :
  A) For congenital ptosis (depends upon LPS action) :
    i) **If levator action is good : LPS is shortened (resection)**
      1) Fasanella-Servat operation
        (Tarso-conjunctivo-Mullerectomy)

2) Blaskovics operation (conjunctival approach)
3) Everbusch's operation (skin approach).

  ii) **If LPS is paralysed :**
    1) Motais operation (superior rectus muscle is used to lift the lid).

  iii) **If both LPS and superior rectus are paralysed :**
    1) Frontalis sling operation (Brow suspension)
    2) Hess operation.

  B) For acquired ptosis :
    i) Treating the underlying cause.
    ii) Conservative treatment.
    iii) Surgery as described for congenital ptosis (however amount of resection required is always less than congenital ptosis of the same degree)
    Fasanella - Servat is adequate.

⬛ **ULCERATIVE BLEPHARITIS :**
  ✍ Blepharitis is subacute or chronic inflammation of lid margin.
  ✍ 5 Clinical Types :
    1) Bacterial (ulcerative) Blepharitis.
    2) Squamous (seborrhoeic) Blepharitis.
    3) Mixed staphylococcal with seborrhoeic Blepharitis.
    4) Posterior Blepharitis (Meibomitis)
    5) Parasitic Blepharitis.

1) **Bacterial (ulcerative) Blepharitis :** (Fig. 11.17)
  ➤ Also known as :
    a) Chronic anterior Blepharitis.
    b) Staphylococcal Blepharitis.
    c) Ulcerative Blepharitis.
  ➤ Chronic infection of anterior part of the lid margin.

Etiology :
Causative organisms :
1) Staphylococci (coagulase positive)

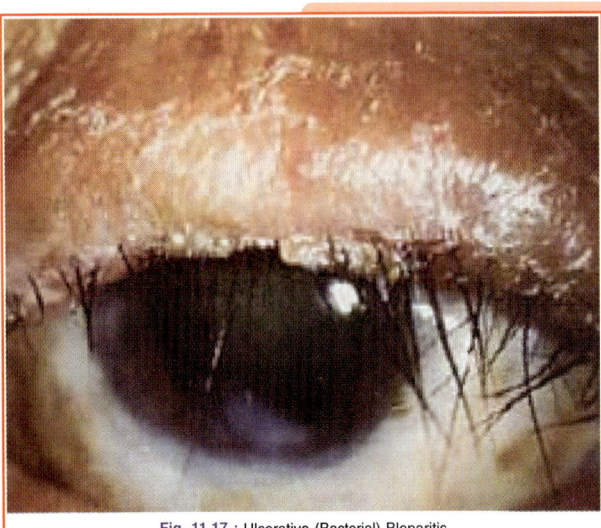

Fig. 11.17 : Ulcerative (Bacterial) Bleparitis

2) Streptococci.
3) Propionibacterium acnes.
4) Moraxella.

Predisposing factors :
1) Chronic conjunctivitis.
2) Dacryocystitis.

Clinical features :

Symptoms :
1) Chronic irritation, itching
2) Lacrimation, Photophobia.
3) Gluing of cilia.
   ⇨ Remissions and exacerbations of symptoms are common.
   ⇨ Symptoms are worse in the morning.

Signs :
1) Yellow crusts at the root of cilia which glue them together.
2) Small ulcers on removing the crust.
3) Rosettes (Red, thickened lid margins with dilated blood vessels).

Complications and Sequelae :

1) *Lash abnormalities :*
   ⇨ Madarosis (sparseness / absence of cilia).
   ⇨ Trichiasis (misdirected cilia).
   ⇨ Poliosis (Graying of lashes).

2) Tylosis (thickening / scarring of lid margin)
3) Eversion of punctum leading to epiphora.
4) Ectropion, eczema of skin.
5) Recurrent stye.
6) Marginal keratitis.
7) Instability of tear film.
8) Secondary inflammatory & mechanical changes in conjunctiva, cornea.

Treatment :

1) *Lid hygiene (twice daily) :*
   ⇨ Warm compress to soften the crusts.
   ⇨ Removal of crusts.
   ⇨ Lid margin cleaning with cotton buds.
   ⇨ Avoid rubbing of eyes.

2) *Antibiotics :*
   ⇨ Eye ointment at the lid margins after crust removal.
   ⇨ Eye drops 4 times a day.
   ⇨ Oral erythromycin, doxycycline.

3) Topical steroids (fluorometholone).
4) Artificial eye drops (methylcellulose)

2) Seborrhoeic (Squamous) Blepharitis : (Fig. 11.18)

Etiology :

1) Dandruff (Seborrhoea of scalp).
2) Corynebacterium acne.

Clinical features :

Symptoms :
1) Deposition of whitish material (soft scales) at the lid margin.

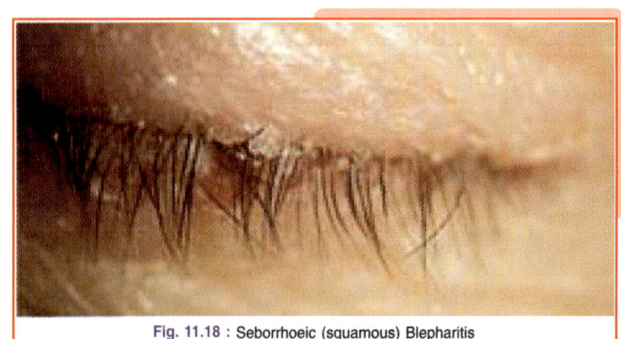

Fig. 11.18 : Seborrhoeic (squamous) Blepharitis

2) Irritation, watering.

3) Falling of eyelashes.

Signs :

1) Accumulation of white dandruff like scales on lid margin, among the lashes.

⇨ On removal of scales, surface is hyperaemic, greasy (no ulcers).

2) Lashes fall off easily.

3) Lid margins are thickened.

4) Signs like bacterial blepharitis.

Complications :

Similar to bacterial blepharitis but of lesser frequency.

Treatment :

1) General measures, balanced diet.

2) Seborrhoea of scalp should be treated.

3) Removal of scales from lid margin.

4) Antibiotics (erythromycin) in mixed type.

▢ SYMBLEPHARON :

☞ Condition where lids become adherent with the eyeball due to adhesions between the palpebral and bulbar conjunctiva. **(Fig. 11.19)**

Etiology :

Due to the healing of kissing raw surfaces upon palpebral and bulbar conjunctiva.

1) Thermal, chemical burns.

2) Membranous conjunctivitis.

3) Conjunctival ulcers.

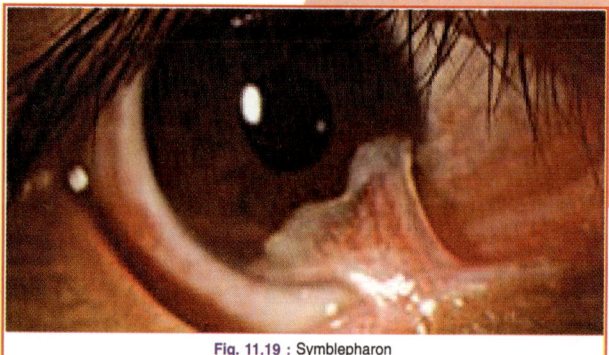

Fig. 11.19 : Symblepharon

4) Stevens-Johnson syndrome.

5) Ocular pemphigus.

6) Injuries.

Clinical features :

1) Restriction of ocular movements.

2) Diplopia due to restricted motility.

3) Lagophthalmos (Inability to close the lid).

4) Cosmetic disfigurement.

Types : (Fig. 11.20)

1) Anterior symblepharon : adhesions anteriorly.

2) Posterior symblepharon : adhesions in fornices.

3) Total symblepharon : involves whole lid.

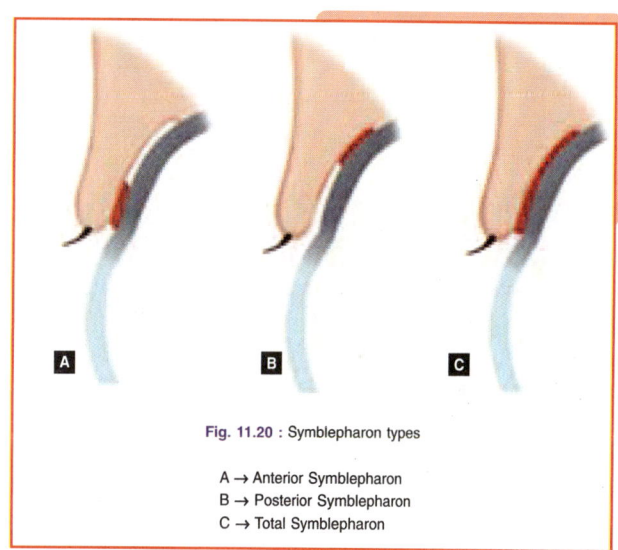

Fig. 11.20 : Symblepharon types

A → Anterior Symblepharon
B → Posterior Symblepharon
C → Total Symblepharon

Complications :

1) Dryness.

2) Thickening / Keratinization of conjunctiva.

3) Corneal ulcer due to exposure keratitis.

Treatment :

A) Curative :

✎ Symblepharectomy, and covering the raw area by surrounding conjunctiva, conjunctival or buccal mucosal graft, amniotic membrane transplantation (AMT).

B) Prophylaxis :

✎ Application of lubricants by sweeping glass rod.

✎ Therapeutic soft contact lenses.

◘ TRICHIASIS :

- ☞ It is inward misdirection of cilia (that rub against eyeball) with normal position of lid margin. **(Figs. 11.21 & 11.22)**
- ☞ If inward turning of eyelashes is along with lid margin (as in entropion) it is called as pseudotrichiasis.

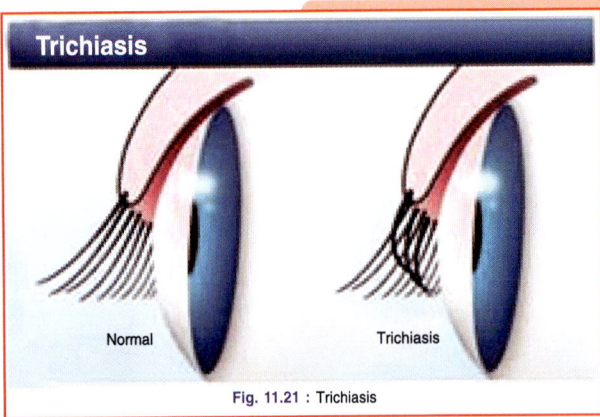

Fig. 11.21 : Trichiasis

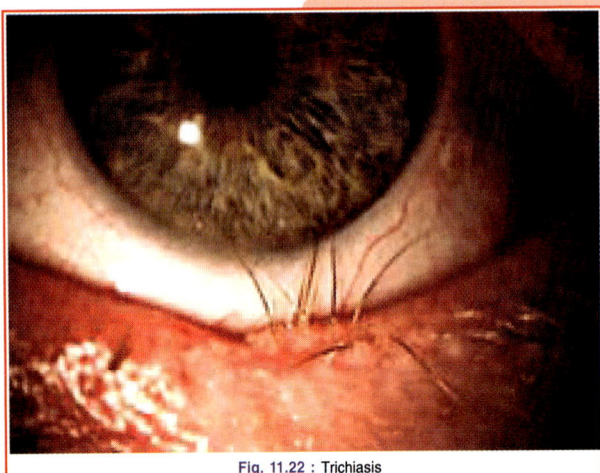

Fig. 11.22 : Trichiasis

Etiology :

1) Cicatrising trachoma.

2) Ulcerative Blepharitis.

3) Healed membranous conjunctivitis.

4) Hordeolum externum.

5) Injuries, burns, operative scars on lid margins.

Clinical features :

Symptoms :

1) Foreign body sensation

2) Photophobia

3) Pain, Irritation

4) Lacrimation

Signs :

1) Misdirected cilia.

2) Congestion of conjunctiva.

3) Signs of causation (Trachoma, Blepharitis).

4) Reflex Blepharospasm.

Complications :

1) Recurrent corneal abrasions.

2) Corneal opacities.

3) Corneal vascularization.

4) Corneal ulcers.

Treatment :

1) Epilation (mechanical removal with forceps)
   - ☞ Temporary measure, recurrence occurs.
2) Electrolysis :
   - ☞ destroying the lash follicle by electric current.
3) Cryoepilation.
4) Surgery :
   - ☞ like cicatrical entropion.

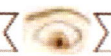

Chapter

12

Ocular Injuries

Most Important (Must Read Topics)	Elective Topics
1) Ocular Injuries, classification	1) Hyphaema
2) Blunt Trauma to eye	2) Penetrating, Perforating Injury
3) Sympathetic ophthalmitis	3) Chemical burns of eye

☐ CLASSIFICATION OF OCULAR INJURIES :

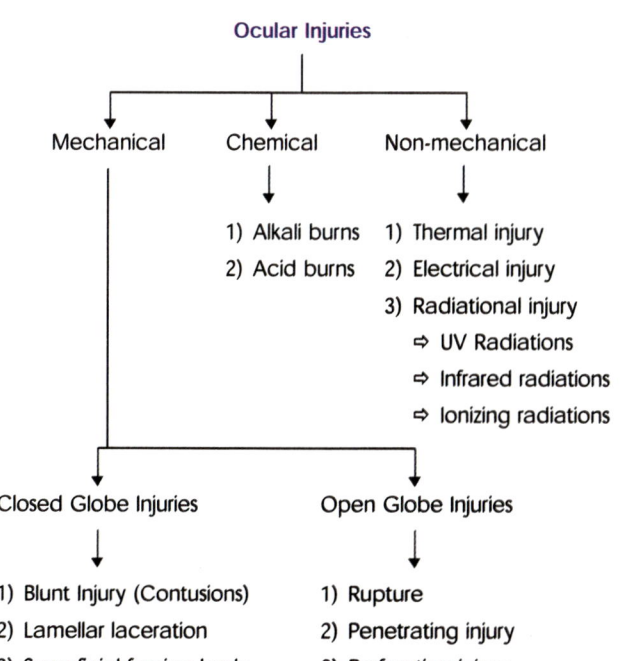

Ocular Injuries

Mechanical — Chemical — Non-mechanical

Chemical
1) Alkali burns
2) Acid burns

Non-mechanical
1) Thermal injury
2) Electrical injury
3) Radiational injury
   ⇨ UV Radiations
   ⇨ Infrared radiations
   ⇨ Ionizing radiations

Closed Globe Injuries
1) Blunt Injury (Contusions)
2) Lamellar laceration
3) Superficial foreign body
4) Mixed
Zone I : Conjunctiva, sclera, cornea are involved.

Open Globe Injuries
1) Rupture
2) Penetrating injury
3) Perforating injury
4) Intraocular foreign body
5) Mixed

Zone II : Anterior chamber, lens is involved.

Zone III : Posterior part is involved.

Zone I : Only cornea is involved.

Zone II : Involvement of Cornea, Sclera upto 5 mm.

Zone III : > 5 mm of sclera is involved.

☐ ILL EFFECTS / OCULAR MANIFESTATIONS OF BLUNT TRAUMA TO EYE & MANAGEMENT :

Blunt Trauma can cause following types of injuries :

A) Closed globe injury.

B) Globe Rupture injury.

C) Extraocular lesions.

A) Closed Globe Injury :

I) Cornea :

1) Corneal abrasions, partial/complete tear in Descemet's membrane, corneal erosions.

   Rx : ⇨ Antibiotic treatment, patching the eye.

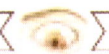

⇨ Loosely attached epithelium should be removed by debridement and 'pad & bandage' is applied for 2 days.

2) Corneal opacity :

   Rx : Keratoplasty to be done.

3) Blood staining of cornea (due to hyphaema and ↑ IOP).

II) Sclera :

1) Rupture (commonly at the limbus or behind the insertion of Recti)

   Rx : ❑ Suturing with reposition of prolapsed uvea.

   ❑ Enucleation if eye is seriously damaged.

2) Intraocular hemorrhage.

III) Iris & ciliary body :

1) Iridodialysis (detachment of iris from ciliary body)

2) Antiflexion of iris.

3) Retroflexion of iris.

4) Angle Recession (leading to Angle Recession Glaucoma).

5) Traumatic miosis.

6) Traumatic mydriasis.

7) Radiating tears.

8) Rupture at pupillary margins.

9) Cyclodialysis

10) Aniridia / Iridemia :

   completely torn iris sinks in the anterior chamber.

11) Iridocyclitis

   Rx : Steroids, Atropine, Antibiotics.

   Atropine is contraindicated if there is pupillary margin rupture & if subluxated lens is present.

IV) Lens :

1) Vossius Ring :

   ⇨ Circular ring of brown pigment on the anterior capsule.

2) Rosette (Traumatic / Concussion) Cataract.

Rx : ❑ If glaucoma occurs, control the IOP with standard medications.

❑ Steroids are given if lens particles cause iritis.

❑ Phacoemulsification if zonules are intact.

❑ ICCE if zonules are lost.

❑ Posterior capsulectomy, Anterior vitrectomy.

❑ Pars plana lensectomy, Vitrectomy.

3) Subluxation / Dislocation of lens :

   ⇨ Subluxation can cause Iridodonesis, phacodonesis.

   Rx : Subluxation :

   ❑ Spectacles/Contact lens wear.

   ❑ Lensectomy & Anterior vitrectomy.

   ❑ Surgery is associated with high risk of Retinal detachment.

V) Retina :

1) Berlin's edema (Commotio retinae) :

   ⇨ It is macular edema characterised by milky white cloudiness in the posterior pole and cherry red spot in the fovea.

   Rx : may resolve spontaneously, if it does't resolve high dose iv steroids are given to reduce retinal swelling and it improves BCVA (Best corrected visual acuity).

2) Macular hole, macular degeneration.

   Rx : Vitrectomy.

3) Retinal tear/Detachment :

   Rx : ❑ Sealing the Retinal tear by laser photocoagulation, diathermy, cryoapplication.

   ❑ Reducing the vitreous traction on retina by scleral buckling, external plombage or encirclage.

   ❑ Vitrectomy & gas injection.

4) Retinal hemorrhages.

5) Proliferative Retinopathy.

VI) Choroid :

1) Choroid Rupture.

2) Choroidal hemorrhage.

3) Choroidal Detachment.

4) Choroiditis.

Rx : 1) for choroidal rupture :

   ❑ anti VEGF therapy (Bevacizumab, Ranibizumab)

   ❑ Laser photocoagulation.

2) for choroidal detachment :

   ❑ Topical steroids, cycloplegics, mydriatics.

   ❑ IOP lowering if there is ↑ IOP.

   ❑ suprachoroidal fluid drainage with AC Reformation.

VII) Vitreous :

1) Pigmentory opacities.

2) Vitreous hemorrhage :

   Rx : Vitrectomy.

3) Vitreal detachment or herniation.

   Rx : Uncomplicated posterior vitreous detachment (PVD) → no treatment is needed. Reassurance is given to the patient.

   ⇨ Retinal tear complicating the PVD :

      Laser photocoagulation.

   ⇨ Vitreous hemorrhage complicating the PVD :

      Vitrectomy.

   ⇨ Retinal detachment complicating the PVD :

      Photocoagulation

VIII) Optic Nerve :

1) Optic atrophy :

   Rx : Stem cells treatment.

IX) Anterior chamber :

1) Traumatic hyphaema :

   Rx : ⇨ If it is absorbed spontaneously, no treatment is needed.

   ⇨ If IOP ↑ → Acetazolamide.

   ⇨ Paracentesis to drain the blood.

X) IOP changes :

1) Traumatic Glaucoma.

   Rx : Acetazolamide, steroids

2) Traumatic hypotony.

XI) Refractive changes :

1) Myopia.

2) Hypermetropia.

B) Globe Rupture Injury :

I) Full thickness scleral, corneal laceration.

II) Prolapse of Iris.

III) Extrusion of ocular contents.

IV) Vitreous loss, Intraocular hemorrhage.

V) Accompanying signs :

   Hyphaema, commotio retinae, choroid rupture, vitreous hemorrhage, retinal tear.

Rx : 1) Repair of the tear under general anaesthesia.

2) Steroids, Atropine, Antibiotics.

3) Enucleation if eyeball is badly damaged, and if salvation is not possible.

C) Extraocular lesions :

I) Lacrimal apparatus lesions :

1) Dislocations

2) Lacerations

II) Conjunctiva :

1) Chemosis.

2) Laceration.

3) Subconjunctival hemorrhages.

III) Eyelids :

1) Ecchymosis :

   ⇨ Black eye.

   ⇨ Appears as bilateral ring hematomas (Panda eye).

2) Lacerations.

3) Avulsion of lids.

4) Traumatic ptosis :

   ⇨ due to the damage to levator.

Rx : Treatment of the cause,

Conservative treatment,

Fasanella-servat operation.

IV) Orbital injury :

1) Blow out fracture.
2) Orbital hemorrhage.
3) Orbital emphysema.

V) Optic Nerve :

1) Traumatic papillitis.
2) Laceration of optic nerve.
3) Optic nerve avulsion.
4) Optic nerve sheath hemorrhage.

Rx : Steroids, surgical decompression.

◻ HYPHAEMA : (Fig. 12.1)

- It is the collection of blood in the anterior chamber.
- Bleeding occurs from conjunctival or scleral vessels and rarely from the root of iris.

Causes of Hyphaema :

1) Intraoperative / Postoperative.
2) Blood dyscrasias.
3) Herpetic Iridocyclitis.
4) Rubeosis iridis (as in diabetics)
5) Intraocular malignancies.
6) Idiopathic.
7) Juvenile xanthogranuloma.
8) Trauma.

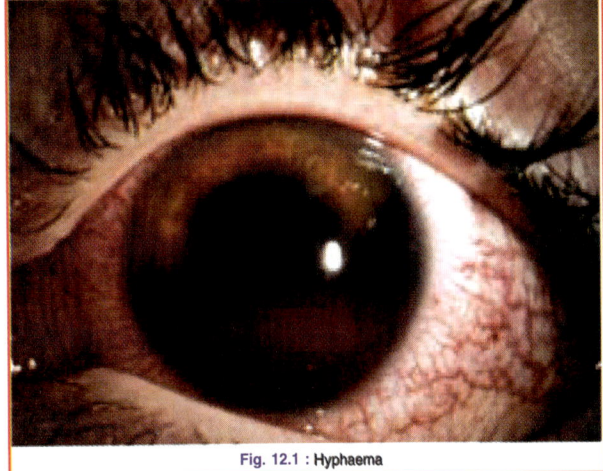

Fig. 12.1 : Hyphaema

Clinical features :

1) Blood usually doesn't get clotted, and gets settled at most dependent part of the anterior chamber & thus fluid meniscus is formed.
2) Blood may get clotted in presence of Iridodialysis, sphincteric tear.
3) '8 ball or blackball' hyphaema : **(Fig. 12.2)**
   - When blood is clotted, hyphaema appears as a small black ball (like number 8 ball in billiards game).
   - This clotted blood causes secondary Glaucoma.

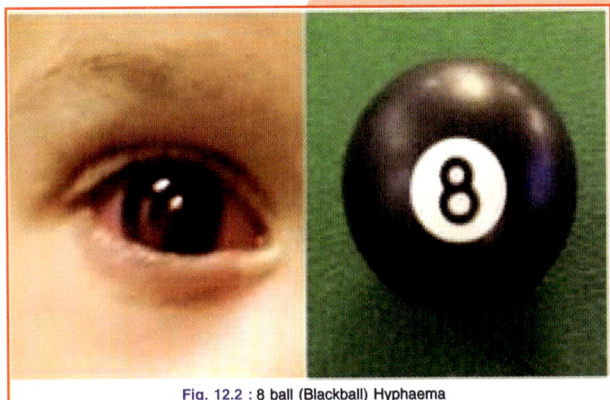

Fig. 12.2 : 8 ball (Blackball) Hyphaema

Complications :

1) Secondary Glaucoma.
2) Blood staining of the cornea.
3) Secondary Optic Atrophy :
   - due to Secondary Glaucoma.

Treatment :

General :

1) Complete bed rest with propped up position.
2) Sedation.
3) Patching of the eyes.

Medical :

1) Local corticosteroids to minimize traumatic uveitis.
   - Mild hyphaema without secondary glaucoma, responds to the above therapy (Aspirin should not be used as it increases the risk of secondary hemorrhage).
2) Secondary Glaucoma :
   - Tab acetazolamide ½-1 tab 4 times daily.
   - Timolol eye drops 2 times daily.

3) Paracentesis :

- ☙ if blood is not absorbed within 5-7 days.
- ☙ if there is persistent high IOP for 3-7 days.
- ☙ if there is blood staining of the cornea.

4) Limbal incision & clot removal in blackball hyphaema.

☐ SYMPATHETIC OPHTHALMITIS :

- ⚘ It is bilateral granulomatous uveitis (panuveitis) and results from penetrating ocular trauma.
- ⚘ Injured eye is called →exciting eye,
- ⚘ fellow eye which →sympathizing eye develops uveitis

Etiology :

Predisposing factors :

1) Penetrating Injury.
2) Ciliary region wounds. (so ciliary body is called dangerous zone / area of the eye).
3) Wounds with incarceration of iris, ciliary body, lens capsule.
4) Common in children than in adults.
5) Rarely, during intraocular surgery.
6) Doesn't occur when suppuration develops in the injured eye.

Pathogenesis :

- ⚘ 'Allergic theory' → most accepted.

    Uveal pigment acts as an allergen and excites hypersensitivity reaction, thus develops plastic uveitis in sound eye (sympathizing).

Pathology :

1) In injured eye (exciting) → Plastic Iridocyclitis.
2) In normal (sympathizing) eye → plastic Iridocyclitis
3) Sympathetic perivasculitis.
4) 'Dalen Fuchs' nodules' **(Fig. 12.3)**

    due to the proliferation of pigment epithelium of iris, ciliary body with invasion by lymphocytes, epitheloid cells.

Clinical features :

I) In exciting eye : **(Fig. 12.4)**

1) 'Keratic precipitates' are present on the back of cornea (first sign) and is dangerous sign.

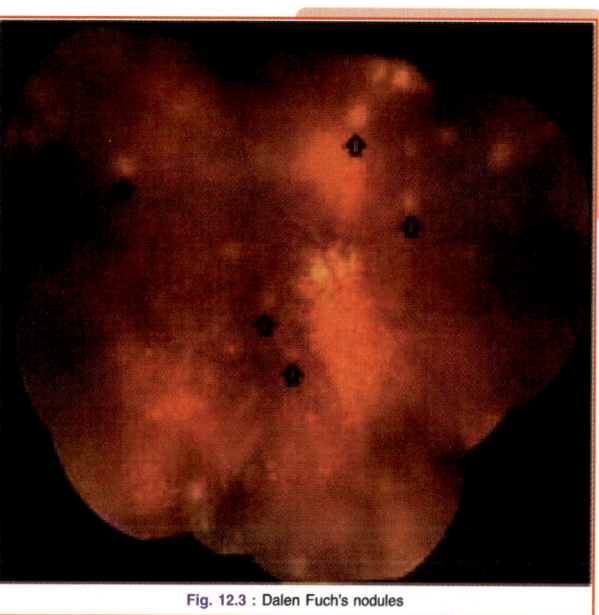

Fig. 12.3 : Dalen Fuch's nodules

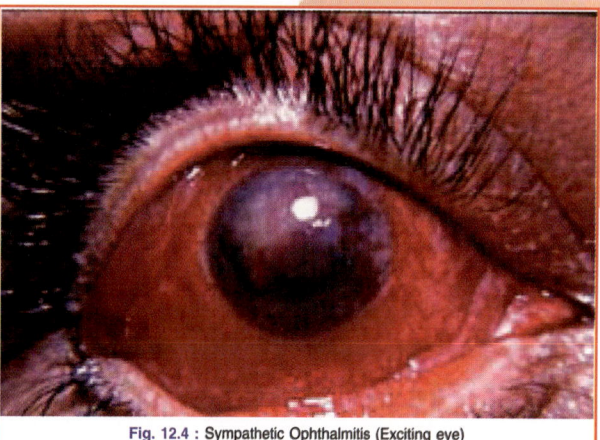

Fig. 12.4 : Sympathetic Ophthalmitis (Exciting eye)

2) Retrolental flare (early sign).
3) Plastic uveitis.
4) Photophobia, lacrimation (early presenting symptoms).
5) Pain, Redness, ciliary congestion.

II) In sympathizing eye :

- ☙ after 4-8 weeks of injury in other eye.
- ☙ earliest reported case : 9 days of injury.
- ☙ mostly occur within 1 year.
- ☙ 2 stages :

    a) Prodromal stage :

    1) Photophobia.

    2) Transient indistinctness of near objects (due to weakening of accommodation).

3) Retrolental flare (first sign)

4) Presence of KP's on the back of cornea.

5) Tenderness, Ciliary congestion.

6) Vitreous haze (opacities)

7) Disc edema occasionally.

b) *Fully developed stage :*

1) Acute plastic Iridocyclitis.

Treatment :

A) *Prophylactic :*

1) Corticosteroids, Antibiotics.

2) Repair of the wounds using microsurgery to free the incarceration of uveal tissue or lens capsule.

3) Evisceration or Frill excision.

Excision of injured eye if there is no chances of saving useful vision.

B) *Curative :*

Just like Iridocyclitis.

1) Topical corticosteroids, and by other routes also.

2) Atropine 3 times a day.

3) Immunosuppressants in severe cases.

This treatment must be given for long time.

C) *Operative :*

in cases where there is organic damage and eye has been quiet for many months.

i) *in milder cases* : Optical Iridectomy.

ii) *in worst cases* (with perception of light and projection of rays.) : Lens may be extracted when other eye is blind or has been removed.

☐ PENETRATING & PERFORATING INJURY : (Fig. 12.5 & 12.6)

⚘ Penetrating injury is single full thickness wound of eyewall by sharp object.

⚘ Perforating injury is two full thickness wounds (one entry and one exit) of eyewall caused by sharp object or missile.

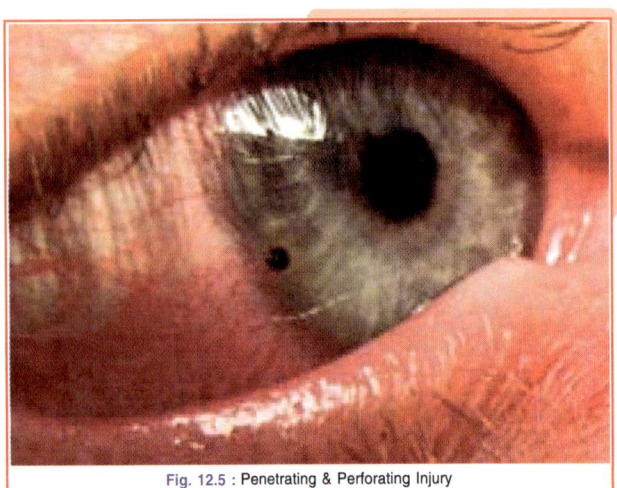

Fig. 12.5 : Penetrating & Perforating Injury

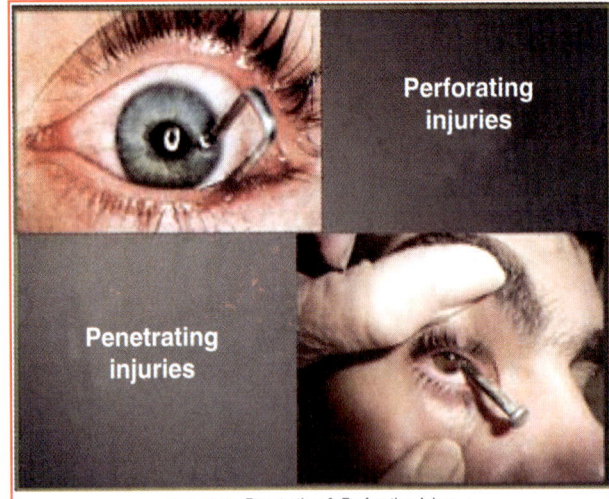

Fig. 12.6 : Penetrating & Perforating Injury

Modes of Injury :

1) Sharp pointed materials (needles, nails, glass pieces, pen, pencils, arrow, screwdriver).

2) Foreign body travelling at very high speed (bullet).

Mechanism of eye damage :

1) Mechanical effects of trauma.

2) Introduction of infection.

3) Post traumatic Iridocyclitis.

Lesions with management :

1) *Conjunctival wounds :*

⚘ leads to subconjunctival hemorrhage.

⚘ *Rx* : Suturing (if wounds are > 3 mm)

2) *Corneal wounds :*

a) Uncomplicated (no prolapse of intraocular contents)

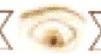

Rx : small wounds : pad and bandage, Atropine, antibiotics

large wounds : sutured.
(> 2 mm)

b) Complicated corneal wounds (prolapse of iris, lens matter, vitreous)

Rx : ➢ Abscising the iris and then suturing (Iris should never be reposited because it may cause infection).

➢ Lensectomy, Anterior vitrectomy.

3) Scleral wounds :

Rx : Suturing.

4) Wounds of Lens :

Small wounds in the anterior capsule seal and then lead to Traumatic cataract.

Rx : Like treatment mentioned in Traumatic cataract.

5) Severely wounded eye :

Corneoscleral tears with prolapse of uvea, lens rupture, vitreous loss, retinal injury, choroidal injury.

Rx : Enucleation.

◻ CHEMICAL BURNS OF EYE :

Etiology :

1) Hot water, steam, hot ashes, explosive powder, molten metals etc. cause burns.

a) Alkali burns (lime, caustic soda, ammonia).

b) Acid burns (H_2SO_4, HCL, HNO_3).

2) Poison gases.

lacrimatory gas, phosgene, mustard gas, arsenical.

3) 'Mica' in coloured powders used in holi.

Clinical features :

Symptoms :

1) Red eye.

2) Swelling of lids, conjunctiva.

3) Reflex Blepharospasm.

4) Photophobia, Lacrimation.

Signs :

1) Severe congestion, chemosis of conjunctiva.

2) Burn marks over the surrounding skin.

3) Dull, opaque cornea or may get sloughed off.

4) Fluorescein staining positive.

Grading of chemical injuries, burns : (Fig. 12.7)

Grade I : Clear cornea, no limbal ischaemia.

Grade II : Hazy cornea with visible iris, < 1/3rd (120⁰) limbal ischaemia.

Grade III : Total corneal epithelium loss, Stromal haze obscuring the iris, 1/3rd to ½ (120⁰-180⁰) limbal ischaemia.

Grade IV : Opaque cornea, >½ (> 180⁰) limbal ischaemia.

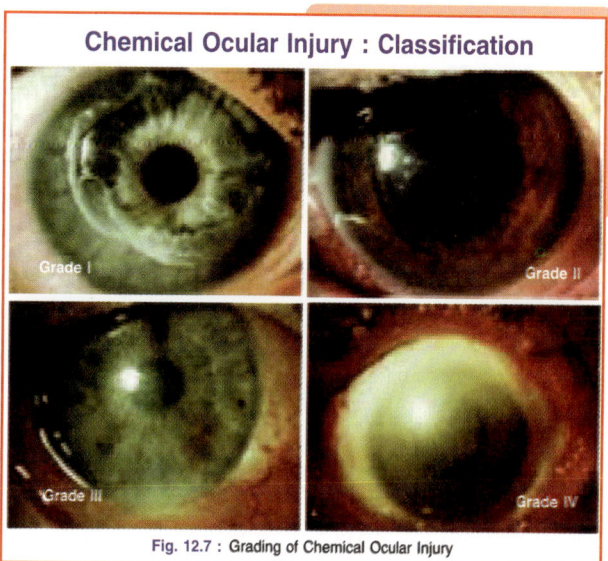

Chemical Ocular Injury : Classification

Fig. 12.7 : Grading of Chemical Ocular Injury

Complications :

1) Symblepharon

2) Corneal ulcer.

Treatment :

1) Immediately wash the eye with plenty of clean water. Acids are neutralized with dilute alkali. Alkali is neutralized with weak acids.

2) Treatment of corneal ulcer if erosions are present.

3) If cornea is not involved : Steroid drops & ointment is given to prevent symblepharon formation, to reduce congestion & chemosis of conjunctiva.

4) Conjunctivitis caused by lacrimatory gases is treated by irrigation with bland lotion, normal saline, clean water, 3% $NaHCO_3$. Use of dark glasses is prescribed.

Chapter

13

Errors of Refraction & Accommodation

Most Important (Must Read Topics)	Elective Topics
1) Hypermetropia	—
2) Myopia	
3) Astigmatism	
4) Presbyopia	
5) Aphakia	
6) Pseudophakia	

❑ HYPERMETROPIA :

✦ Also known as 'Long sightedness' or 'Hyperopia'.

✦ Refractive error in which the parallel rays of light coming from infinity are focused behind the retina with accommodation being at rest.

✦ Person cannot *see* near objects clearly.

Etiology :

<u>5 types</u> :

1) Axial Hypermetropia :

⮞ commonest form.

⮞ due to axial shortening of eyeball.

   a) Physiological axial hypermetropia : All newborns are invariably hypermetropic (+ 2.5D) due to the shortness of globe.

   b) Pathological axial hypermetropia :

When retina is displaced forwards (Retinal detachment, retinal tumor etc.)

⮞ High axial hypermetropia is also present in microphthalmos/nanophthalmos (axial length < 20 mm)

2) Curvature Hypermetropia :

⮞ Curvature of cornea, lens or both is flatter than the normal, resulting in decrease in refractive power.

⮞ Due to cornea plana (after corneal injury), lens plana.

3) Index hypermetropia :

⮞ due to decrease in refractive index of lens in old age due to cortical sclerosis.

⮞ also in diabetics under treatment.

4) Positional hypermetropia :

⮞ due to posteriorly placed lens.

5) Aphakia :

- In Aphakia there occurs high hypermetropia.

Clinical types :

1) *Simple/Developmental/Physiological Hypermetropia :*

- due to biological variations in development of eyeball.

    a) Developmental axial hypermetropia.

    b) Developmental curvatural hyper- metropia.

2) *Non-physiological hypermetropia :*

Congenital :

a) Microphthalmos

b) Nanophthalmos

c) Microcornea

d) Congenital lens subluxation

e) Congenital aphakia

Acquired :

a) Senile hypermetropia (Index type)

b) Positional hypermetropia (subluxation of lens)

c) Aphakia.

d) Consecutive (due to overcorrected myopia surgically).

e) Pseudophakia (due to underpowered IOL implantation)

3) *Functional hypermetropia :*

Paralysis (IIIʳᵈ nerve) of accommodation.

Optics : (Fig. 13.1)

Clinical features :

Symptoms :

1) Blurred vision (more for near than distant).

2) Asthenopic symptoms :

   eye strain

3) Convergent squint :

   due to continuous efforts of accommodation → excess convergence → dissociation of muscle balance → Convergent squint.

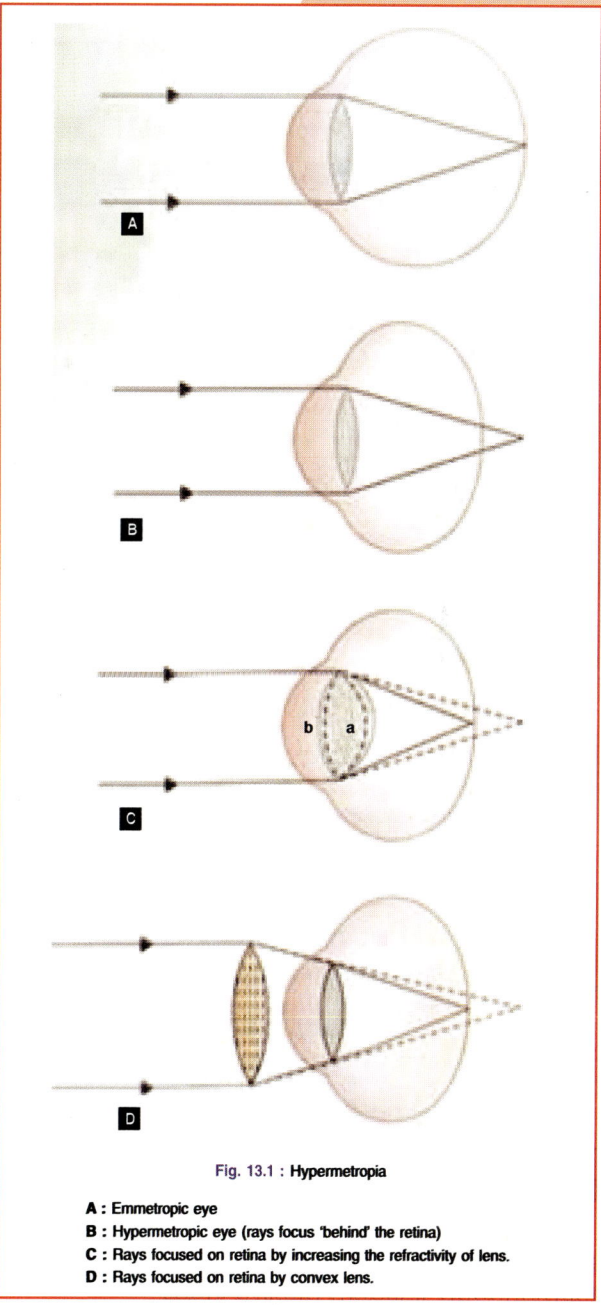

Fig. 13.1 : Hypermetropia

A : Emmetropic eye
B : Hypermetropic eye (rays focus 'behind' the retina)
C : Rays focused on retina by increasing the refractivity of lens.
D : Rays focused on retina by convex lens.

Signs :

1) Small eyeball.

2) Smaller cornea.

3) Shallow anterior chamber

   - predispose to angle closure glaucoma.

4) Apparent divergent squint :

   (due to large positive angle α) as macula is relatively far from the disc.

5) Ophthalmoscopy :

   - Pseudopapillitis (optic disc is smaller, hyperaemic).

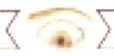

☞ Shot silk appearance of Retina : **(Fig. 13.2)** a peculiar sheen.

☞ Degenerative retinoschisis.

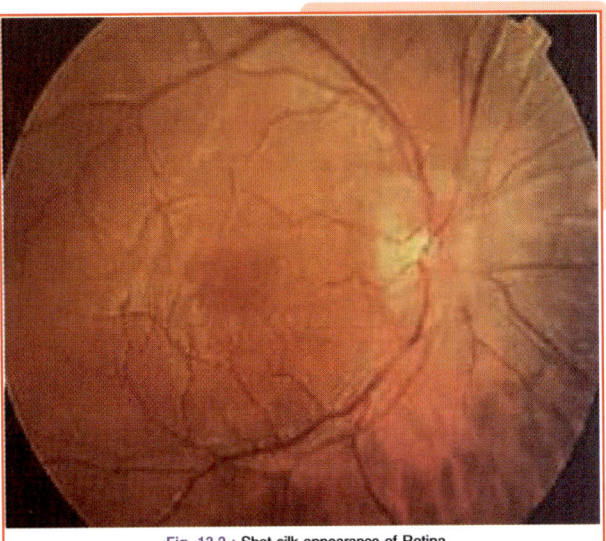

Fig. 13.2 : Shot silk appearance of Retina.

Treatment :

𝕮 Mild hypermetropia without any symptom doesn't require treatment (for young).

𝕮 Treatment is given in high hypermetropia & if patient have symptoms (for middle aged).

A) Optical :

☞ Convex (plus) lens are prescribed after full cycloplegic correction.

☞ In presence of accommodative convergent squint, full atropine correction must be given.

☞ Contact lenses (power is little more than spectacle power)

B) Surgical :

☞ Clear lens extraction with (mono/ multifocal) IOL implantation.

☞ Mostly in aphakic hypermetropia.

C) Laser :

☞ Photorefractive keratoplasty (PK) with excimer laser.

(Cornea is made thinner with laser, so it becomes more convex)

⬛ MYOPIA :

𝕮 also known as 'Short sightedness'.

𝕮 Refractive error in which the parallel rays of light coming from infinity are focused infront of the retina with accommodation being at rest.

𝕮 Person cannot *see* far objects clearly.

Etiology :

5 types :

1) Axial myopia :

☞ commonest form.

☞ due to axial lengthening of eyeball (↑ anteroposterior length of eyeball).

2) Curvatural myopia :

☞ curvature of cornea, lens or both is increased (keratoconus, keratoglobus, megalocornea, lenticonus), resulting in increase in refractive power.

3) Index myopia :

☞ due to increase in refractive index of the lens due to nuclear sclerosis.

4) Positional myopia :

☞ due to anteriorly placed lens.

5) Myopia due to excessive accommodation.

Clinical Types :

1) *Congenital myopia :* (2-3 years of age)

☞ Child is born with elongated eyes.

☞ Refraction upto – 10 D.

☞ Megalocornea may also cause it.

2) *Simple / Developmental Myopia :*

☞ most common.

☞ occurs in 8-12 years of age so also known as school myopia.

☞ Refraction upto -5 to -6D.

☞ associated with axial type due to physiological variation in length of eyeball, or associated with precocious neurological growth in childhood.

☞ Curvatural type is due to underdevelopment of eyeball.

☞ Due to excessive near work in childhood.

3) *Pathological Myopia : (Progressive / degenerative myopia)*

☞ occurs in 5-10 years of age.

- Refraction upto -15 D to -25 D.
- Degenerative changes occurs in fundus.
- It is strongly hereditary (more common in females) and due to general growth processes.

Genetic factors
(major role)　　General growth
processes
(minor role)

↓

More growth of the Retina

↓

Stretching of the sclera

↓

features of
Pathological
Myopia
{
➢ Increased axial length
➢ Choroid, Retina, Vitreous degeneration
}

4) <u>Acquired / secondary myopia</u> :

post traumatic, post keratitic, drug induced, pseudomyopia, consecutive myopia, space myopia, night myopia.

Optics : (Fig. 13.3)

Clinical features :

Symptoms :

1) Blurred vision (more for distant than near).
2) Asthenopic symptoms
   eye strain.
3) Divergent squint
   due to less accommodation → less convergence → Divergent squint.
4) Black floaters, flashes of light (due to vitreous degeneration)
5) Sudden loss of vision (due to Retinal Detachment)
6) Delayed dark adaptation.

Signs :

1) Prominent eyeball (pseudoproptosis).
2) Large cornea, large pupil.
3) Deep anterior chamber.
4) Apparent convergent squint.
5) Vitreous degeneration.

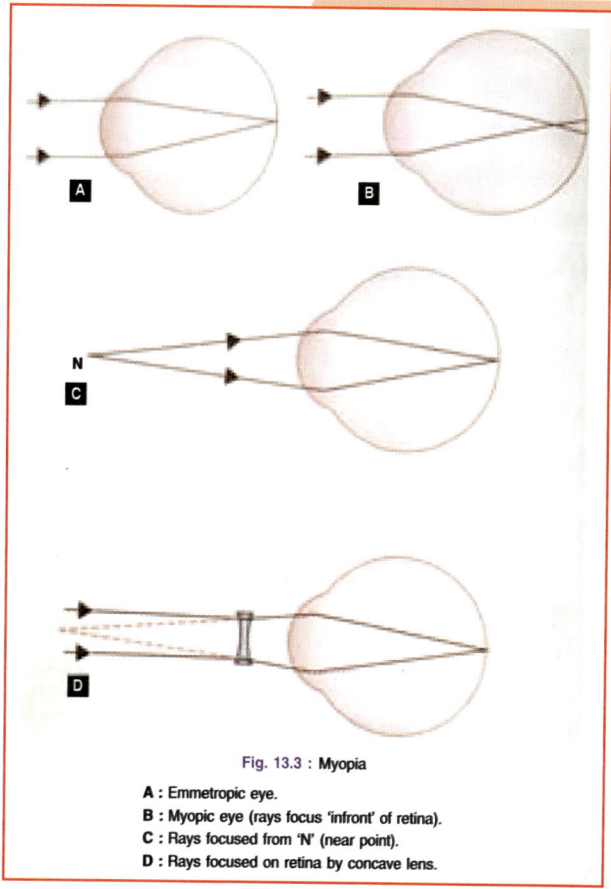

Fig. 13.3 : Myopia

A : Emmetropic eye.
B : Myopic eye (rays focus 'infront' of retina).
C : Rays focused from 'N' (near point).
D : Rays focused on retina by concave lens.

6) *Ophthalmoscopy :*

a) <u>Simple myopia</u> : Normal, only large disc.

b) <u>Pathological myopia</u> :

➢ Optic disc is large with mild pallor.

➢ large physiological cup.

➢ Temporal crescents, Annular crescents are seen (mostly on nasal side) **(Fig. 13.4)**.

➢ Macula : Foster's - fuch's spots are seen, cystoid macular degeneration **(Fig. 13.5)**.

➢ Peripheral Retina : Lattice & snail track degeneration.

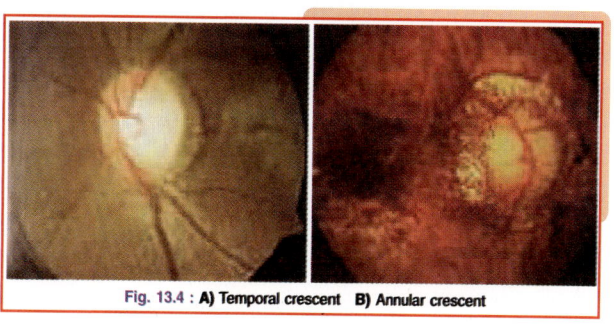

Fig. 13.4 : **A) Temporal crescent　B) Annular crescent**

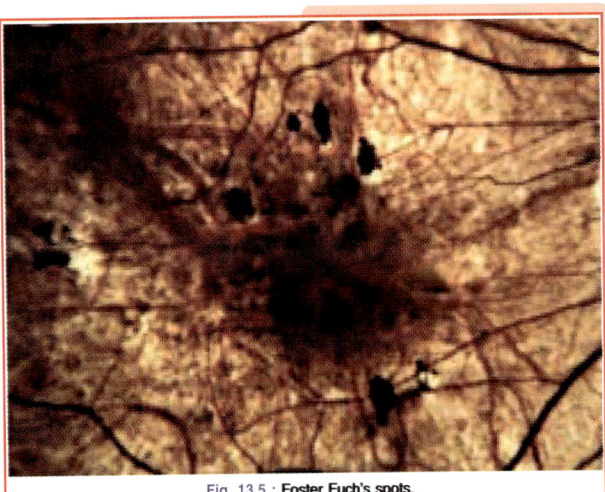

Fig. 13.5 : **Foster Fuch's spots.**

➢ Vitreous : Shows liquefication, opacities, posterior vitreous detachment (Weiss reflex).

Grading of Myopia : (American optometric Association) :

1) Low myopia (≤ -3D).

2) Moderate myopia (-3D to -6D)

3) High myopia (≥ -6D)

Treatment :

A) General measures :

1) Balanced diet rich in protein, vitamins.

2) Visual hygiene :

➢ proper posture for near work.

➢ early management of associated disease.

3) Avoidance of outdoor sports & strenous activities (reading in dark, can lead to ocular fatigue).

B) Optical :

✍ Concave (minus) lens are prescribed.

✍ Myopia must never be overcorrected :

a) In low/moderate myopia (upto -6D)

full correction is given for constant use, especially in children.

b) In high Myopia (> -6D)

Slight under correction is done.
Problems of high minus glass :

i) Minification of object.

ii) Image distortion (barrel distortion).

iii) Reduced peripheral field of vision.

iv) Cosmetically, eyes appear smaller behind the glasses.

✍ Contact lenses :

preferred in myopic correction. (but commonly used are spectacles)

Advantages : i) Image distortion is eliminated.

ii) Field of vision is increased

Disadvantages : i) Not tolerated by all.

ii) Needs extreme accuracy/hygiene.

iii) Costly.

iv) Coneal infections, abrasions.

C) Surgical :

a) Corneal based :

1) Radial Keratomy.

by laser

2) Photorefractive keratectomy.

3) Laser in situ keratomileusis (LASIK)

4) ReLEx (Refractive lenticule extraction) also called ('All - femtolaser vision correction')

5) ICR implantation (Intracorneal Rings).

6) Orthokeratology.

b) Lens based :

1) Clear lens extraction with PC IOL implantation.

2) Minus phakic IOL in AC, even in presence of clear crystalline lens.

D) Laser :

1) Photorefractive keratoplasty.

2) LASIK.

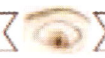

E) LVA (Low vision Aids) :

- Prescribed in progressive myopia & in advanced degenerative changes, where vision cannot be obtained with spectacles and contact lenses.

F) Prophylactic :

- Genetic counselling (not to marry two individuals with progressive myopia).

☐ ASTIGMATISM :

- Type of Refractive error wherein the refraction varies in different meridian of the eye.
- So, rays of light entering the eye cannot converge to a point focus but form focal lines.

Two types :

i)   Regular Astigmatism.

ii) Irregular Astigmatism.

I) Regular Astigmatism :

Astigmatism is regular when the refractive power changes uniformly from one meridian to other (there are two principal meridians).

Etiology :

1) *Corneal Astigmatism :*
   - ⇨ Abnormalities in the curvature of cornea.

2) *Lenticular Astigmatism :*
   - a) Curvatural (lenticonus)
   - b) Positional (subluxation/oblique placement of the lens)
   - c) Index (different refractive index of lens in different meridian)

3) *Retinal Astigmatism* (oblique placement of macula).

Types of Regular Astigmatism :

1) *WTR (With the Rule) Astigmatism :*
   - ⇨ Principal meridians are placed at right angle to each other but vertical meridian is more curved than horizontal.

2) *ATR (Against the Rule) Astigmatism :*
   - ⇨ Horizontal meridian is more curved than vertical meridian and are at right angle.

3) *Oblique Astigmatism :*
   - ⇨ Two principal meridian are not horizontal and vertical, though these are at 90°. *e.g.* 45° & 135°.

4) *Bioblique Astigmatism :*
   - ⇨ Two principal meridian are not at right angle to each other *e.g.* 30° & 100°.

Optics :

Configuration of rays refracted from a toric surface is called as 'Strum's conoid'. **(Fig. 13.6)**

Point A	: Vertical rays are converging more than horizontal rays, so section here is horizontal oval or an oblate ellipse.
Point B (first focus)	: Vertical rays have come to the focus, while horizontal rays are still converging, so section formed here is horizontal line.
Point C	: Vertical rays are diverging and their divergence is less than the convergence of horizontal rays, so horizontal oval is formed.
Point D	: Divergence of vertical rays is equal to the convergence of horizontal rays. Section here is

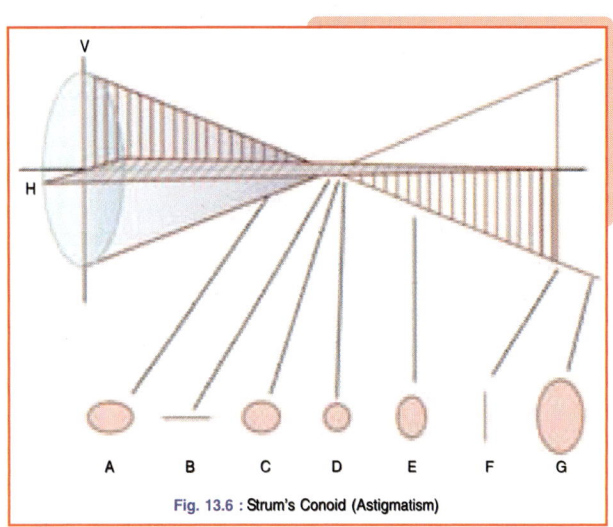

Fig. 13.6 : Strum's Conoid (Astigmatism)

circle which is called 'circle of least diffusion'.

Point E : Divergence of vertical rays is more than the convergence of horizontal rays, so section here is vertical oval.

At Point F : Horizontal rays have came to (second the focus while vertical rays focus) are diverging, so here vertical line is formed.

Point G : Both horizontal, vertical (Beyond F) rays are diverging, so section will be vertical oval or prolate ellipse.

'Focal interval of strum' :

Distance between two foci (B and F).

Refractive types of Regular Astigmatism :

1) *Simple Astigmatism :*
   ⇨ Rays are focused on retina in one meridian and in other meridian either in front (simple myopic astigmatism) or behind (simple hypermetropic astigmatism) the retina.

2) *Compound Astigmatism :*
   ⇨ Rays of light in both the meridian are focused either in front or behind the retina (compound myopic / compound hypermetropic Astigmatism).

3) *Mixed Astigmatism :*
   ⇨ Rays of light in one meridian are focused in front and in other meridian behind the retina.
   ⇨ Thus, in one meridian eye is myopic and in other hypermetropic.
   ⇨ Patient have less symptoms as circle of diffusion is formed on the retina.

Clinical features :

Symptoms :

1) Blurred vision, defective vision.

2) Asthenopic symptoms
   ⇨ eye strain

3) Elongation of objects :
   proportionate to the degree and type of Astigmatism.

4) Keeping reading material close to the eyes.

Signs :

1) Half closure of lid.

2) Head tilt.

3) Oval or tilted optic disc.

4) Different power in two meridians (on Retinoscopy).

Management :

Investigations :

1) Retinoscopy : different power in two meridians

2) Keratometry : different corneal curvature in two meridians in corneal Astigmatism.

3) Astigmatism fan test.

4) Jackson's cross cylinder test.

Treatment :

1) *Optical :*
   ⇨ Appropriate cylindrical lens.
   ⇨ Spectacles with full correction of cylindrical power and appropriate axis for distant, near vision.
   ⇨ Contact lens : Rigid contact lens for upto 2-3 D. (Soft contact lens correct only little astigmatism).
   ⇨ For higher degrees of Astigmatism, Toric contact lens are needed. To maintain the correct axis of toric lens, Ballasting / Truncation is required.

2) *Surgical :*
   1) Astigmatic keratotomy (AK).
   2) PARK (Photo Astigmatic Refractive Keratotomy).
   3) LASIK.
   4) SMILE procedure.

II) Irregular Astigmatism :

Irregular change of Refractive power in two meridians.

Etiological types :

1) *Curvatural :*

Keratoconus, corneal scar.

2) *Index :*

Variable refractive index in different part of the lens (in cataract).

Clinical features :

Symptoms :

1) Defective vision.

2) Distortion of objects

3) Polyopia.

Signs :

1) Irregular pupillary reflex on Retinoscopy.

2) Keratoconus on slit lamp examination.

3) Distorted circles on Placido's disc.

4) Irregular corneal curvature on photo keratoscopy & corneal topography.

Treatment :

1) *Optical :*

⇨ Contact lens which replace the anterior surface of cornea.

2) *Laser :*

⇨ Phototherapeutic keratectomy with excimer laser.

3) *Surgery :*

⇨ is done in extensive corneal scarring.

⇨ Penetrating keratoplasty OR

Deep anterior lamellar keratoplasty (DALK)

❏ PRESBYOPIA (Eye Sight of Old Age) :

✍ It is not an error of refraction, but a condition of Physiological insufficiency of accommodation leading to progressive fall in near vision.

Etiology :

1) Age related changes in lens :

⊾ decrease in lens capsule elasticity.

⊾ progressive increase in size and sclerosis of the lens.

2) Age related decline in ciliary muscle power.

Symptoms :

1) Difficulty in near vision :

difficulty in reading small prints,

difficulty in threading a needle.

2) Asthenopic symptoms :

eye strain due to ciliary muscle fatigue.

3) Intermittent diplopia.

Treatment :

1) *Optical :*

⊾ Appropriate convex glasses for near work.

⊾ Rough guide for providing presbyopic glasses :

45 years – +1 to +1.25 D

50 years – +1.5 to +1.75 D

55 years – +2.0 to +2.25 D

60 years – +2.5 to +3.0 D

⊾ Exact presbyopic addition required, should be estimated individually in each eye.

⊾ Basic principles for presbyopic correction:

1) Find out refractive error for distant & correct it first.

2) Find out presbyopic correction in each eye separately and add it to the distant correction.

3) Near point should be fixed by taking due consideration for profession of the patient.

4) Weakest convex lens with which an individual can *see* clearly at near point should be prescribed, since overcorrection result in asthenopic symptoms.

⊾ Presbyopic spectacles can be unifocal, bifocal, varifocal.

2) *Surgery :*

i) Cornea based :

➢ Monovision conductive keratoplasty.

➢ Monovision LASIK.

➢ Presbyopic bifocal LASIK.

➢ LASIK - PARM (Presbyopia Avalos Rozakis Method)

ii) *Lens based:*
   ➢ Multifocal / Accommodating IOL
   ➢ Monovision with IOL.

iii) *Sclera based :*
   ➢ Anterior ciliary sclerotomy.
   ➢ Scleral spacing & ablation.
   ➢ Scleral expansion.

▢ APHAKIA :

✒ It is absence of crystalline lens from the eye.

✒ From optical point of view, it may be considered as a condition in which lens is absent from pupillary area.

✒ It produces high degree of hypermetropia.

Etiology :

1) Congenital absence (rare).
2) Surgical aphakia (most common) after lens removal.
3) Due to absorption of lens matter after trauma.
4) Traumatic extrusion of lens from the eye.
5) Posterior dislocation into the vitreous.

Optics : (Fig. 13.7 & 13.8)

1) High degree hypermetropia.
2) Total power of the eye is reduced to +44 D from normal of + 60 D.
3) Accommodation is lost fully.
4) Anterior focal point : is 23.2 mm infront of the cornea.
5) Posterior focal point : is 31 mm behind the cornea (*i.e.* 7 mm behind the eyeball).

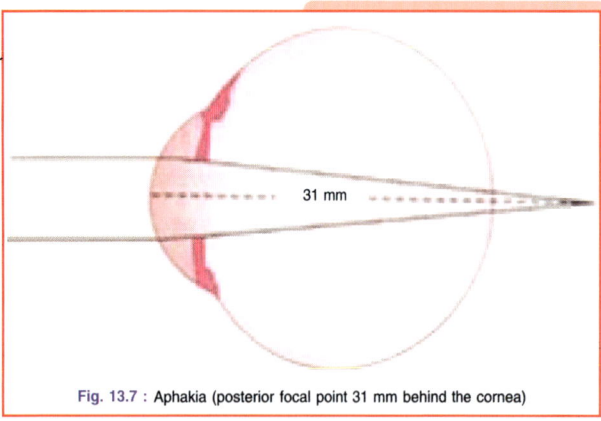

31 mm

Fig. 13.7 : Aphakia (posterior focal point 31 mm behind the cornea)

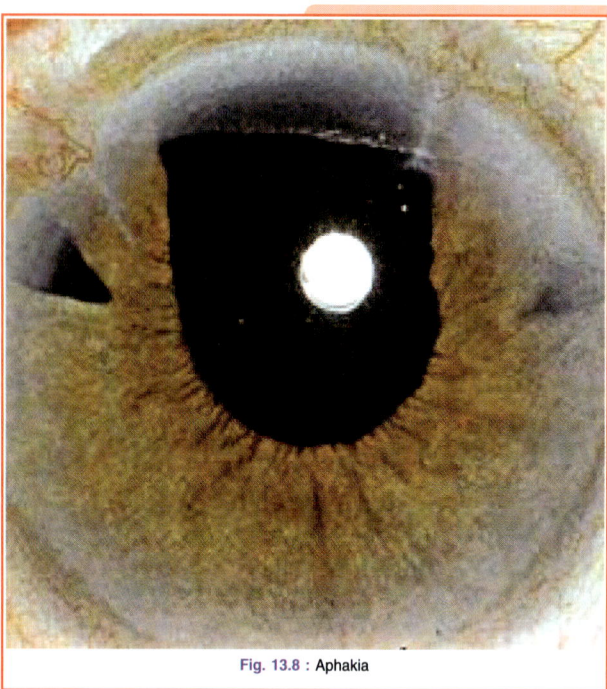

Fig. 13.8 : Aphakia

Clinical features :

Symptoms :

1) Defective vision : for both far & near.

   due to high hypermetropia & absence of accommodation.

2) Erythropsia ⎰
3) Cyanopsia ⎱ Seeing Red & Blue images

   These two occurs due to the excessive entry of UV & IR rays in absence of crystalline lens.

Signs :

1) Limbal scar.
2) AC is deeper than the normal.
3) Iridodonesis.
4) Jet black pupil.
5) Purkinje's image test shows only 2 images (normally 4 images are seen)
6) Fundus examination :

   Hypermetropic small disc.
7) Retinoscopy :

   High hypermetropia.

Treatment :

1) Optical :

   ➢ Spectacles

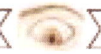

- ✎ Contact lenses.
- ✎ IOL.

2) Surgery :

- ✎ Refractive corneal surgery :
  - i) Keratophakia
  - ii) Epikeratophakia } have less success

3) Laser :

- ✎ Hypermetropic LASIK (it is done when IOL cannot be implanted).

☐ PSEUDOPHAKIA :

- ✐ A condition of Aphakia when corrected with IOL implant is referred to as pseudophakia.
- ✐ also called Artephakia.

Refractive status of pseudophakic eye :

1) Emmetropia (most ideal)

- ✎ Power of IOL implanted is exact.

2) Consecutive myopia :

- ✎ due to overcorrection.
- ✎ IOL which is implanted overcorrects the refraction.

3) Consecutive hypermetropia :

- ✎ undercorrection leads to this.
- ✎ occurs when under power of IOL is implanted.

Signs of Pseudophakia : (with PC IOL) **(Fig. 13.9)**

1) Surgical scar near the limbus.
2) Deep anterior chamber.

3) Iridodonesis (mild).
4) Jet black pupil,

    but when light is thrown,

    shining reflex is observed.

5) Purkinje's image test shows 4 images.
6) Presence of IOL on slit limp examination after dilatation of pupil.
7) Visual status & Refraction depending upon the power of IOL implanted (described above).

Management :

1) Spectacles for :
   a) near vision alone (in pseudophakia with emmetropia).
   b) both near & distance (in pseudophakia with consecutive refractive error).

2) LASIK or Advanced surface ablation.
3) IOL exchange or Pigiback IOL.

- ✎ when consecutive refractive error is large.

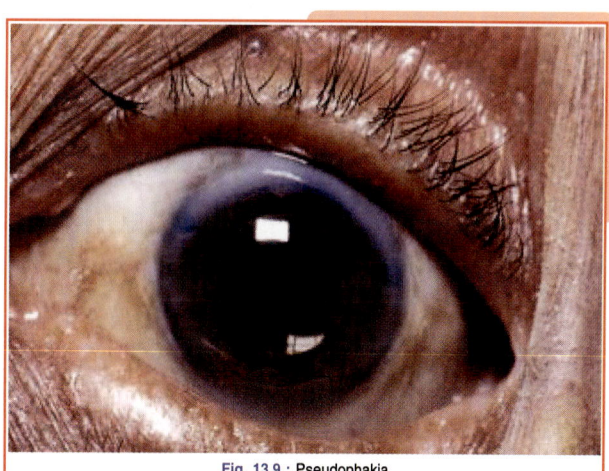

Fig. 13.9 : Pseudophakia

Chapter

14

Ocular Pharmacology

Most Important (Must Read Topics)	Elective Topics
1) Atropine	1) Steroids
2) Cyclopentolate	2) Antiviral's
3) Timolol Maleate	3) Viscoelastics
4) Pilocarpine	4) Artificial tears
5) Antifungal's	5) NSAID's
6) Acyclovir	6) Antiallergic's
7) Antibacterial's	7) Local Anesthetic's
	8) Ophthalmology Dyes
	9) Immunosuppressants
	10) Anti VEGF drugs

☐ ATROPINE :

☞ Anticholinergic agent.

☞ It is Mydriatic & Cycloplegic.

   1) *Mydriatic* : dilates the pupil

   2) *Cycloplegic* : paralyse the ciliary muscle.

MOA :

Dilates the pupil by prevention of contraction of ciliary muscle.

☞ **Strongest (longest) Cycloplegic :**

   effect lasts for 10-14 days.

Uses :

I) *As an mydriatic :* In :

   1) Fundus examination, Retinoscopy.

   2) To test posterior synechiae.

   3) To break posterior synechiae.

   4) For pre-operative assessment of cataract.

   5) During ECCE.

   6) During posterior segment surgery.

II) *As an cycloplegic :*

   1) For perfect refraction in children.

   2) Refraction where pupil is small.

3) Iridocyclitis, Endophthalmitis.

4) In accommodative spasm.

5) In accommodative convergent squint.

6) Penalization treatment in Amblyopia.

Contraindications :

1) Glaucoma

2) Iris supported IOL

Side effects :

1) Temporary blurring of vision.

2) Burning, Irritation of the eye.

Preparation :

Atropine sulphate ointment or drops.

☐ CYCLOPENTOLATE :

ᴵᴲ It is mydriatic & cycloplegic.

ᴵᴲ Short acting cycloplegic :

effect lasts for 6 hours to 18 hours.

ᴵᴲ Anticholinergic agent.

Uses :

Same as that of Atropine.

Side effects :

Same as that of Atropine.

Preparation :

Cyclopentolate hydrochloride

☐ TIMOLOL MALEATE :

ᴵᴲ It is β adrenergic blocker.

MOA :

Non-selective (β-1 & β-2 blocker)

↓

Blocks β-2 receptor in ciliary processes

↓

Decreases aqueous production

↓

So, used in Glaucoma
(Infact are 1ˢᵗ DOC in POAG).

Indications :

1) All types of Glaucoma.

2) 1ˢᵗ DOC in POAG & all secondary Glaucoma.

Contraindications :

1) Bronchial Asthma, Emphysema, COPD.

2) Heart block, CHF, Cardiac myopathy.

Side effects :

A) *Ocular* :

1) Burning, Itching.

2) Conjunctival hyperemia.

3) Superficial punctate keratopathy.

B) *Systemic* :

CVS : 1) Bradycardia

2) Arrhythmias.

3) Heart failure, syncope

RS : 1) Bronchospasm.

CNS : 1) Anxiety, Depression

2) Confusion, Drowsiness

3) Hallucinations.

Misc. : 1) Diarrhoea

2) Rashes, etc.

Preparations :

ᴵᴲ 0.25%, 0.5% eyedrops.

ᴵᴲ exerts phenomena of :

i) Short term escape : marked fall in IOP

ii) Long term drift : slow rise in IOP in those who were controlled with many months of therapy.

☐ PILOCARPINE : (Miotics)

ᴵᴲ It is Parasympathomimetic (Cholinergic) (directly acting)

ᴵᴲ Used as Miotics.

MOA :

1) ↑ Aqueous outflow by contraction of longitudinal fibres of ciliary muscle.

↓

Changes in Trabecular meshwork

↓

↓ IOP (so used in POAG)

2) Opens Iridocorneal angle,
    so used in PACG.

Uses :
1) POAG
2) PACG
3) Chronic synechial angle closure glaucoma.

Contraindications :
1) Inflammatory glaucoma.
2) Malignant glaucoma.
3) Known allergy

Side effects :
A) *Ocular* : due to miosis itself :
    1) Reduced visual acuity in polar cataract, Contraction of visual field.
    2) Spasm of accommodation leading to myopia, frontal headache, RD etc.
    3) Iritis, lacrimation, conjunctivitis.

B) *Systemic* : 1) Bradycardia.
    2) ↑ Sweating, diarrhoea, salivation.
    3) Scoline Apnoea (mostly not with pilocarpine).

Preparations :
1) 1%, 2%, 4% eyedrops.
2) Ocuserts as pilo-20 & pilo-40
3) Pilocarpine gel 4%.

▢ ANTIFUNGAL'S :

Classified as : 1) Polyenes.
    2) Imidazole
    3) Pyridines.
    4) Silver compounds

I) Polyenes :
    ⌦ Mainstay of antifungal therapy.

MOA :

Fungal cell membrane have sterols

↓

Polyenes bind to the sterols and makes the membrane permeable

↓

Lethal imbalances in fungal cell contents.

Preparations :
1) *Nystatin 3.5% ointment (fungistatic)*
    Use : Aspergillus, Candida eye infections (Fungal eye infections).

2) *Amphotericin B :*
    It is fungistatic or fungicidal depending upon the concentration of drug & sensitivity of the fungus.

    ➢ intravitreally / iv for use in :
    Candida, Histoplasma, Cryptococcus, Aspergillus eye infections.

3) *Natamycin :*
    ➢ Broad spectrum antifungal against Candida, Aspergillus, Fusarium, Cephalosporium.
    ➢ <u>DOC</u> : For Fusarium Solani keratitis.

II) Imidazole :

Miconazole, clotrimazole, ketoconazole, Econazole, itraconazole.
1) *Miconazole (Topical / Subconjunctival application)*
    ➢ Broad spectrum against Candida, Fusarium, Aspergillus, Cryptococcus, Trichophyton, Cladosporium.

2) *Clotrimazole :*
    ➢ DOC for Aspergillus eye infections.
    ➢ also used against candida.

3) *Oral ketoconazole :*
    ➢ in fungal keratitis complicated by endophthalmitis.

III) Pyridine :
    ⌦ Flucytosine (fluorinated salt of pyrimidine).

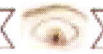

- Used as aqueous drops, orally, iv.
- very effective against Candida, yeasts.

IV) Silver compounds :

- Silver sulphadiazine.
- Very effective against Aspergillus, fusarium.

ACYCLOVIR (Acycloguanosine)

- It is an Antiviral Drug.
- Extremely safe & effective against Herpes simplex and Herpes Zoster infections.

MOA :

- Inhibits the viral DNA by preferentially entering into the infected cells, with little effect on normal cells.
- Penetrates into the deeper layers and thus is very effective in stromal keratitis.

Preparations :

1) 3% ointment.
2) Tablet for oral use
3) Injection for iv use.

Indications :

1) Topical 3% ointment for stromal Herpes simplex keratitis.
2) Oral acyclovir :
   - after penetrating keratoplasty in patients of herpes simplex keratitis.
   - in Recalcitrant stromal/uveal disease caused by HSV.
   - to reduce the ocular complications of keratitis/uveitis in Herpes zoster ophthalmicus.

Side effects :

Punctate epithelial keratopathy.

STEROIDS :

Properties : 1) Anti inflammatory
2) Anti allergic
3) Anti fibrotic

Classification :

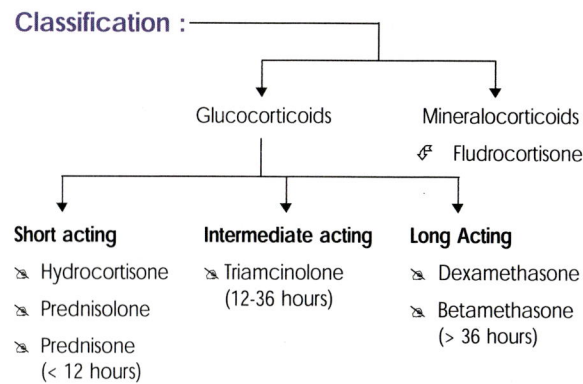

	Glucocorticoids		Mineralocorticoids
			Fludrocortisone

Short acting	Intermediate acting	Long Acting
Hydrocortisone	Triamcinolone (12-36 hours)	Dexamethasone
Prednisolone		Betamethasone (> 36 hours)
Prednisone (< 12 hours)		

Mode of Administration :

A) Topical steroids :

- Dexamethasone
- Betamethasone
- Hydrocortisone
- Fluorometholone
- Cortisone acetate

B) Systemic steroids :

- Prednisolone
- Dexamethasone
- Betamethasone

Indications :

A) Topical Steroids :

1) Allergic conjunctivitis (Vernal catarrh, phlyctenular conjunctivitis)
2) Allergic keratitis.
3) Uveitis.
4) Scleritis, Episcleritis.
5) Cystoid macular edema.
6) After intraocular surgery. (Cataract, Pterygium, Keratoplasty)

B) Systemic steroids :

1) Optic Neuritis, Traumatic Optic Neuropathy.
2) Sympathetic ophthalmitis.
3) Posterior, Anterior Uveitis.
4) Vogt-Koyanagi-Harada Syndrome (VKH).
5) Retrobulbar neuritis, papillitis.
6) Scleritis.
7) Corneal graft rejections.

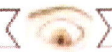

Side effects :

A) Topical steroids :

1) Glaucoma (due to mucopolysaccharide deposition in the trabecular meshwork).

2) Cataract.

3) Dry eye.

4) Activation of infection (if it is given in herpetic, fungal, bacterial keratitis).

5) Ptosis.

B) Systemic steroids :

1) Peptic ulcer.

2) Osteoporosis

3) Hypertension.

4) Psychiatric disturbances (mild euphoria is common)

Contraindications :

Infective conditions (due to bacteria, virus, fungi).

⬛ ANTIBACTERIAL'S :

A) Sulfonamides :

➣ Bacteriostatic, structural analogue of PABA acts by inhibiting bacterial folate synthetase.

➣ *Indications :*

1) Chlamydial infections like Trachoma, inclusion conjunctivitis.

2) Ocular Toxoplasmosis.

B) β lactams :

1) Penicillins :

a) Benzyl penicillin.

b) Procaine penicillin.

c) Methicillin, Cloxacillin, Flucloxacillin :

⇨ for staphylococcal infections.

d) Carbenicillin.

e) Ampicillin (broad spectrum antibiotic)

f) Amoxicillin

2) Cephalosporins :

a) *1st generation (narrow spectrum) :*

⇨ Cefazolin, Cephalexin.

⇨ effective against Gram positive, staphylococci.

b) *2nd generation (intermediate spectrum) :*

⇨ Cefuroxime, Cefoxitin.

⇨ effective against Gram negative, staphylococci.

c) *3rd generation (wide spectrum) :*

⇨ Cefixime, Cefotaxime.

⇨ effective mainly against gram negative but not staphylococci.

C) Aminoglycosides :

➣ Streptomycin, Gentamicin, Tobramycin, Amikacin, Neomycin, Framycetin.

D) Tetracyclines (broad spectrum) :

➣ Bacteriostatic, active against Gram positive, Gram negative, fungi, chlamydia, Rickettsiae.

E) Polypeptides :

➣ Bactericidal.

➣ Polymixin B, Bacitracin, colistin, Neosporin.

➣ Polymixin B is used mainly against Pseudomonas.

F) Fluoroquinolones (Bactericidal) :

1) 1st generation (Ciprofloxacin, Norfloxacin).

2) 2nd generation (Ofloxacin)

3) 3rd generation (Sparfloxacin).

4) 4th generation (Gatifloxacin, Moxifloxacin)

Indications :

1) Bacterial conjunctivitis.

2) Bacterial Corneal Ulcer.

3) Post surgeries (cataract, keratoplasty)

⬛ ANTIVIRAL'S :

A) For Herpes Simplex (Idoxuridine, Acyclovir, Vidarabine, Trifluridine, Famiciclovir).

B) For Herpes Zoster (Acyclovir, Famiciclovir, Valaciclovir, Vidarabine, Sorvudine)

C) For CMV Retinitis (Ganciclovir, Foscarnet, Zidovudine).

D) Non-selective (Interferons, Immunoglobulins).

Acyclovir is most commonly used and is already discussed.

VISCOELASTICS :

- These are substances with dual properties (viscous liquids as well as elastic solids).

Properties :

1) Chemically inert, iso osmotic, non pyrogenic, non antigenic, non toxic, sterile.
2) Optically clear.
3) Viscosity should be enough to provide space for manipulation within the eye.
4) Hydrophilic and dilutable.
5) Protectability.

Preparations :

1) Methylcellulose (most commonly used)
2) Sodium hyaluronate.
3) Hypromellose.
4) Chondroitin sulfate.

Alternatives to Viscoelastics :

Air, serum, Blood products, balanced salt solution (none of them match the above properties)

Uses :

1) Cataract surgery (with or without IOL implantation)
   for : i) maintenance of anterior chamber.
   ii) Protection of corneal endothelium.
   iii) Coating the IOL.
   iv) Preventing the entry of blood, fluid in anterior chamber.
2) Other surgeries (Glaucoma surgery, Keratoplasty, Retinal Detachment surgery, Perforating injury).

Side effects :

1) Post operative rise in IOP if considerable amount is left inside the anterior chamber.

ARTIFICIAL TEARS / LUBRICATING AGENTS :

- Lubricating agents are also known as tear substitute.
- Artificial tears are used for the treatment of dry eye.

Ingredients :

1) Inorganic electrolytes (salts) to maintain the ocular tonicity.
2) Buffers like boric acid to adjust the pH.
3) Viscosity agents (main constituent of artificial tears) enhances viscosity and promote tear film stability :
   a) Cellulose esters (methylcellulose).
   b) Polyvinyl alcohol.
   c) Mucoadhesives (Hyaluronidase, Dextran).
   d) White petrolatum and lanolin (Lacrigel).
4) Additional ingredients (vit. A, lipids)
5) Preservatives (benzal konium chloride)

Preparations :

1) Eye drops (solutions) (most common).
2) Lubricating gel solutions.
3) Lubricating ointment (2nd most common).
   - Preferred for bed time use.
4) Slow release ocular insert (solid devices).
   - Used for Severe Drug Eye Syndrome.
   - Very costly.

NSAIDs :

- Commonly used are Ketorolac, Flurbiprofen.

Mechanism of action :

Inhibits prostaglandin synthesis by inhibiting cycloxygenase.

Indications :

1) To prevent CME after surgery (cataract)
2) To maintain pupillary dilatation during cataract surgery.
3) Before surgery and then in post operative period upto 6 weeks.
4) Allergic conjunctivitis.
5) Inflamed Pterygium.
7) Uveitis.

ANTIALLERGIC DRUGS :

They include :
1) Antihistaminics :
   - Azelastine, Chlorpheniramine maleate, Olopatadine.

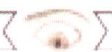

2) *Mast cell stabilizers :*
  ✎ Sodium cromoglycate, ketotifen.

3) *Topical NSAIDs :*
  ✎ Flurbiprofen, Ketorolac.

4) *Oral antihistaminics :*
  ✎ Fexofenadine, Cetrizine.

5) *Immunomodulators :*
  ✎ Tacrolimus, Cyclosporine.

Indications :

1) Allergic conjunctivitis.
2) Other allergic eye conditions.

▢ LOCAL ANESTHETIC DRUGS :

Commonly used are :
1) Lignocaine.
2) Bupivacaine.
3) Proparacaine.

Mechanism of Action :

Decreases the entry of sodium ions during upstroke of action potential.

Administration :

1) Topical Anesthesia (Lignocaine, Proparacaine).
2) Infiltration Anesthesia (2% Lignocaine, Bupivacaine).

Indications :

1) *Surface Anesthesia :*
  ✎ For the removal of Corneal, conjunctival foreign body.
  ✎ For procedures like Tonometry, Lacrimal syringing, corneal scraping.

2) *Infiltration Anesthesia :*
  ✎ For doing intraocular surgeries like cataract surgery, Trabeculectomy, squint surgery, keratoplasty, pterygium excision.

▢ DYES IN OPHTHALMOLOGY :

✐ They are used as a tool for diagnosis and management of ocular diseases.

✐ These are :
1) Fluorescein sodium.
2) Fluorexone.
3) Indocyanine green.
4) Trypan blue.
5) Rose Bengal.
6) Lissamine green.
7) Methylene blue.
8) Verteporfin.

A) Fluorescein Sodium :

  ✎ most essential and commonly used.

Preparations :
1) Fluorescein impregnated strips (preferred)
2) 2% aqueous solution.

Uses : ☺ **RASCAL**

For : 1) Rigid contact lens fitting.
  2) Applanation tonometry.
  3) Seidel's test (Tear film is stained to detect the aqueous leakage from anterior chamber).
  4) Corneal staining (to detect the abrasions and ulcer)
  5) A : —
  6) Lacrimal tests.

IV fluorescein uses :
1) Fundus fluorescein angiography.
2) Vitreous fluorophotometry.
3) Iris angiography.

B) Fluorexone :

  ✎ Used when fluorescein is contraindicated.
  ✎ It does not stain soft contact lenses.

Uses :

For : 1) Evaluation of corneal integrity in patients wearing soft (hydrogel) contact lenses.
  2) Applanation tonometry without removing soft contact lens.
  3) Tear film BUT test.

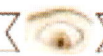

C) Indocyanine Green (ICG) :

Uses :

For : 1) ICG fundus angiography.

2) ICG enhanced anterior capsulo-rrhexis.

3) ICG enhanced posterior capsulo-rrhexis.

D) Rose Bengal & Lissamine green :

Uses :

1) For staining devitalised, degenerated, dead cells of conjunctiva, cornea.

2) In ocular surface disorders like dry eyes (keratoconjunctivitis sicca KCS).

E) Trypan Blue :

Uses :

1) To enhance the visualisation of anterior lens capsule before anterior capsulotomy/capsulorrhexis in cataract surgery.

F) Verteporfin :

Uses :

1) Photodynamic therapy (PDT) for wet type ARMD (age related macular degeneration) in patients with subfoveal choroidal neovascularization.

▢ IMMUNOSUPPRESSANTS & ANTIMITOTIC'S:

A) Immunomodulators :

➤ Cyclosporine, Tacrolimus.

B) Cytotoxic :

1) Antimetabolites (Azathioprine, Methotrexate).

2) Alkylating drugs (Cyclophosphamide).

Indications :

1) *Uveitis :*

➤ Vogt Koyanagi Harada Syndrome.

➤ Sympathetic Ophthalmia.

➤ Behcet's Syndrome.

2) Corneal graft rejections.

3) Immune mediated corneal ulcer (Mooren's ulcer)

4) Glaucoma filtration surgery.

5) Recurrent pterygium.

6) Scleritis.

7) Cicatrical pemphigoid.

8) Grave's Ophthalmopathy.

9) Ocular myasthenia gravis.

▢ ANTI VEGF DRUGS :

Commonly used are : 1) Ranibizumab

2) Bevacizumab

3) Pegaptanib

Indications :

1) Neovascular Age related macular degeneration (commonest indication).

2) Diabetic Retinopathy.

3) CRVO.

4) Neovascular Glaucoma.

5) Retinopathy of Prematurity.

6) Central serous retinopathy.

Complications :

1) Cataract.

2) Glaucoma.

3) Vitreous hemorrhage.

4) Retinal detachment.

5) Endophthalmitis.

Chapter

15

Darkroom Procedures

Most Important (Must Read Topics)	Elective Topics
1) Retinoscopy, Objective Refraction 2) Subjective Refraction 3) Ophthalmoscopy 4) Direct vs Indirect Ophthalmoscopy	1) Slit Lamp Biomicroscopy

☐ OBJECTIVE REFRACTION :

☞ The procedure of determining and correcting the refractive errors is called clinical Refraction.

☞ Two methods :
1) Objective Refraction
2) Subjective Refraction.

OBJECTIVE REFRACTION :

It includes :

I) Retinoscopy.
II) Refractometry
III) Photorefraction
IV) Keratometry

I) Retinoscopy :

✍ also called skiascopy or shadow test.

✍ it is an objective method of finding the error of refraction by method of neutralization.

Principle :

Retinoscopy is based on the fact that when the light is reflected from mirror into the eye, the direction in which light will travel across the pupil, depends upon the refractive state of the eye.

Pre requisites : (Fig. 15.1)
1) Dark Room.
2) Trial box (+/–, cyl/sph lens) (pinhole, occluder, prism)
3) Trial frame.
4) Vision box (Snellen's).
5) Retinoscope :
   a) Mirror Retinoscope.
   b) Self illuminated retinoscope.

Procedure :
1) Patient is made to sit at a distance of 1 metre from the examiner.
2) With the help of Retinoscope light is thrown onto patient's eye who is instructed to look at the far point (to relax accommodation).

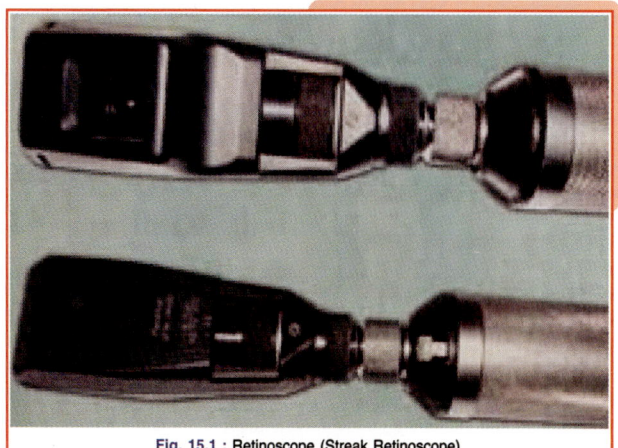

Fig. 15.1 : Retinoscope (Streak Retinoscope)

3) When cycloplegic has been used, patient can look directly into the light and have refraction assessed along the actual visual axis.

4) Through the hole in the retinoscope's mirror, examiner observes red reflex in pupillary area of the patient.

5) Then the retinoscope is moved in vertical and horizontal meridia keeping watch on red reflex (which also moves when retinoscope is moved).

6) Speed & brilliance
   Width of the Reflex } are noted
   Swirling of the Reflex

Observation & inferences : (Fig. 15.2)

1) No movement of Red Reflex : Myopia of 1D.

2) With movement of Red Reflex along the movement of Retinoscope : Emmetropia/ Myopia/ Hypermetropia of less than 1D

3) Against movement of Red Reflex to the movement of Retinoscope : Myopia of greater than 1D

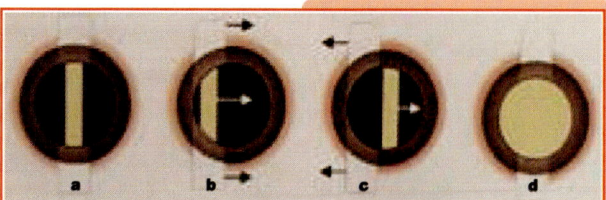

Fig. 15.2 : Inferences of Retinoscopy

a) No movement of Red reflex
b) With movement of Red reflex, along the movement of Retinoscope.
c) Against movement of Red reflex to the movement of Retinoscope
d) Reflex at point of neutralization

Neutralization :

1) When the red reflex moves with or against the movement of retinoscope we do not exactly know the amount of Refractive error.

2) When it doesn't move, we know for certain that patient has myopia of 1D.

3) To estimate the degree of Refractive error, movement of red reflex is neutralized by addition of :

Spherical
  a) (+) convex → for with movement
  b) (−) concave → against the movement

4) When simple spherical error alone is present, movement of red reflex will be neutralized in both vertical & horizontal meridia.

5) In presence of Astigmatic refractive error, one meridian is neutralized by adding appropriate cylindrical lens with its axis right angle to the meridian being neutralized.

Problems :

1) Red reflex may not be visible or may be poor (in small pupil, hazy media, high refractive error)

2) Changing Retinoscopy findings.

3) Scissors shadow may be seen.

4) Conflicting shadows.

5) Triangular shadows.

II) Autorefractometry : (Fig. 15.3)

- based on Scheiner/Optometer principle.
- carried out by computerized autorefractometer (optometer).

III) Photorefraction :

- Allows refraction measurement in both the eyes simultaneously using an infrared camera from 1 meter distance.
- *Advantages :*
  - Results are not influenced by accommodation. So cycloplegia with atropine is not required.
  - Portable, hand held instrument.

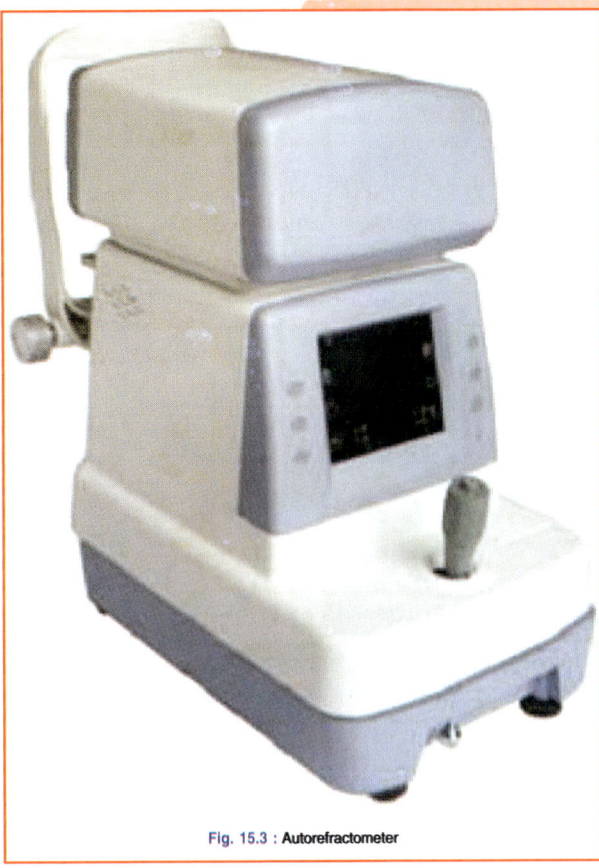

Fig. 15.3 : **Autorefractometer**

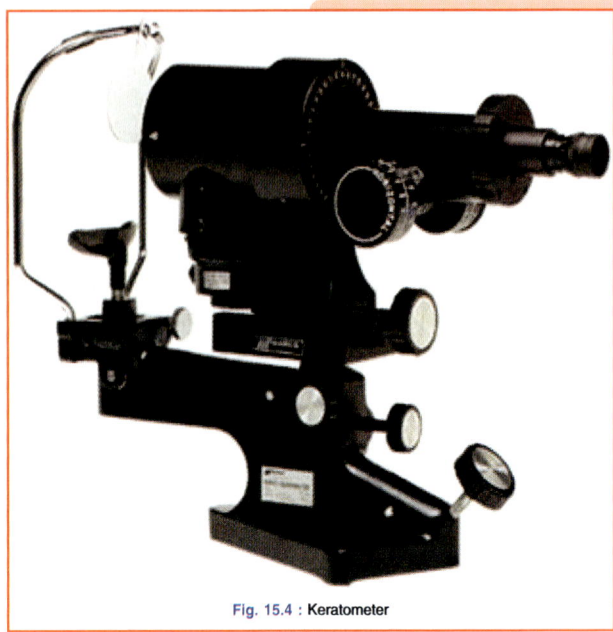

Fig. 15.4 : **Keratometer**

IV) Keratometry : (Fig. 15.4)

- also called Ophthalmometry.
- It is an objective method of estimating corneal Astigmatism by measuring the curvature of central cornea.

Principle :

Anterior surface of the cornea acts as a convex mirror; so the size of image produced varies with its curvature. Therefore, from size of image formed by the anterior surface of cornea (First Purkinje image), Radius of curvature of cornea can be calculated.

2 types of Keratometer :

1) Javal-Schiotz keratometer
2) Bausch & Lomb keratometer.

☐ SUBJECTIVE REFRACTION :

- ✐ It means finding out the most suitable lenses to be prescribed.
- ✐ It should always be carried out after getting a rough estimate of refractive error by Objective Refraction as described above.

It includes three steps :

I) Subjective verification of baseline refraction.

II) Subjective refinement of Refraction.

III) Subjective binocular balancing.

I) Subjective verification of baseline refraction :

- ➤ By 'trial and error' method.
- ➤ Patient is seated at the distance of 6 metre from Snellen's chart. Trial frame is put on the face of the patient and visual acuity is noted for both eyes separately.
- ➤ Occluder is put infront of the one eye & appropriate lens combination (as indicated by retinoscopy or automated refractometry) is placed in other eye.
- ➤ By increasing/decreasing the power of lens, most suitable spherical lens is chosen. (Strongest convex in hypermetropia & weakest concave in myopia).
- ➤ Cylindrical axis should be finalized by same 'trial & error' method.
- ➤ Similar procedure is repeated for the second eye.

II) Subjective Refinement of Refraction :

- ➤ Most suitable combination of lenses chosen after subjective verification of baseline refraction, are then refined before final prescription is made.

➢ It is always best to refine cylinder first and then sphere.

Refining the Cylinder	Refining the Sphere
1) Jackson's cross cylinder test	1) Fogging technique
2) Astigmatic fan test	2) Duochrome test
3) Staenopic slit test	3) Pin hole test.

III) Subjective binocular balancing :

➢ also known as 'equalizing the accommodative effort'. OR 'equalization of vision'.

➢ final step in subjective refraction.

➢ This allows both the eyes to have retinal image simultaneously in focus.

☐ OPHTHALMOSCOPY (Fundoscopy) :

✴ Ophthalmoscopy is clinical examination of interior of the eye (fundus), by means of an ophthalmoscope.

✴ It is the method for examining posterior segment of the eye (vitreous compartment, retina, optic disc, macula).

✴ It is done to assess the state of fundus and to detect opacities of ocular media.

<u>3 types</u> of Ophthalmoscopy :

1) Direct Ophthalmoscopy.
2) Indirect Ophthalmoscopy
3) Distant direct Ophthalmoscopy.

1) Direct ophthalmoscopy : (Fig. 15.5 & 15.6)

☙ most commonly done method for routine fundus examination.

☙ Image is formed on the observer's retina and has following characteristics : ☺ 15 EV.

1) 15 times magnified image
2) Erect
3) Virtual.

2) Indirect ophthalmoscopy : ☺ 5 IR (Fig. 15.7 & 15.8)

☙ *Principle :*

Make the eye highly myopic by placing a convex lens in front of the patients eye.

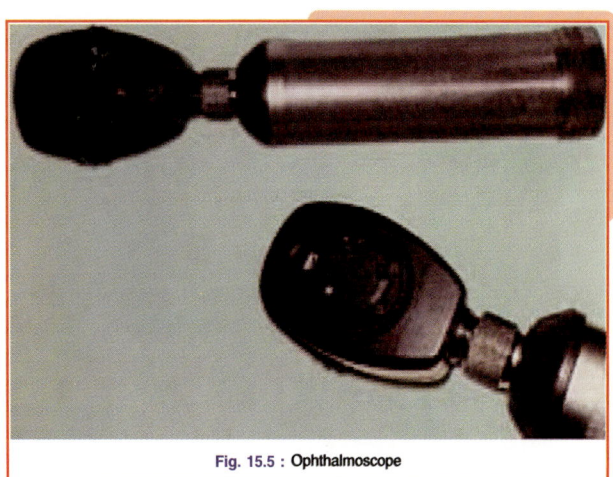

Fig. 15.5 : Ophthalmoscope

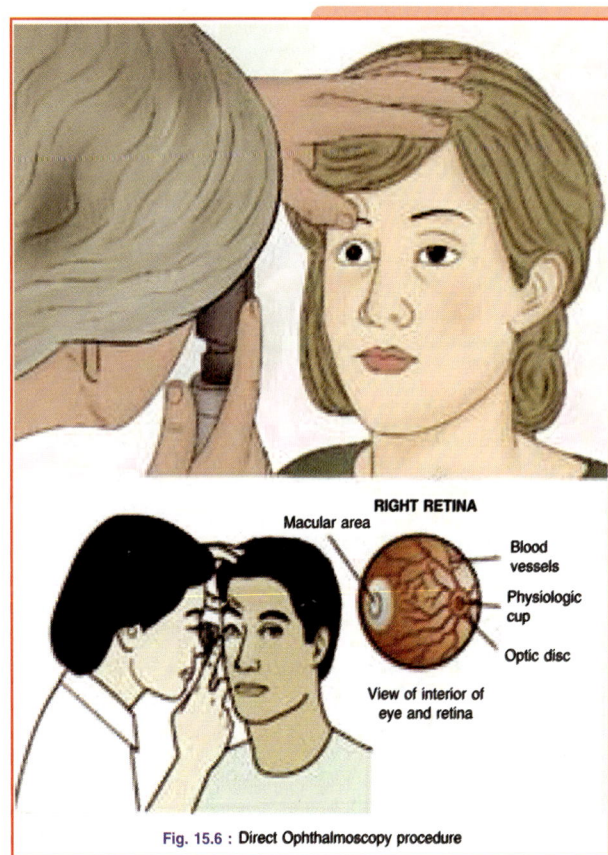

RIGHT RETINA
Macular area
Blood vessels
Physiologic cup
Optic disc
View of interior of eye and retina

Fig. 15.6 : Direct Ophthalmoscopy procedure

☙ *Advantage :*

Examination through hazy media is possible. (not possible in Direct Ophthalmoscopy).

☙ *Image has following characteristics :*

1) 5 times magnified image.
2) Inverted.
3) Real

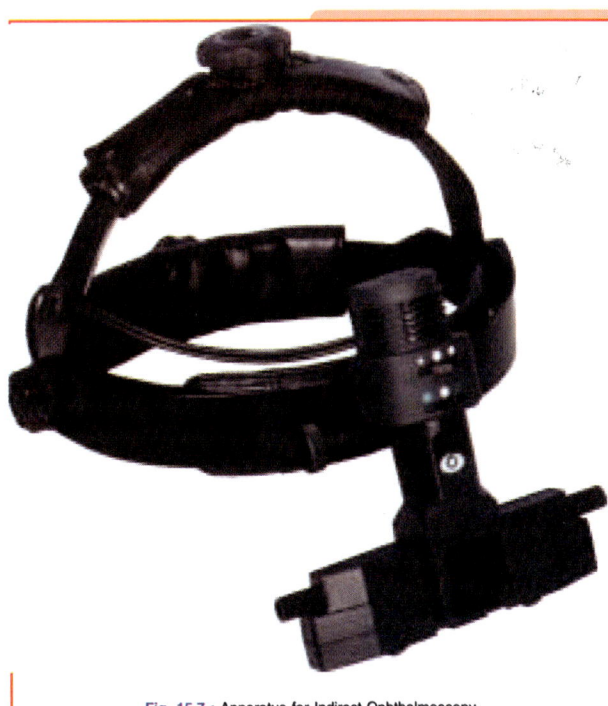

Fig. 15.7 : Apparatus for Indirect Ophthalmoscopy

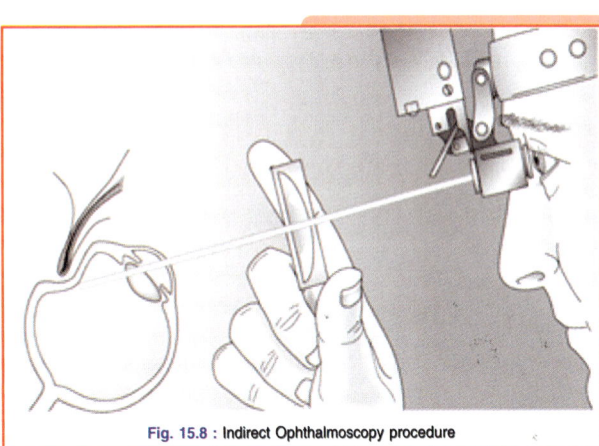

Fig. 15.8 : Indirect Ophthalmoscopy procedure

Direct ophthalmoscopy uses :

1) To evaluate the details of optic disc, fovea centralis, retinal fixation, retinal vasculature.

Indirect ophthalmoscopy uses :

1) Examination of fundus as far as to the periphery.
2) Examination of peripheral retinal lesions.
3) Management of retinal detachment.

3) Distant Direct Ophthalmoscopy :

- Should be routinely performed before

direct Ophthalmoscopy, as it gives lot of information.

- Light is thrown into patient's eye from a distance of 20-25 cm and the features of red glow in pupillary area are noted.

Uses :

To : 1) Diagnose opacities in refractive media.

2) Differentiate between mole and hole of iris.

3) Recognize detached retina or a tumor arising from the fundus.

◻ DIRECT vs INDIRECT OPHTHALMOSCOPY :

Feature	Direct Ophthalmoscopy	Indirect Ophthalmoscopy
1) Condensing lens	Not required	Required
2) Examination distance	As close to the patient's eye	At an arm's length
3) Image	Virtual, erect	Real, inverted
4) Magnification	15 times	5 times
5) Illumination	Not so bright, not useful in hazy media	Bright, useful in hazy media
6) Area of field	2 disc dioptres	8 disc dioptres
7) Stereopsis	Absent	Present
8) Fundus view	Slightly beyond the equator	Upto ora serrata
9) Examination through hazy media	Not possible	Possible

◻ SLIT LAMP EXAMINATION / BIOMICROSCOPY : (Fig. 15.9)

- Slit lamp is low power microscope (biomicroscope) combined with a high intensity light source (slit lamp) that can be focused in a thin beam.

- Biomicroscopic examination of fundus can be performed after full mydriasis using a slit lamp and any one of the following lenses :

1) Indirect slip lamp biomicroscopy :

  ➢ Using + 78 D or + 90 D small diameter lens.

  ➢ image formed is inverted, real, magnified.

2) Hruby lens biomicroscopy :

  ➢ a plano concave lens of 58.6 D is used.

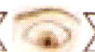

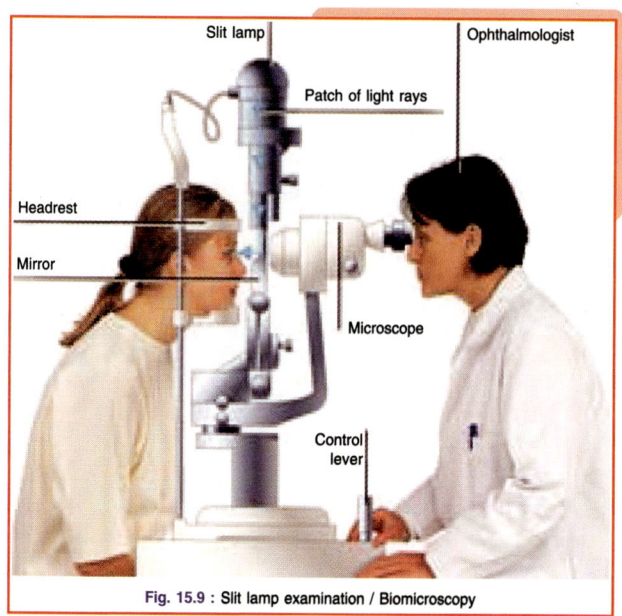

Fig. 15.9 : Slit lamp examination / Biomicroscopy

3) Constant lens biomicroscopy :

➤ by : a) posterior fundus contact lens
    (modified Koeppe's lens)

   b) Goldmann's three mirror
      contact lens.

Uses :

1) To examine anterior segment :

   ✍ eyelids, cornea, conjunctiva, sclera,
     anterior chamber, lens, capsule.

   ✍ for anterior segment examination above
     3 types of lenses are not required.

2) For fundus examination (above 3 types of
   lenses are required).

Methods of Illumination using slit lamp :

7 methods as described by Berliner :

1) Diffuse Illumination.

2) Direct illumination.

3) Indirect illumination

4) Retroillumination

5) Specular reflection

6) Sclerotic scatter

7) Oscillatory illumination of Koeppe.

Chapter

16

Community Ophthalmology

Most Important (Must Read Topics)	Elective Topics
1) Vision 2020 : The Right to sight	1) Eye Banking 2) Eye Donation 3) Rehabilitation of the Blind

☐ VISION 2020 : THE RIGHT TO SIGHT :

WHO definition of Blindness :

✒ 'Visual acuity of less than 3/60, or a corresponding visual field loss to less than 10⁰, in the better eye with best possible correction'.

✒ 'Inability to count the fingers in daylight at a distance of 3 metres'.

'Vision 2020 : The right to sight' is a global initiative launched by WHO in Geneva on 18th February, 1999 in a broad coalition with a 'Task Force of International NGOs' to combat the gigantic problem of blindness in the world.

A) Partners of Vision 2020 : The Right to Sight :

1) WHO
2) Task force of International NGOs.

B) Objectives of Vision 2020 : The Right to Sight :

1) To eliminate avoidable blindness by 2020.
2) To reduce global burden of blindness which currently affects 45 million people worldwide.

C) Implementation of Vision 2020 : The Right to Sight :

1) Through four phases of five year plans, first one started in 2000, then 2005, 2010 and last phase commenced in 2015.

D) Strategic Approaches : Global Perspective :

1) Disease prevention and control.
2) Training of eye health personnel.
3) Strengthening of existing eye care infrastructure.
4) Use of appropriate & affordable technology.
5) Mobilisation of resources.

1) Disease prevention & control :

➢ Globally WHO has identified five major blinding eye conditions :
  i) Cataract.
  ii) Childhood blindness.
  iii) Trachoma.
  iv) Refractive errors and low vision.
  v) Onchocerciasis.

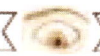

➤ These conditions have been chosen on the basis of their contribution to the burden of blindness and the feasibility and affordability of intervention to control them.

➤ Disease control programmes :

i) Cataract → YAG capsulotomy at all district hospitals

ii) Childhood blindness → School eye screening programmes, vit. A prophylaxis.

iii) Trachoma → SAFE strategy

S → Surgery for lid deformity

A → Antibiotics

F → Facial hygiene

E → Environmental sanitation

iv) Refractive errors and low vision → Refraction centre in all PHC, low vision centre in all tertiary care centres.

v) Onchocerciasis → Annual doses of Ivermectin.

E) Strategic plan for Vision 2020 : The Right to Sight :

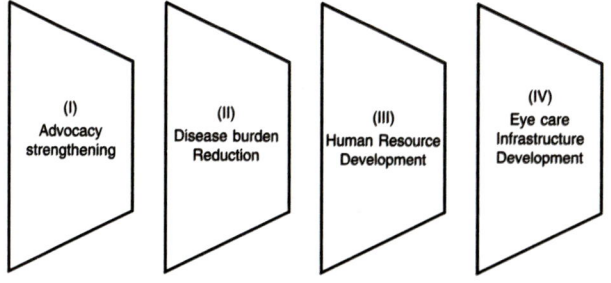

(I) Advocacy strengthening
(II) Disease burden Reduction
(III) Human Resource Development
(IV) Eye care Infrastructure Development

I) Advocacy strengthening :

➤ Public awareness and information about the eye care & prevention of blindness.

➤ Introduction of eye care topics in school curriculum.

➤ Involvement of professional organizations such as AIOS, EBAI, IMA.

➤ Strengthening the functioning of DBCS.

➤ Enhance the involvement of NGOs, Community leaders.

➤ Strengthen the hospital programmes for eye donation through counselling by volunteers.

II) Disease burden Reduction :

➤ by operating Disease Control Programmes (as mentioned above) plus

➤ for : Corneal blindness → Eye banking

Glaucoma → Eye camps, screening at eye care institutions.

Diabetic Retinopathy → Awareness generation by health workers, laser treatment at tertiary level.

III) Human Resource Development :

➤ Uniform curriculum in UG medical education.

➤ Training of Postgraduates, increase in seats.

➤ Assessment of potential DNB institutions.

➤ CME for Ophthalmologists.

➤ Increase in the number of paramedical personnel.

➤ Development of dedicated district programme managers.

IV) Infrastructure Development : (Fig. 16.1)

❑ EYE BANKING :

✍ Eye bank is an organization which deals with the collection, storage and distribution of cornea for the purpose of corneal grafting, research and supply of eye tissue for other ophthalmic purposes.

Functions of an eye bank :

1) Promotion of eye donation.

2) Registration of eye pledger for donation.

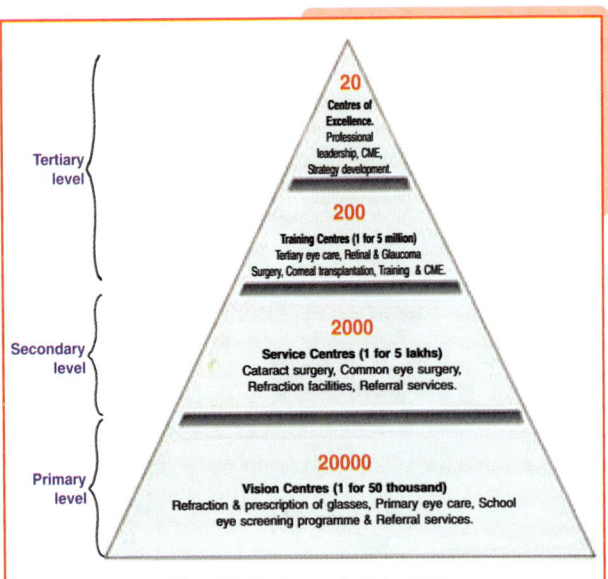

Fig. 16.1 : Infrastructure for Vision 2020

3) Collection of donated eyes from deceased.

4) Receiving & processing the donor eyes.

5) Preservation of tissue for short, intermediate, long or very long term.

6) Distribution of donor tissues to corneal surgeons.

7) Research activities for improvement of preservation methodology, corneal substitute and utilisation of other eye components.

Eye bank personnel :

1) Eye bank incharge who is qualified Ophthalmologist.

2) Eye bank technician.

3) Clerk cum storekeeper.

4) Medical social worker or Public relation officer.

5) Driver cum projectionist.

Eye Collection centres :

✐ These are peripheral satellites of an eye bank for better functioning.

✐ 1 collection centre in urban area for population > 2,00,000.

✐ 4-5 collection centres are associated with each eye bank.

Functions of eye collection centres :

1) Local publicity for eye donation.

2) Registration of voluntary donors.

3) Arrangements for eye collection after death.

4) Initial processing, packaging, transportation of collected eyes to the attached eye banks.

Personnel for eye collection centres :

1) Ophthalmic technician trained in an eye bank.

2) Local honorary workers / voluntary agencies like Lions Club, Rotary Club etc.

3) Honorary Ophthalmic surgeon or medical officer trained in enucleation.

☐ EYE DONATION :

✐ "After your die,

   Donate your Eye".

✐ Eye donation is an act of donating one's eyes after his/her death.

Facts about eye donation :

1) Anyone at any age can pledge to donate the eyes after death, all that is needed is a clear healthy cornea.

2) Eyes have to be removed within six hours of death.

3) Eye donation gives sight to two blind persons as one eye is transplanted to one blind person.

4) Eyes can be pledged and donated to any nearest eye bank.

5) Donated eyes are never bought or sold. Eye donation is never refused.

6) Eyes cannot be removed from a living human being in spite of consent of oneself and wish.

7) Families can donate the eyes of their dear departed even if it has not been pledged before.

✐ Who can't donate eyes : ☺ RASH CELL

   People suffering from :

   1) Retinoblastoma.

   2) AIDS.

   3) Septicemia.

   4) Hepatitis.

5) Creutzfeldt - Jacob Syndrome.

6) Encephalitis

7) End stage cancer.

8) Leukemia.

9) Lymphoma.

⬛ REHABILITATION OF THE BLIND :

1) Medical Rehabilitation :

- ✎ By LVA (low vision aids)

2) Training & Psychosocial Rehabilitation :

- ✎ Mobility training with the help of stick.
- ✎ Training in daily living skills such as bathing, washing, putting on clothes, shaving, cooking and other household work.

3) Educational Rehabilitation :

- ✎ In blind schools by Braille system.

4) Vocational Rehabilitation :

- ✎ In making handicrafts, canning, book binding, candle, chalk making, etc.

Chapter

17

Systemic Ophthalmology

Most Important (Must Read Topics)	Elective Topics
1) Xerophthalmia / Vit A deficiency / Night Blindness / Bitot's spots	1) Ocular Manifestations in AIDS.
	2) Ocular Manifestations in Diabetes Mellitus.
	3) Ocular Manifestations / Eye signs in Thyrotoxicosis.

☐ XEROPHTHALMIA/VITAMIN A DEFICIENCY / NIGHT BLINDNESS / BITOT'S SPOTS :

ᕲ The term xerophthalmia covers all the ocular manifestations of vitamin A deficiency.

ᕲ These usually develop before 2 years of age.

Etiology :

1) Dietary deficiency of vitamin A.

2) Defective absorption from the gut.

3) It is almost invariably accompanied by PEM and infections.

WHO classification : (1982)

XN : Night Blindness.

X1A : Conjunctival xerosis.

X1B : Bitot's spots

X2 : Corneal xerosis

X3A : Corneal ulceration/keratomalacia affecting < 1/3rd of the corneal surface.

X3B : Corneal ulceration/keratomalacia affecting > 1/3rd of the corneal surface.

X5 : Corneal scar due to Xerophthalmia.

XF : Xerophthalmic fundus.

Clinical features :

1) *XN (Night blindness)* – earliest symptom.

2) *X1A (Conjunctival xerosis)* : **(Fig. 17.1)**

   ᕲ one or more patches of dry, lustreless non-wettable conjunctiva, which is described as 'emerging like sand banks at receding tide' when child ceases to cry.

3) *X1B (Bitot's spots)* : **(Fig. 17.2)**

   ᕲ It is the extension of xerotic process as seen in stage X1A.

   ᕲ Raised, silvery white, foamy, triangular patch of keratinised epithelium, situated on bulbar conjunctiva in interpalpebral area.

   ᕲ Usually bilateral & temporal.

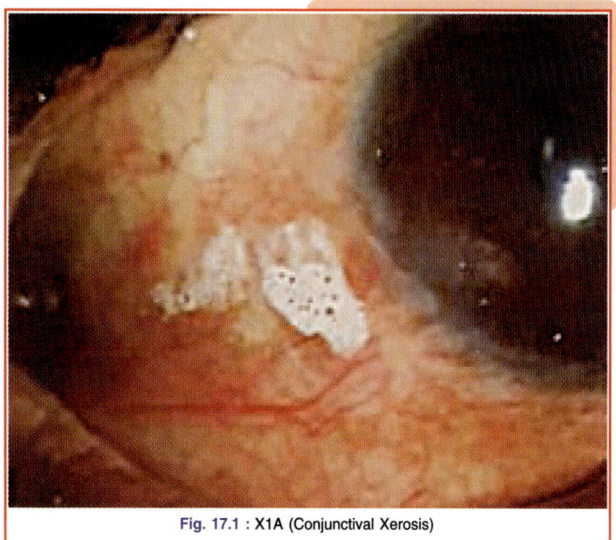

Fig. 17.1 : X1A (Conjunctival Xerosis)

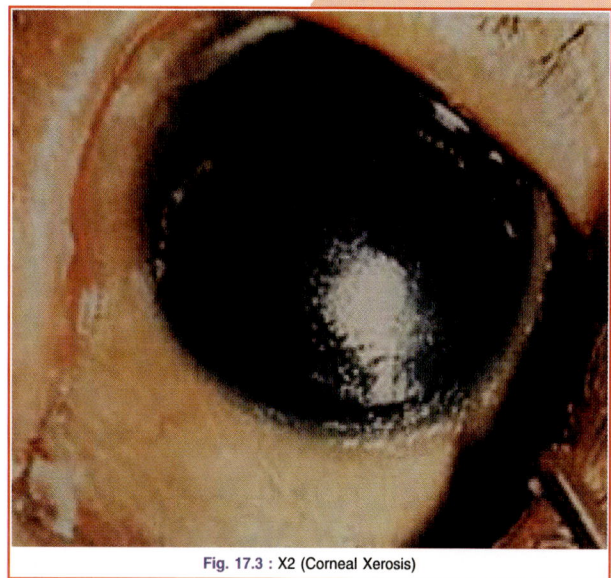

Fig. 17.3 : X2 (Corneal Xerosis)

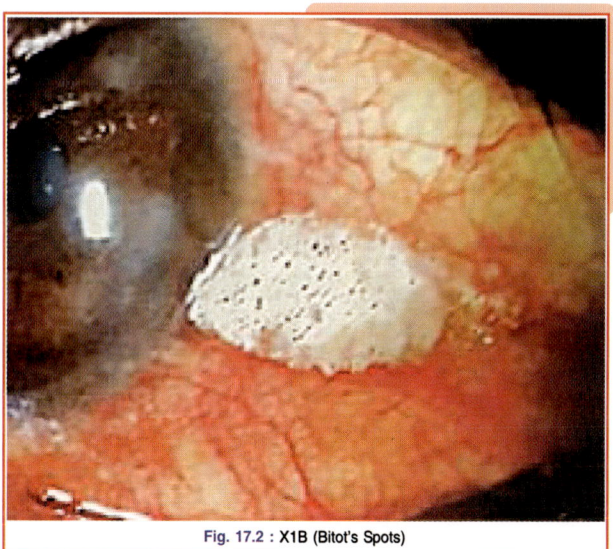

Fig. 17.2 : X1B (Bitot's Spots)

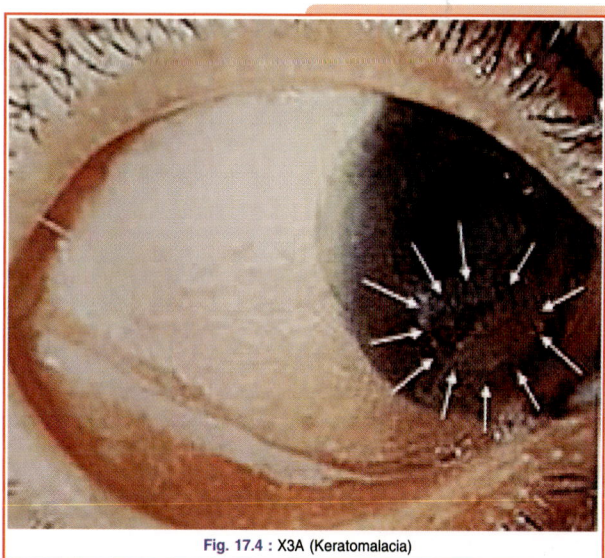

Fig. 17.4 : X3A (Keratomalacia)

4) X2 (Corneal xerosis) : (Fig. 17.3)

- Punctate keratopathy in lower nasal quadrant, followed by haziness and/or granular pebbly dryness, lacks the lustre.

5) X3A & X3B (Corneal ulceration/ keratomalacia) : (Fig. 17.4 & 17.5)

- Small ulcers (1-3 mm) situated peripherally. They are circular with steep margins and are sharply demarcated.

- Large ulcers extends centrally or involve the entire cornea.

6) X5 (Corneal scars) : (Fig. 17.6)

- due to healing of stromal defects of different densities and sizes.

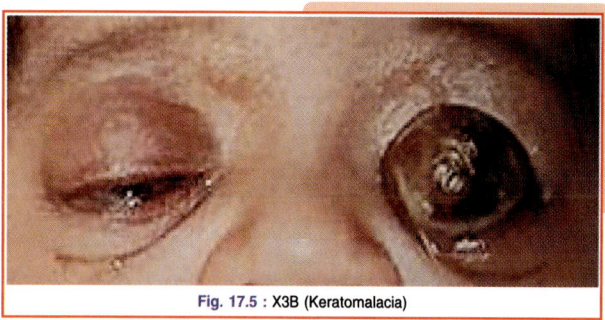

Fig. 17.5 : X3B (Keratomalacia)

7) XF (Xerophthalmic fundus) :

- Typical seek like, raised, whitish lesions scattered uniformly over the part of fundus at level of optic disc.

- Also known as Uyemura's fundus.

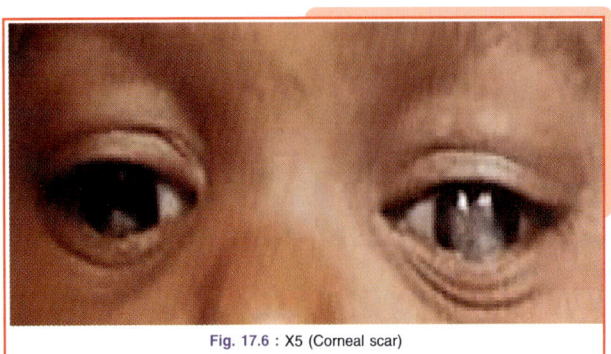

Fig. 17.6 : X5 (Corneal scar)

Treatment :

1) Ocular Therapy.

2) Vitamin A Therapy.

3) Treatment of underlying general disease.

1) Local Ocular Therapy :

   a) for X1A   → Artificial tears (methyl cellulose) every 3-4 hours.

   b) for X3A/X3B → Fullfledged treatment of bacterial corneal ulcer (as mentioned)

2) Vitamin A Therapy :

   ✑ For XN, X1A, X1B, X2, X3A, X3B.

   ✑ Oral administration is given (if vomiting/ diarrhoea exists → im)

   a) All patients > 1 year of age except women of reproductive age :

   $\left\{ \begin{array}{l} \text{orally 2,00,000 IU of vit. A.} \\ \text{im 1,00,000 IU of vit. A} \end{array} \right.$

   immediately on diagnosis,

   then on next day, then after 4 weeks.

   b) Children < 1 year & children of any age who weigh < 8 kg.

   half the doses of patients more than 1 year of age.

   c) Reproductive age, pregnant women :

   i) not having XN, X1A, X1B :

   daily dose of 10,000 IU orally for 2 weeks.

   ii) for corneal xerophthalmia :

   full dosage schedule as for patients > 1 year of age.

3) Treatment of underlying conditions such as PEM, diarrhoea, dehydration, electrolyte imbalance, infections.

Prophylaxis :

1) Short-term approach :

   Administration of vit. A supplements, Recommended are :

   a) Infants 6-12 months & children of any age less than 8 kg :

   1,00,000 IU orally every 3-6 months

   b) Children > 1 year & < 6 years :

   2,00,000 IU orally every 6 months.

   c) Lactating mothers :

   20,000 IU orally once at the delivery or during next 2 months.

   d) Infants < 6 months, not being breastfed

   50,000 IU orally before they attain 6 months of age.

   Revised schedule of vit. A under the programme CSSM (Child survival & Safe Motherhood) :

   1st dose → 1 lakh IU at 9 months of age along with measles.

   2nd dose → 2 lakh IU at 18 months of age along with DPT/OPV booster.

   3rd dose → 2 lakh IU at 2 years age.

2) Medium-term approach :

   ✑ food fortification with vitamin A.

3) Long-term approach :

   ✑ Adequate intake of vit. A rich foods such as green leafy vegetables, papaya, drumsticks.

   ✑ Nutritional health education should be included in curriculum of school children.

❑ OCULAR MANIFESTATIONS IN AIDS :

   ✔ AIDS is caused by HIV which is an RNA retrovirus.

   ✔ **Modes of spread :**

   1) Sexual intercourse with infected person.

   2) Transfusion of infected blood.

3) By infected needles, syringes.

4) Transplacental spread.

⚘ **Ocular manifestations : (Fig. 17.7)**

1) Retinal microvasculopathy :

- ✍ Due to the direct toxic effect of virus on vascular endothelium or immune complex deposits in arterioles.

- ✍ 'Cottonwool spots' in 50% cases.

- ➢ Superficial & deep retinal hemorrhages.

- ➢ Microaneurysms & Telangiectasia.

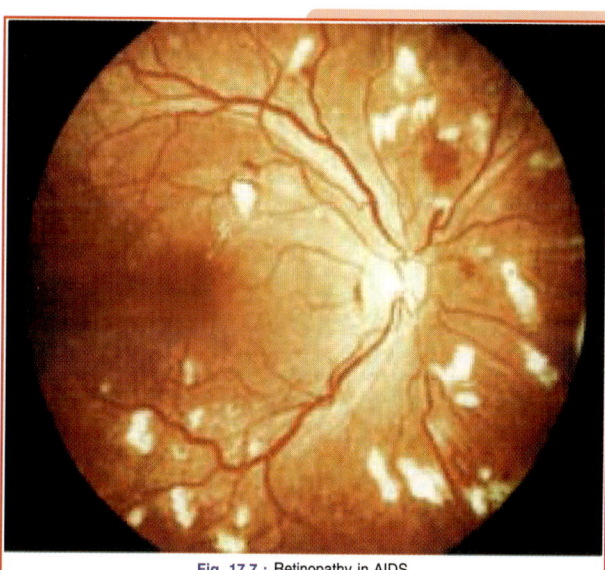

Fig. 17.7 : Retinopathy in AIDS

2) Usual ocular infections :

- ➢ Herpes zoster ophthalmicus.

- ➢ Herpes simplex infections.

- ➢ Toxoplasmosis.

- ➢ Ocular Tuberculosis, syphilis, fungal corneal ulcer.

3) Opportunistic infections :

- ➢ CMV retinitis.

- ➢ Candida endophthalmitis.

- ➢ Cryptococcal infections.

- ➢ Pneumocystis carinii.

- ➢ Choroiditis.

4) Unusual neoplasms :

- ➢ Kaposi sarcoma.

- ➢ Burkitt's lymphoma of orbit.

5) Neurophthalmic lesions :

- ➢ Cranial nerve palsies.

- ➢ Loss of sensory supply to the eye.

- ➢ Optic nerve involvement.

Management :

1) CMV infections → Zidovudine, Ganciclovir, Foscarnet

2) Kaposi sarcoma → Radiotherapy.

3) Herpes infections → Acyclovir.

◻ **OCULAR MANIFESTATIONS IN DIABETES MELLITUS :**

1) **Lids** → Stye, Internal hordeolum, Xanthelasma.

2) **Conjunctiva** → Telangiectasia, subconjunctival hemorrhage.

3) **Cornea** → Pigments on back of the cornea, decreased corneal sensations, Punctate keratopathy, Descemet's folds, Corneal ulcer.

4) **Iris** → Rubeosis iridis (neovascularization)

5) **Lens** → Snowflake cataract in IDDM, Early onset & early maturation of senile cataract.

6) **Vitreous** → Vitreous hemorrhage, fibrovascular proliferation.

7) **Retina** → Diabetic Retinopathy, lipaemia retinalis.

8) **IOP** → POAG, neovascular glaucoma.

9) **Optic nerve** → Optic neuritis

10) **Extra ocular muscles** → Ophthalmoplegia.

11) **Refraction changes** → Hypermetropic shift in hypoglycemia, myopic shift in hyperglycemia.

◻ **OCULAR MANIFESTATIONS/SIGNS IN THYROTOXICOSIS / HYPERTHYROIDISM/ THYROID EYE DISEASE :**

⚘ The term 'Thyroid eye disease' denotes typical ocular changes which include lid retraction, lid lag, proptosis.

These changes have been labelled as :

a) Endocrine exophthalmos.

b) Malignant exophthalmos.

c) Dysthyroid ophthalmopathy.

d) Ocular Grave's disease (OGD)

e) Grave's Ophthalmopathy.

f) Thyroid associated ophthalmopathy (TAO)

Clinical features :

1) *Lid signs :*

a) *Dalrymple's sign (most common sign)*

⇨ 'Retraction of upper lids' produces staring & frightened appearance.

b) *Von Graefe's sign :*

⇨ Globe moves downward, upper lid lags behind.

c) *Enroth's sign :*

⇨ fullness of eyelids due to puffy, edematous swelling.

d) *Gifford's sign :*

⇨ difficulty in eversion of upper lid.

e) *Stellwag's sign :*

⇨ Infrequent blinking.

2) *Conjunctival signs :*

➤ deep injection, chemosis.

3) *Pupillary signs :*

➤ Inequality in pupil dilatation.

4) *Ocular motility defects :*

➤ Mobius sign (Convergence weakness).

➤ Partial / complete immobility of one or all extraocular muscles.

➤ Most common : Unilateral elevator palsy (due to inferior rectus involvement), followed by Abduction palsy (due to medial rectus involvement).

5) *Exophthalmos :*

➤ Classical sign of Thyroid eye disease.

➤ Both eyes are symmetrically affected.

6) *Exposure keratitis and ocular surface discomfort :*

➤ Sandy, grity sensation.

➤ Lacrimation, photophobia.

7) *Optic Neuropathy.*

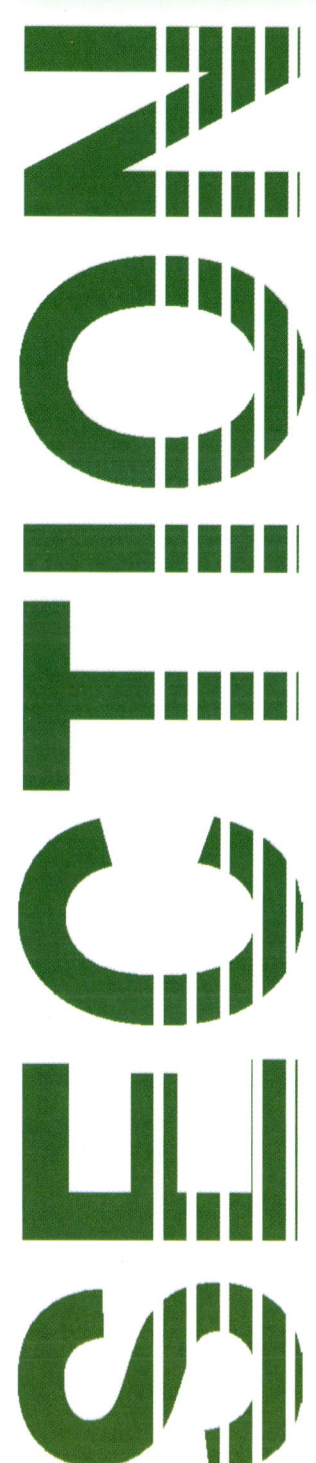

SECTION

II

Instruments
&
Lens

Ophthalmic Instruments

I. EYE SPECULUMS :

1) Universal Eye Speculum : (Fig. 18.1)

➢ Called as Universal Speculum because it can be used for both right and left eyes.

➢ While inserting, open end should face medial canthus and closed end should face lateral canthus.

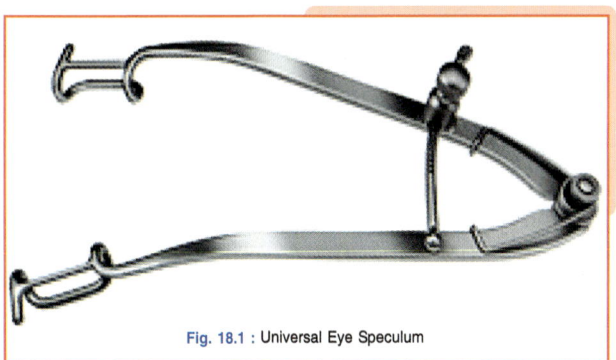

Fig. 18.1 : Universal Eye Speculum

2) Guarded Eye Speculum : (Fig. 18.2)

➢ It has solid blades which keep the lashes away from the field of operation.

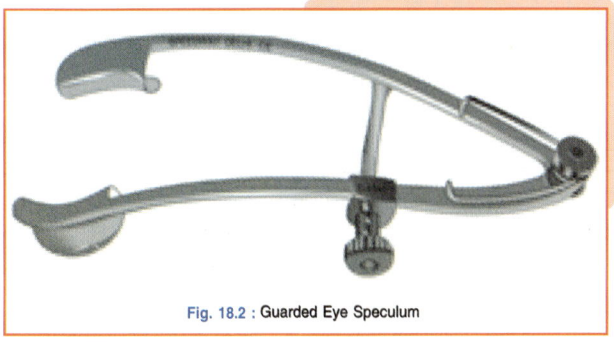

Fig. 18.2 : Guarded Eye Speculum

3) Wire Speculum : (Fig. 18.3)

➢ It is also universal (can be used for both right and left eyes).

➢ Very light in weight and so exerts minimal pressure on the eyeball.

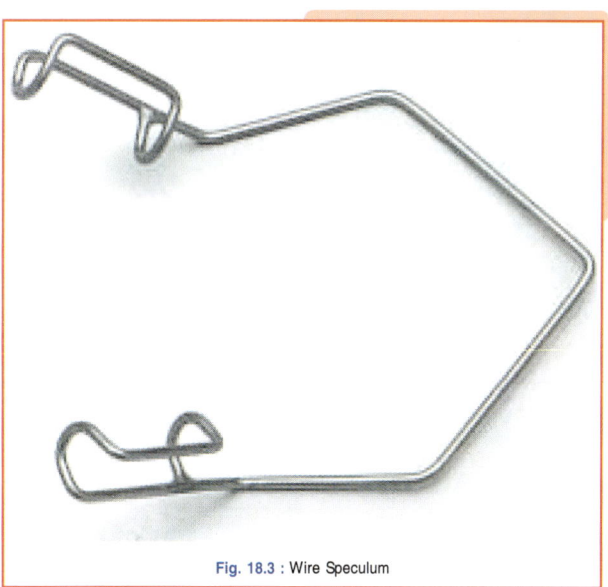

Fig. 18.3 : Wire Speculum

Uses of eye Speculums :

To keep the lids apart during :

i) Extraocular surgery (pterygium excision, squint surgery).

ii) Intraocular surgery (Cataract, Glaucoma etc.)

iii) Outpatient procedures (corneal foreign body removal, scraping of corneal ulcer).

iv) Enucleation, Evisceration operation.

v) Eye examination in patient with blepharospasm.

II. NEEDLE HOLDERS :

4) Barraquer's spring action needle holder : (Fig. 18.4)

➤ Tip may be straight or curved.

➤ Jaws are finely serrated to hold the fine needles firmly.

Uses :

i) for holding the needles and passing the sutures in surgeries on conjunctiva, cornea, sclera and extraocular muscles.

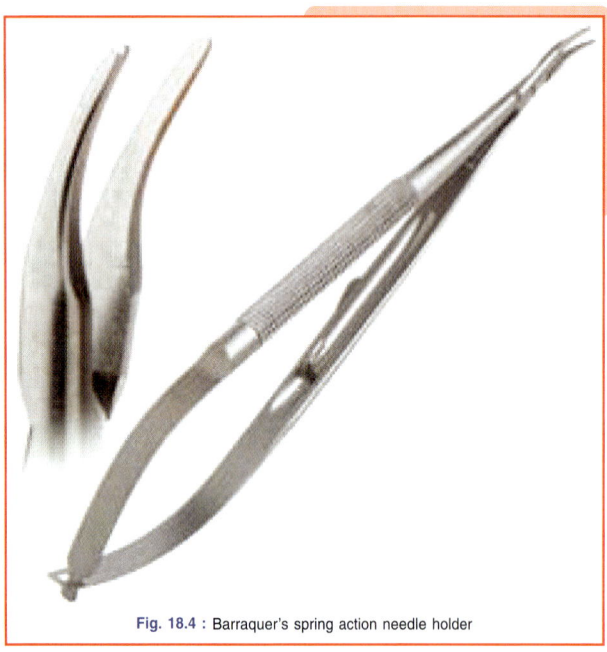

Fig. 18.4 : Barraquer's spring action needle holder

5) Arruga's, Steven, Silcock's and Kelt needle holder : (Fig. 18.5)

➤ Large needle holders.

➤ Upper part has a flat and broad plate to accommodate surgeon's thumb.

Uses :

i) for passing superior rectus suture.

ii) very commonly for lid surgery.

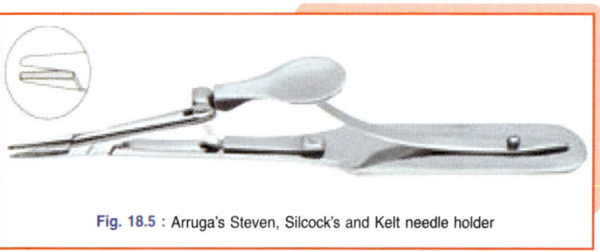

Fig. 18.5 : Arruga's Steven, Silcock's and Kelt needle holder

6) Castroviejo's needle holder : (Fig. 18.6)

➤ medium sized, has S-shaped locking system.

Uses :

i) commonly for extraocular surgery (passing conjunctival sutures, squint surgery).

ii) can be used for intraocular surgery also.

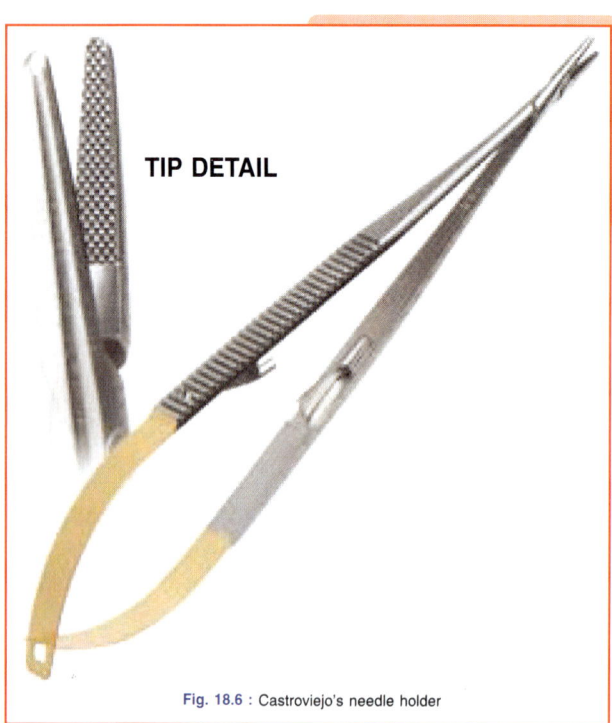

TIP DETAIL

Fig. 18.6 : Castroviejo's needle holder

III. FORCEPS :

7) Plain forceps : (Fig. 18.7)

➤ Serrations are present near the tip.

➤ Absence of teeth.

Uses :

i) To hold skin during eyelid surgery.

ii) To hold nasal mucosal flaps and lacrimal sac flaps in DCR.

iii) To hold conjunctiva in various surgeries.

iv) To hold scleral flap in Trabeculectomy.

v) To tie the sutures.

vi) To hold small sponge swabs.

8) Globe (eyeball) fixation forceps : (Fig. 18.8)

➤ Medium size.

➤ Presence of teeth (2:3 or 3:4).

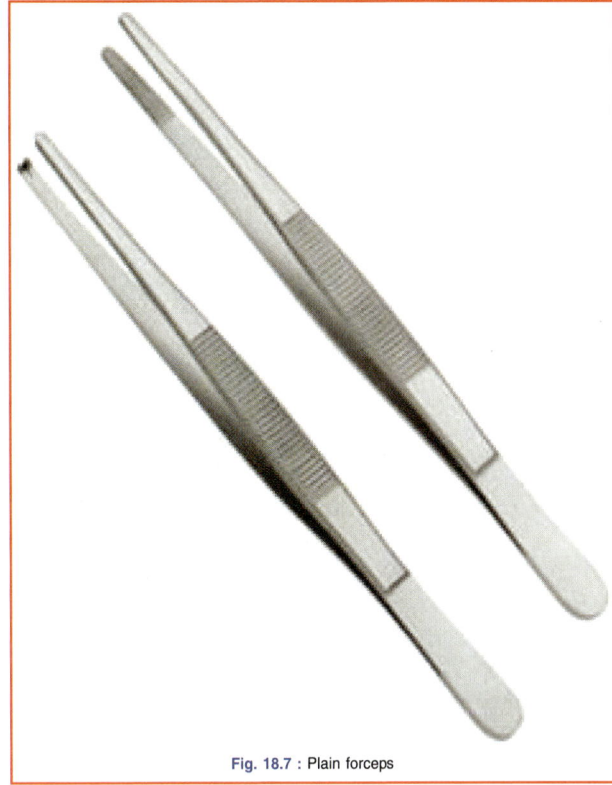

Fig. 18.7 : Plain forceps

Uses :

i) To fix the eyeball during surgeries on eyeball.

ii) In FDT (forced duction test) in case of squint to know if mechanical restriction is present or not.

iii) To catch superior rectus muscle to pass bridle suture under it.

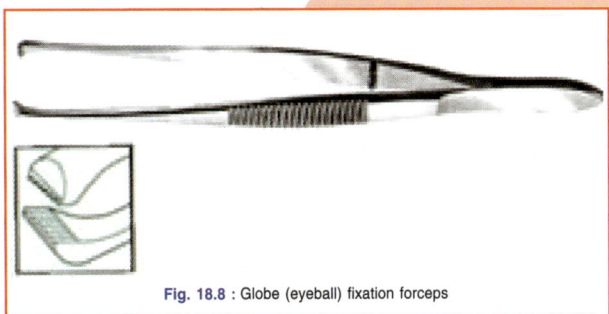

Fig. 18.8 : Globe (eyeball) fixation forceps

9) Superior Rectus holding forceps : (Fig. 18.9)

➢ has S-shaped double curve near the tip.

➢ Presence of teeth (1:2).

Uses :

i) To catch superior rectus muscle to pass bridle suture under it.

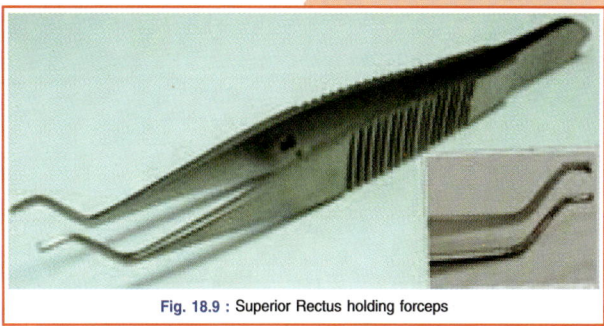

Fig. 18.9 : Superior Rectus holding forceps

ii) To make eyeball stable during surgeries like cataract, Glaucoma etc.

10) Colibri Corneoscleral forceps : (Fig. 18.10)

➢ C-shaped curve near the tip.

➢ Presence of very fine teeth (1:2).

Uses :

i) To hold cornea or sclera for suturing during surgeries such as Cataract, Glaucoma, Keratoplasty, repair of corneal and scleral tears.

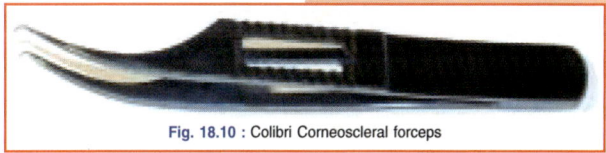

Fig. 18.10 : Colibri Corneoscleral forceps

11) Lim's Corneoscleral forceps : (Fig. 18.11)

i) has a tying platform at the tip.

Uses :

i) Same as Colibri Corneoscleral forceps.

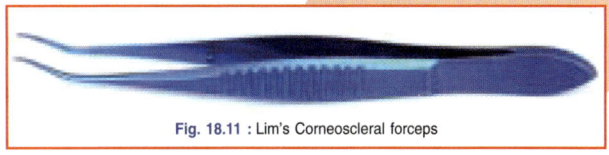

Fig. 18.11 : Lim's Corneoscleral forceps

12) Kelman-McPherson forceps : (Fig. 18.12)

➢ Has bent limbs.

Uses :

i) To hold superior haptic of IOL during IOL insertion.

ii) To tear off anterior capsular flap in ECCE.

iii) Can also be used for tying the sutures.

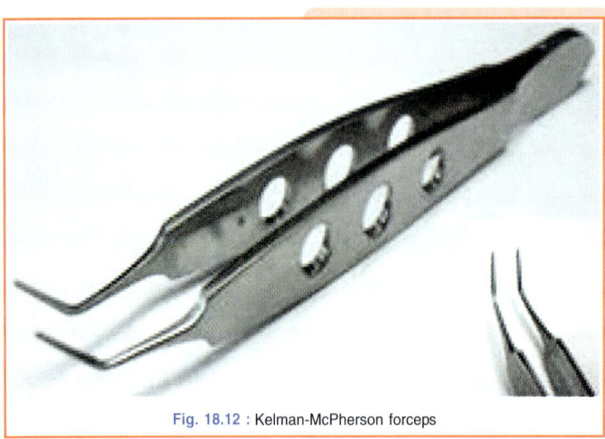

Fig. 18.12 : Kelman-McPherson forceps

13) Iris forceps : (Fig. 18.13)

Uses :

i) To hold the iris for doing iridectomy during trabeculectomy.

ii) Excision for iris prolapse, tumours, entangled foreign bodies.

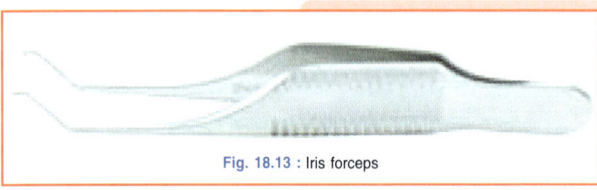

Fig. 18.13 : Iris forceps

14) Artery (Haemostatic) forceps : (Fig. 18.14)

➢ Scissor like appearance.

➢ Presence of multiple straight grooves near the tip.

➢ Locking mechanism near ringed end.

➢ Size may be large, medium, small.

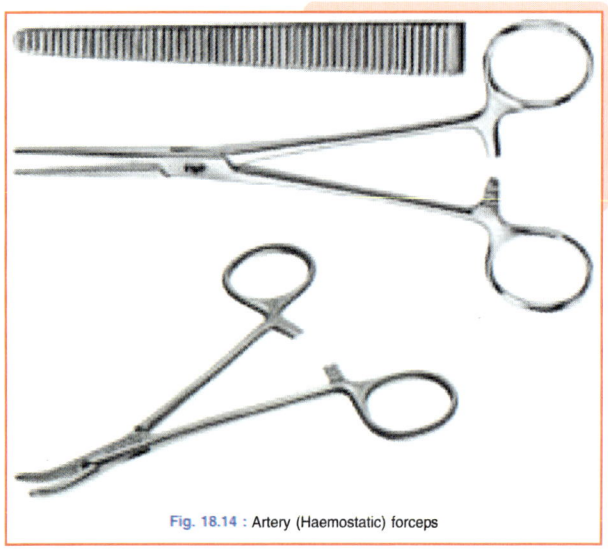

Fig. 18.14 : Artery (Haemostatic) forceps

➢ Small one is called mosquito artery forceps (more commonly used in Ophthalmology).

Uses :

i) To catch the bleeding vessels to prevent bleeding during lid surgeries and lacrimal sac surgeries.

ii) To hold the skin and muscle sutures.

iii) To hold gauze pieces while packing the socket after enucleation or exenteration operation.

15) Epilation (Cilia) forceps : (Fig. 18.15)

➢ Small in size, blunt and flat ends.

Uses :

i) To epilate the cilia in trichiasis and stye.

ii) To remove cilia after electrolysis and cryolysis.

iii) To remove cilia lodged in the punctum.

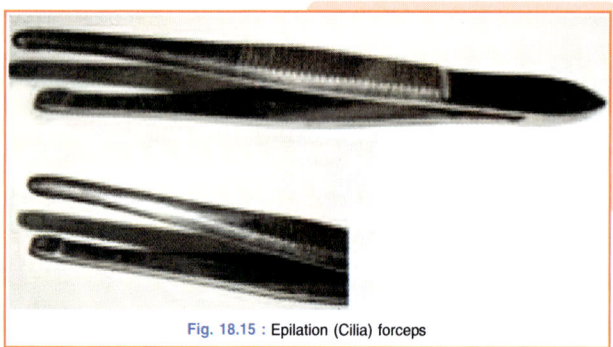

Fig. 18.15 : Epilation (Cilia) forceps

16) Jaffe Tying forceps : (Fig. 18.16)

Uses :

i) for tying the sutures.

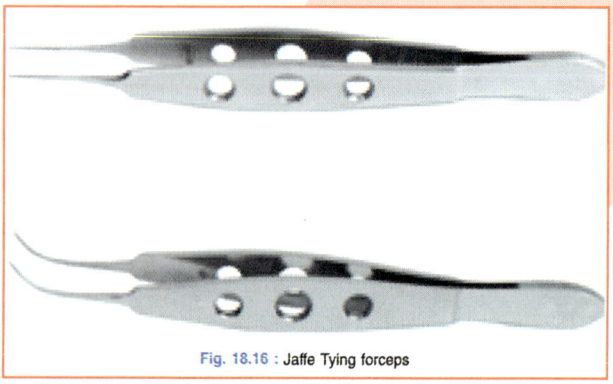

Fig. 18.16 : Jaffe Tying forceps

IV. SCISSORS :

17) Plain straight scissor : (Fig. 18.17)

➤ Has sharp cutting blades.

Uses :

i) To cut conjunctival sutures, eyelashes, muscles.

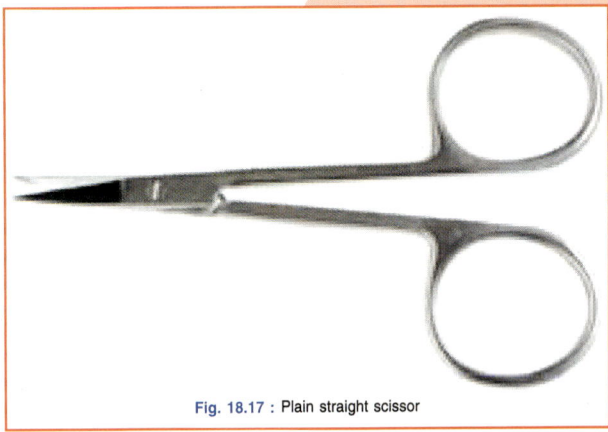

Fig. 18.17 : Plain straight scissor

18) Plain Curved Scissor : (Fig. 18.18)

➤ Has curved, sharp cutting blades.

Uses :

i) To cut and undermine conjunctiva.

ii) To undermine skin during lid and lacrimal sac surgeries.

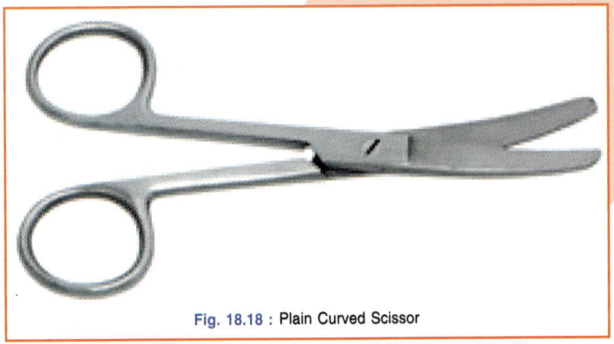

Fig. 18.18 : Plain Curved Scissor

19) Corneal section enlarging scissor : (Fig. 18.19)

➤ Fine, curved scissor having sharp tip.

➤ Blades of the scissors are kept apart by spring action.

Uses :

i) To enlarge corneal or corneoscleral incision for conventional ECCE.

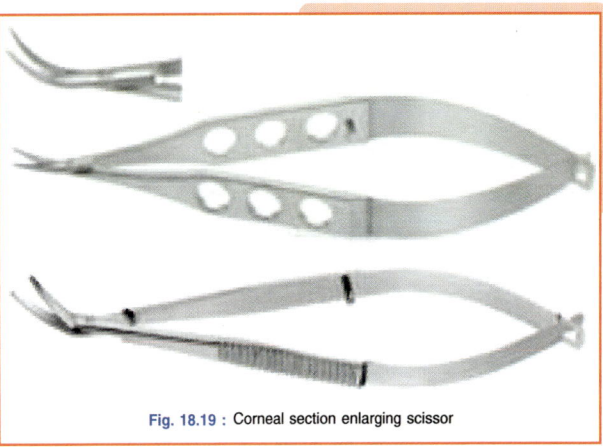

Fig. 18.19 : Corneal section enlarging scissor

ii) To enlarge corneal incision in keratoplasty.

iii) To cut scleral and trabecular tissue in trabeculectomy.

iv) Can also be used to cut undermining conjunctiva in ocular surgeries.

20) Westcott's Conjunctival spring scissor : (Fig. 18.20)

➤ Fine, curved scissor having blunt tip or sharp tip.

➤ May be straight or curved.

➤ Blades are kept apart by spring action.

Uses :

i) As an handy alternative to plain straight and plain curved scissor for cutting and undermining conjunctiva in surgeries like pterygium excision, ECCE, SICS, trabeculectomy, squint surgery.

ii) To cut the sutures.

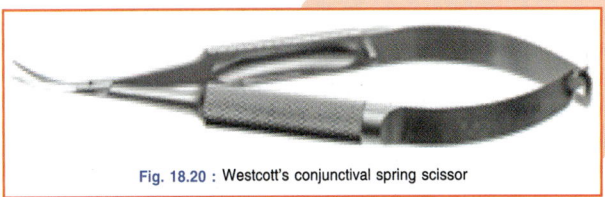

Fig. 18.20 : Westcott's conjunctival spring scissor

21) Vannas scissor : (Fig. 18.21)

➤ Fine, delicate scissor with sharp cutting blades that are kept apart by spring action.

➤ May be straight or curved.

Uses :

To cut :

i) Anterior capsule during ECCE.

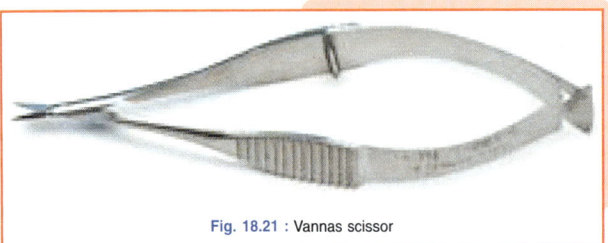

Fig. 18.21 : Vannas scissor

ii)   to cut 10-0 and 9-0 nylon sutures.

iii) to cut sphincter pupillae for sphincterotomy.

iv)   to cut iris for doing Iridectomy.

v)   to cut pupillary membrane.

22) de Wecker's Scissor : (Fig. 18.22)

➢ fine scissor with small blades perpendicular to the arms.

Uses :

i)   To cut iris for iridectomy.

ii) To perform iridotomy.

iii) To cut prolapsed vitreous during vitreous loss in surgeries such as ECCE, ICCE, SICS with vitreous loss.

iv) To cut pupillary membrane.

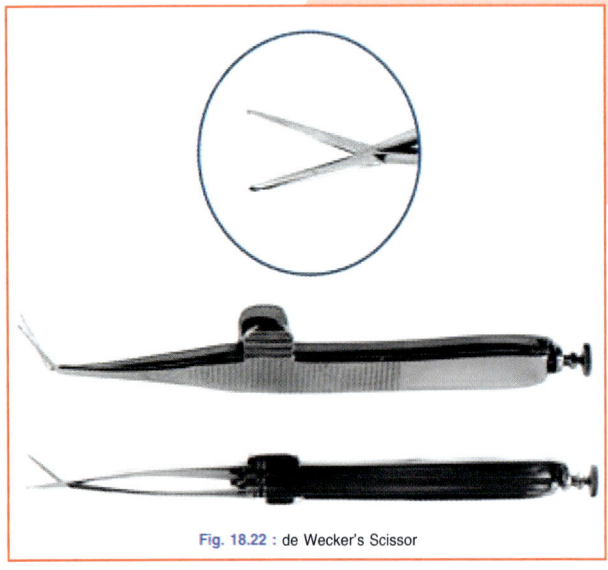

Fig. 18.22 : de Wecker's Scissor

23) Enucleation scissor : (Fig. 18.23)

➢ Long, stout, strong curved scissor with sharp blades and blunt ends.

Use :

i)   To cut optic nerve during enucleation.

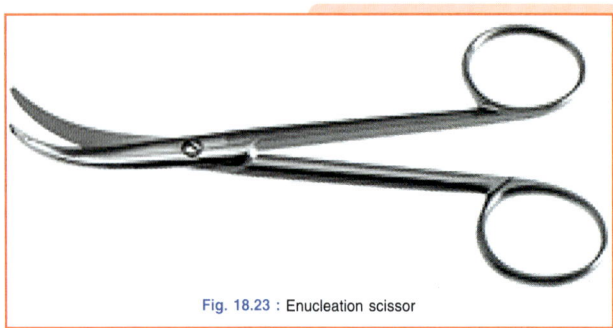

Fig. 18.23 : Enucleation scissor

24) Tenotomy (Strabismus) Scissor : (Fig. 18.24)

➢ Plain, straight or curved scissor with blunt ends.

Uses :

i)   To cut extraocular muscles during squint surgery and enucleation.

ii) To cut delicate tissues without damaging surrounding area in squint surgery and other operations.

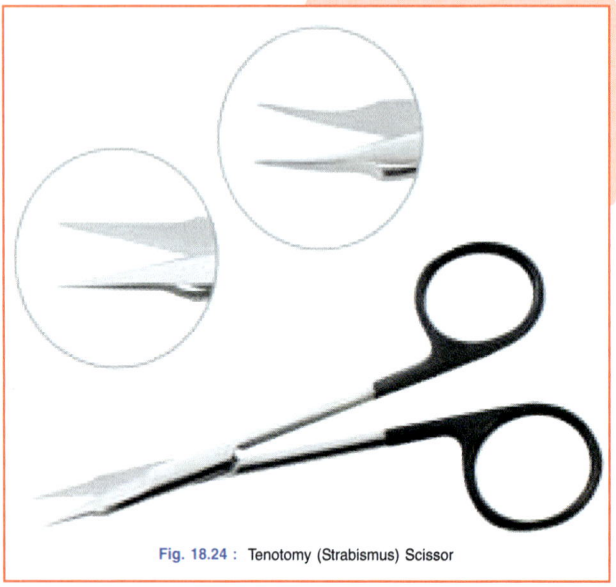

Fig. 18.24 : Tenotomy (Strabismus) Scissor

V. KNIVES (BLADES) :

25) Keratome : (Fig. 18.25)

➢ Has a diamond shaped blade with two cutting edges and a sharp tip.

Uses :

i)   To make valvular corneal incisions for entry into the anterior chamber for Phacoemulsification, SICS, conventional ECCE, Paracentesis, Iridectomy.

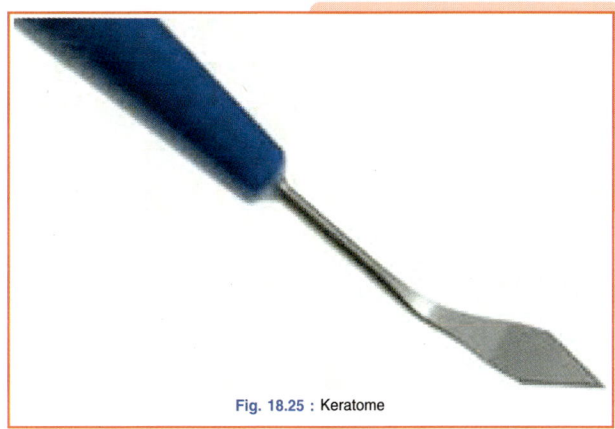

Fig. 18.25 : Keratome

26) 15⁰ Side port entry blade : (Fig. 18.26)

➤ Fine straight knife with pointed tip and single cutting edge.

Uses :

i) To make side port incision (small valvular clear corneal incision) in Phacoemulsification, pars plana vitrectomy.

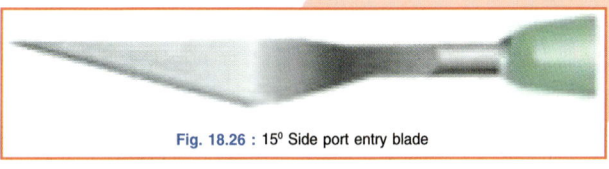

Fig. 18.26 : 15⁰ Side port entry blade

27) Crescent blade : (Fig. 18.27)

➤ also known as Sclerocorneal Splitter.

➤ Has a thin crescentic blade which is sharp at the sides with blunt tip.

Uses :

i) To make tunnel incision in sclera and cornea for phacoemulsification, manual SICS.

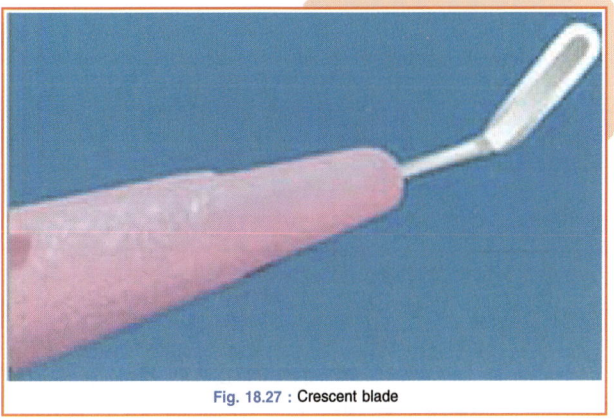

Fig. 18.27 : Crescent blade

ii) Far lamellar dissection of cornea in lamellar keratoplasty.

28) Tooke's knife : (Fig. 18.28)

➤ Flat blade with semicircular blunt dissecting edge.

Uses :

i) To seperate corneal lamellae in lamellar keratoplasty.

ii) To seperate head of pterygium from cornea.

iii) To seperate Tenon's tissue from sclera in surgeries like SICS, ECCE, Trabeculectomy.

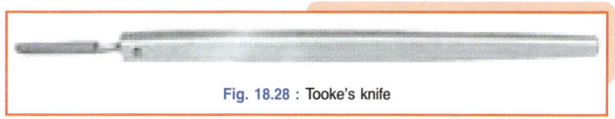

Fig. 18.28 : Tooke's knife

29) Cystitome or Capsulotome : (Fig. 18.29)

➤ Small needle knife with a bent tip, sharp on both the edges.

Uses :

i) For performing capsulorrhexis or anterior capsulotomy during ECCE.

30) Bard-Parker blade holder : (Fig. 18.30)

➤ Flat handle with short grooved neck.

➤ Handle no.3 is used in Ophthalmic surgery.

Uses :

i) Abexterno corneoscleral incision for cataract surgery.

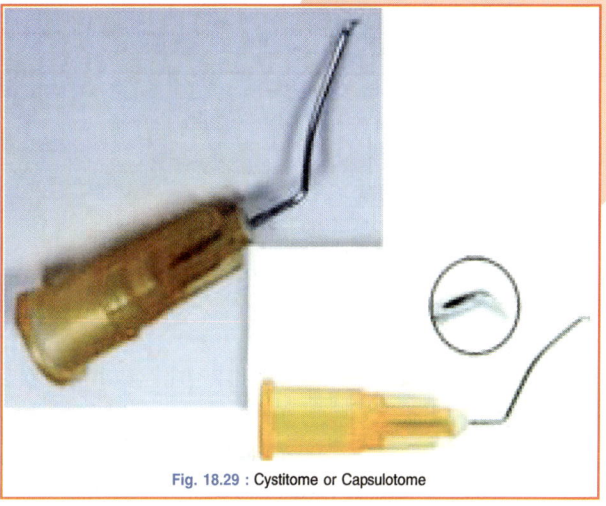

Fig. 18.29 : Cystitome or Capsulotome

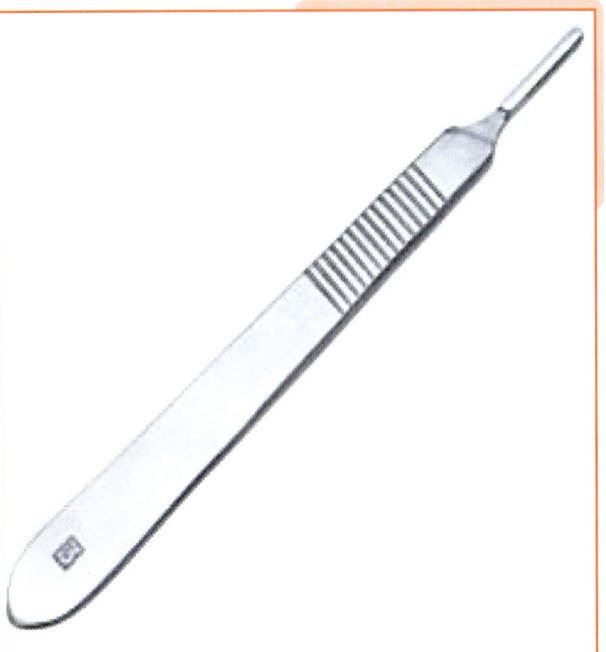

Fig. 18.30 : Bard-Parker blade holder

ii) To make incision in Trabeculectomy.

iii) For incision in DCR, ptosis, lid surgery.

iv) To give incision in Chalazion.

v) To dissect the pterygium head from cornea.

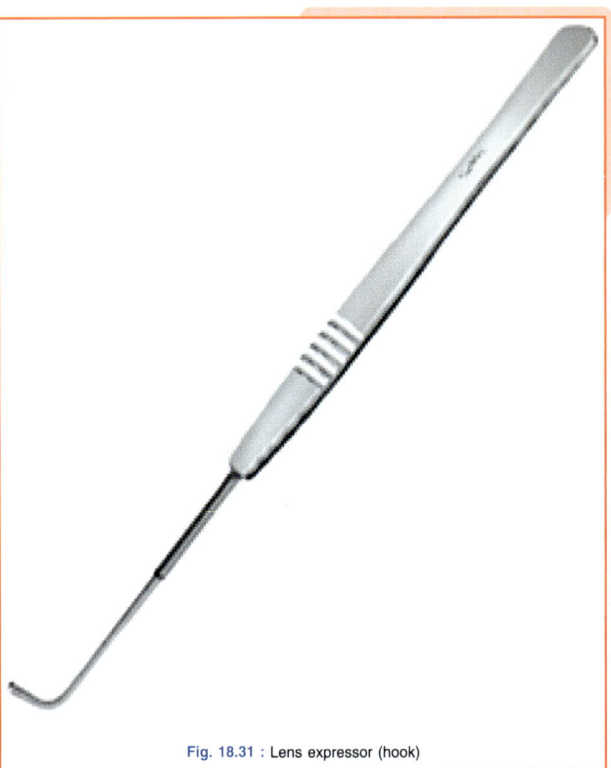

Fig. 18.31 : Lens expressor (hook)

VI. HOOKS AND RETRACTORS :

31) Lens expressor (hook) : (Fig. 18.31)

➢ Has flat metal handle with curved blunt tip.

➢ Plane of the handle is right angle to the curvature of hook.

Uses :

i) To express the nucleus in ECCE.

ii) Can also be used as muscle hook, if muscle hook is not available.

iii) Along with wire vectis to extract out dislocated lens.

iv) As a fine tissue retractor in DCR to retract lacrimal sac during punching or breaking the bone.

32) Muscle (Strabismus) hook : (Fig. 18.32)

➢ Like lens expressor in appearance but has a hook with blunt knob to prevent slippage of muscle.

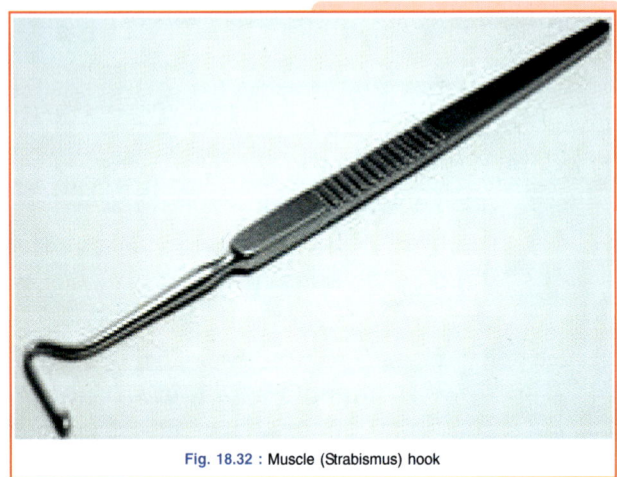

Fig. 18.32 : Muscle (Strabismus) hook

Uses :

i) To hook extraocular muscles during surgery for squint, enucleation, Retinal detachment.

ii) Can be used in place of lens expressor, if lens expressor is absent.

33) Cat's Paw Lacrimal Wound retractor : (Fig. 18.33)

➢ Fork like, resembles cat's paw with tip bent inwards.

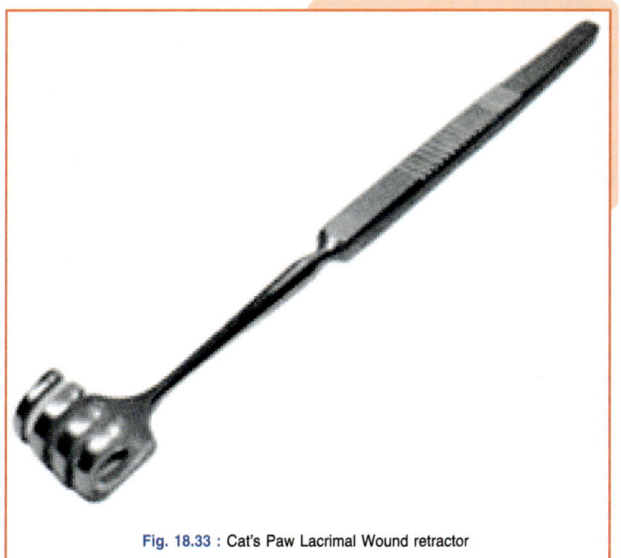

Fig. 18.33 : Cat's Paw Lacrimal Wound retractor

Uses :

i)   To retract skin during lacrimal sac surgery (DCT, DCR) and lid surgery.

34) Desmarre's Lid Retractor : (Fig. 18.34)

➢ Saddle shaped instrument.

➢ Tip has a smooth fold which is folded inwards.

Uses :

i)   To retract lid for eyeball examination in blepharospasm, marked swelling, ecchymosis.

ii) For removal of corneoscleral suture, corneal foreign body.

iii) For double eversion of upper lid to examine superior fornix.

iv) Can be used as a tissue retractor.

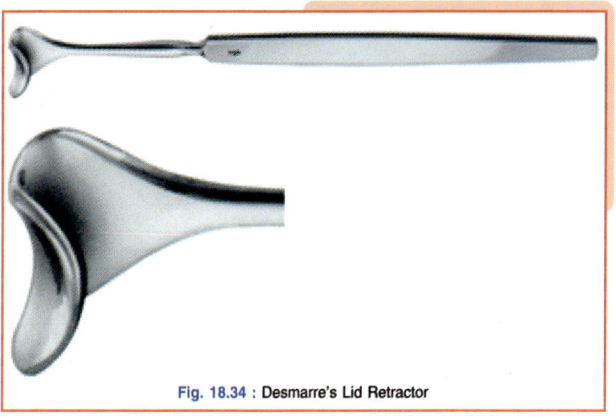

Fig. 18.34 : Desmarre's Lid Retractor

35) Muller's self retaining lacrimal wound Retractor : (Fig. 18.35)

➢ Has two limbs, each limb has 2 or 3 pointed pins (hooks) for engaging incised edges of skin and deeper tissue.

Uses :

i)   To retract incised edges of skin and deeper tissues during DCT, DCR.

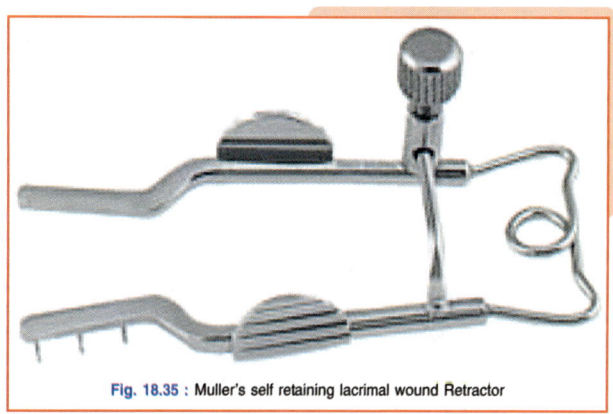

Fig. 18.35 : Muller's self retaining lacrimal wound Retractor

VII. CALLIPER :

36) Castroviejo Calliper : (Fig. 18.36)

➢ Divider like instrument, has 2 arms.

➢ On one arm graduated scale (in mm) is attached and other arm can be moved by a screw over the scale.

Uses :

i)   Measurement of corneal size.

ii) Measurement during squint surgery to calculate amount of recession, resection.

iii) Measurement to locate pars plana during pars plana surgeries.

iv) Measurement of visible horizontal iris diameter.

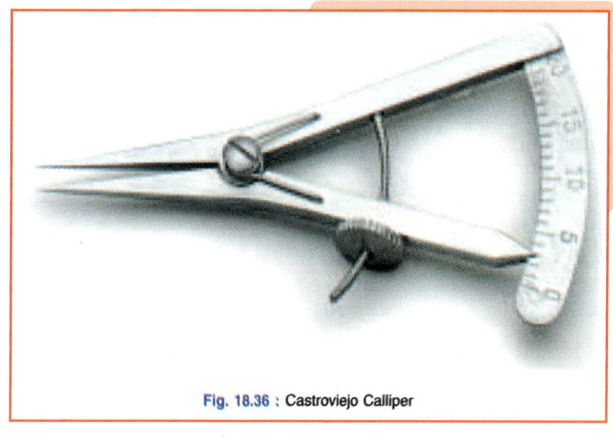

Fig. 18.36 : Castroviejo Calliper

VIII. CLAMPS :

37) Lambert's Chalazion Clamp : (Fig. 18.37)

➢ Has two circular blades one of which is open and has screw which can be tightened.

➢ Solid blade is placed on the skin side, open side is placed on the conjunctival side of chalazion.

Uses :

i) To fix the chalazion and achieve haemostasis during incision and curettage operation.

ii) To fix the chalazion and then to give intralesional injection of steroids.

iii) For excision of a small granuloma or papilloma of the lid.

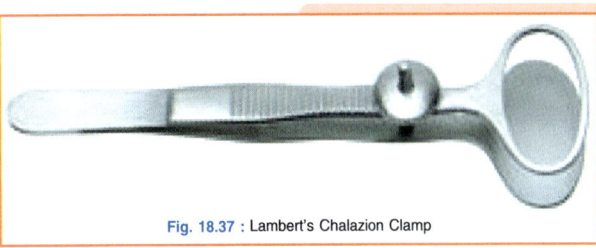

Fig. 18.37 : Lambert's Chalazion Clamp

38) Snellen's Entropion/lid clamp : (Fig. 18.38)

➢ Has D-shaped plate opposed by U-shaped rim when tightened with screw, clamps the tissues.

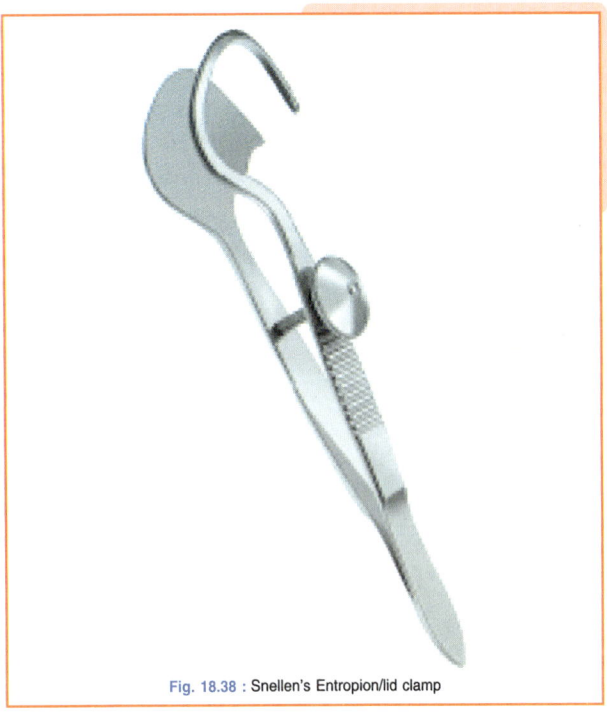

Fig. 18.38 : Snellen's Entropion/lid clamp

➢ D-shaped plate is kept towards conjunctiva, U-shaped rim on skin side, handle towards temporal side.

Uses :

i) In lid surgeries (entropion, ectropion).

ii) Helps in haemostasis during surgery.

39) Berke Ptosis Clamp : (Fig. 18.39)

➢ J-shaped ends, presence of internal serrations.

Uses :

i) To hold LPS (Levator palpebrae superioris) during ptosis surgery.

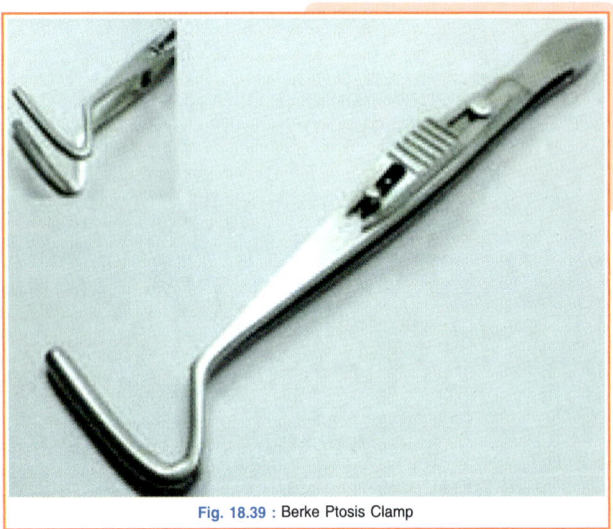

Fig. 18.39 : Berke Ptosis Clamp

IX. INSTRUMENTS FOR CATARACT SURGERY :

40) Wire vectis : (Fig. 18.40)

➢ Has metallic handle to which a wire loop is attached.

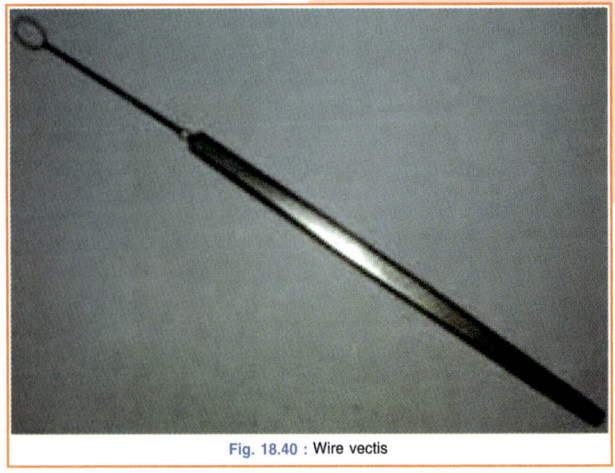

Fig. 18.40 : Wire vectis

Uses :

i) To remove subluxated lens and anteriorly dislocated lens in ICCE.

ii) To remove nucleus in ECCE.

iii) To remove nucleus from anterior chamber by Phacosandwich method in SICS.

41) Simcoe's two way irrigation and aspiration cannula : (Fig. 18.41)

➤ Open end is for irrigation and other for aspiration.

Uses :

i) Far irrigation and aspiration of lens matter in ECCE.

ii) For aspiration of Hyphaema.

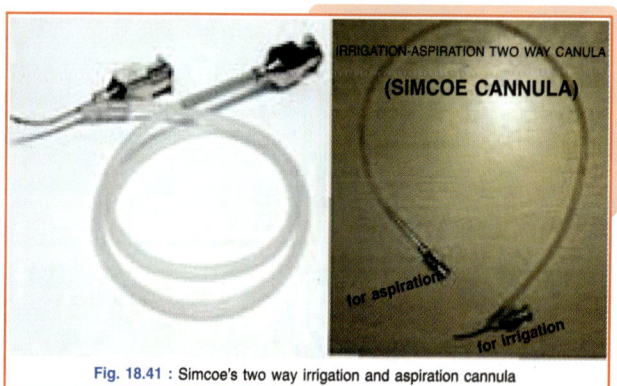

Fig. 18.41 : Simcoe's two way irrigation and aspiration cannula

42) Iris Repositor : (Fig. 18.42)

➤ Has delicate, flat, malleable, straight or bent blade with blunt edges and tip attached to a handle.

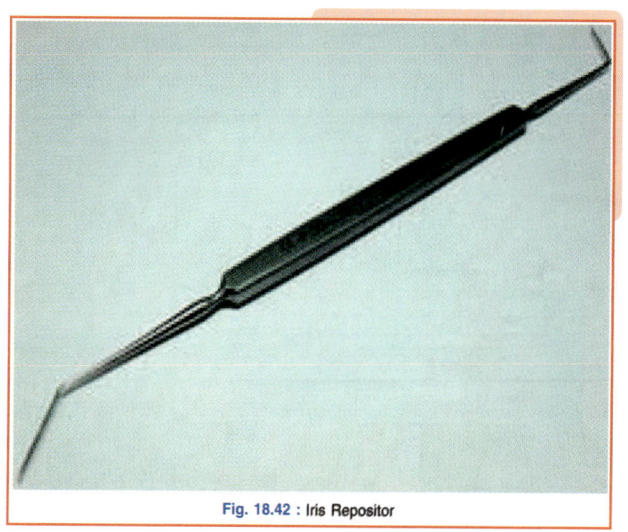

Fig. 18.42 : Iris Repositor

Uses :

i) To reposit the iris in anterior chamber in any surgery.

ii) To break synechiae at pupillary margin.

43) Sinskey hook or IOL dialer : (Fig. 18.43)

➤ Fine, strong instrument with bent tip.

Uses :

i) To dial the PMMA non foldable IOL for proper positioning in capsular bag or ciliary sulcus.

ii) As a left hand instrument during Phacoemulsification to rotate the lens, to chop the nucleus.

iii) To break posterior synechiae during ECCE.

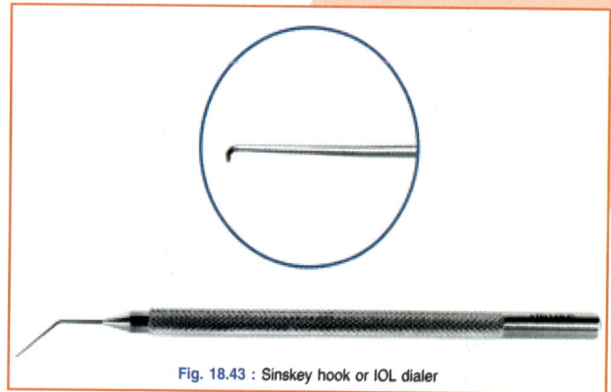

Fig. 18.43 : Sinskey hook or IOL dialer

44) Hydrodissection cannula : (Fig. 18.44)

➤ Single bore cannula with 45⁰ angulation from free end.

Uses :

i) For hydrodissection and hydrodelineation in Phacoemulsification and manual SICS.

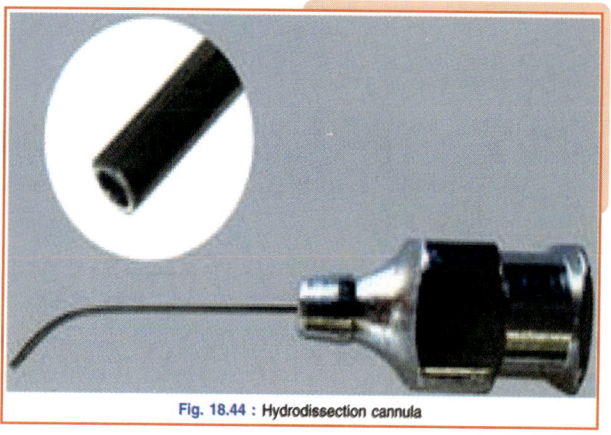

Fig. 18.44 : Hydrodissection cannula

45) Irrigation vectis : (Fig. 18.45)

➢ Has a wire loop at its end with irrigating ports.

➢ Anterior end of loop has three 0.3 mm openings, posterior end of loop is continuous with hollow handle.

Uses :

i) To push the nucleus out of the anterior chamber in SICS.

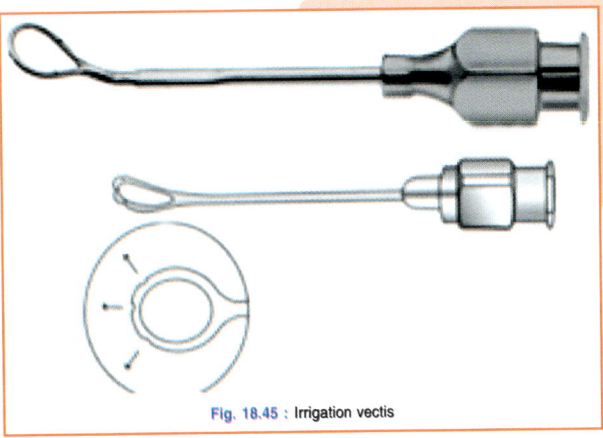

Fig. 18.45 : Irrigation vectis

46) McNamara's Lens Spatula : (Fig. 18.46)

➢ Straight long instrument with two flat spoons or spatula at the two ends.

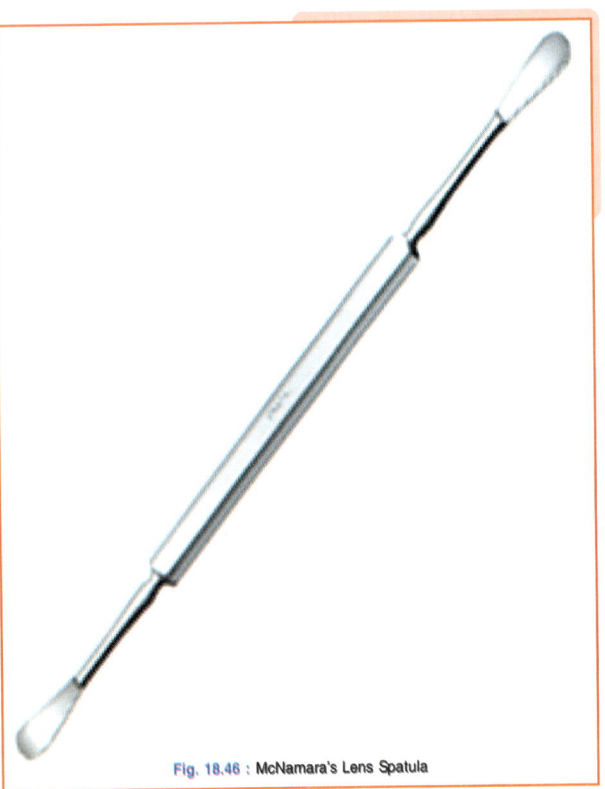

Fig. 18.46 : McNamara's Lens Spatula

Uses :

i) To apply counter pressure (smith Indian technique) at 12 O'clock position.

47) Chopper : (Fig. 18.47)

➢ Resembles Sinskey hook in shape.

➢ Has a bent tip of which inner edge is cutting.

Uses :

i) To chop the nucleus into smaller pieces.

ii) For manipulation of nucleus in Phacoemulsification.

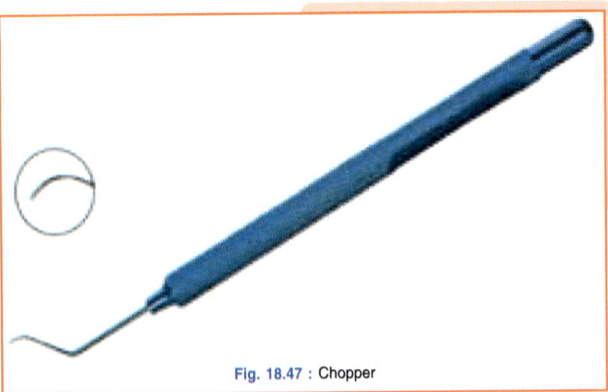

Fig. 18.47 : Chopper

X. INSTRUMENTS FOR LACRIMAL SAC SURGERY (DCT AND DCR) :

48) Nettleship's Punctum Dilator : (Fig. 18.48)

➢ Long narrow cylindrical instrument with conical pointed tip.

➢ Has corrugated metal handle for better gripping with thumb and index finger.

Uses :

i) For dilating the punctum and canaliculus during syringing, probing in congenital dacryocystitis, dacryocystography (DCG), DCT, DCR.

49) Bowman's Lacrimal Probe : (Fig. 18.49)

➢ Metal wire with blunt rounded ends.

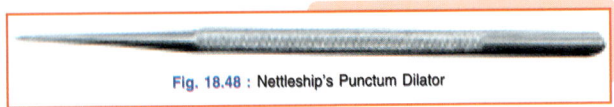

Fig. 18.48 : Nettleship's Punctum Dilator

Uses :

i) To probe nasolacrimal duct in congenital dacryocystitis.

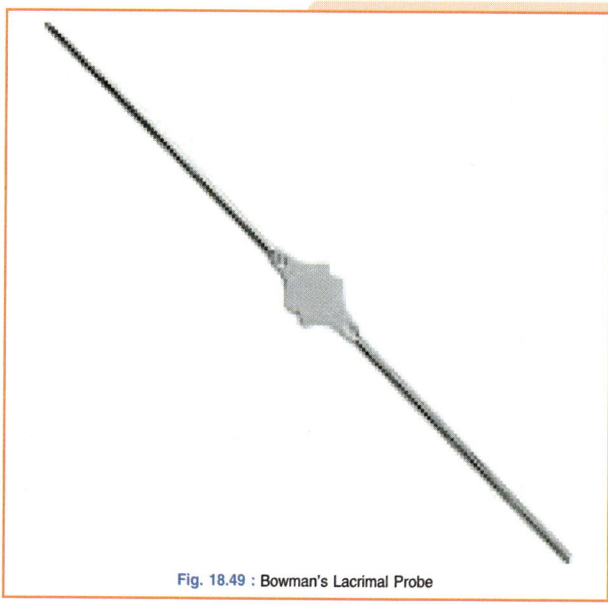

Fig. 18.49 : Bowman's Lacrimal Probe

ii) To identify lacrimal sac in surgeries such as DCT and DCR.

50) Citelli's Bone punch : (Fig. 18.50)

- ➤ Large instrument which has a spring handle and two long blades.
- ➤ Upper blade has a hole with sharp cutting edge.
- ➤ Lower blade has a cup like depression with sharp edge.

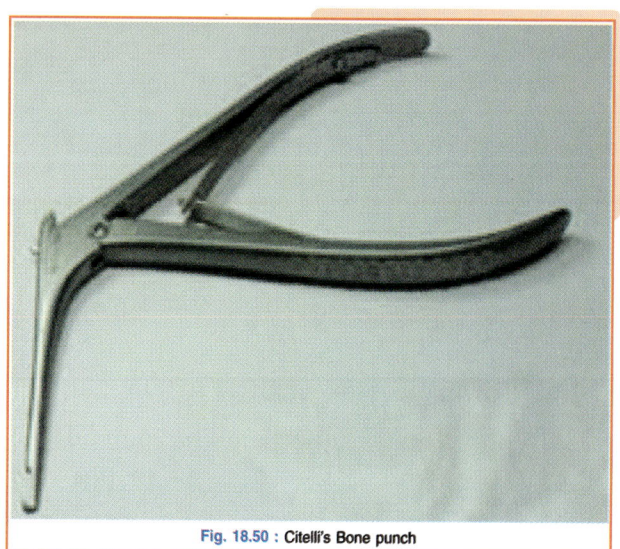

Fig. 18.50 : Citelli's Bone punch

Uses :

i) To punch or break the bones (lacrimal bone, adjacent nasal bone, frontal process of maxilla) in DCR to create a bone ostium between lacrimal sac and middle meatus.

51) Lacrimal cannula : (Fig. 18.51)

- ➤ Long curved hypodermic needle with blunt tip.

Uses :

i) For lacrimal syringing.

ii) As an anterior chamber cannula for putting air, tryphan blue dye, balanced salt solution in the anterior chamber during intraocular surgery.

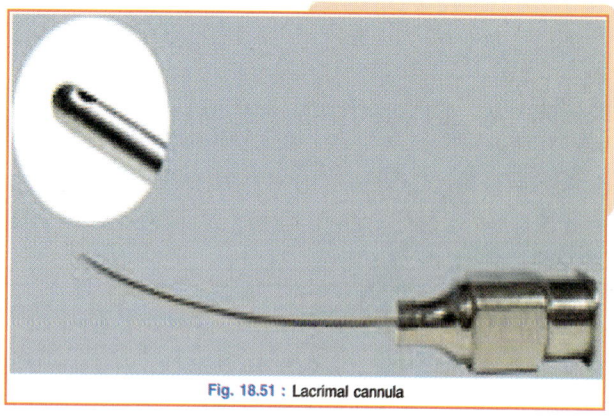

Fig. 18.51 : Lacrimal cannula

52) Chisel : (Fig. 18.52)

- ➤ Has a blade with straight sharp cutting edge with one surface bevelled.
- ➤ Has a long and stout handle.

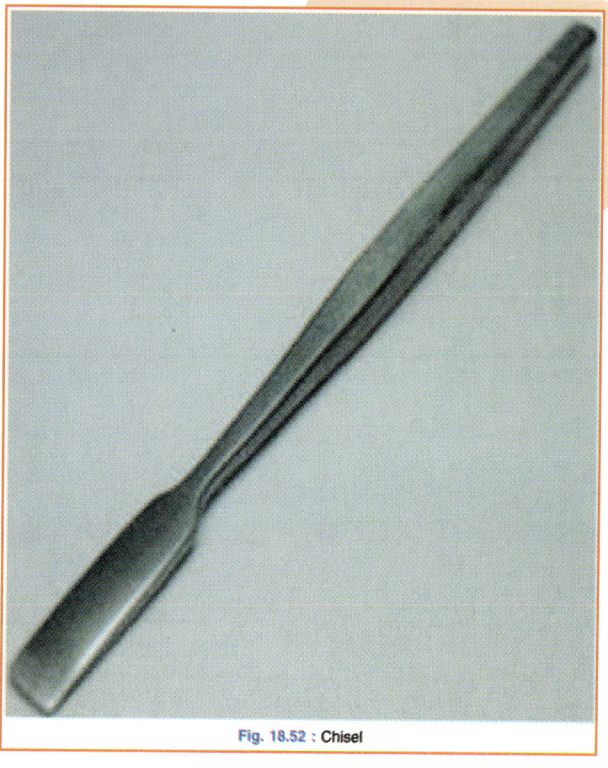

Fig. 18.52 : Chisel

Uses :

i)   To cut the bone during DCR, orbitotomy.

53) Hammer : (Fig. 18.53)

➢   Small steel hammer with a corrugated handle.

Uses :

i)   To hammer the chisel during DCR, orbitotomy.

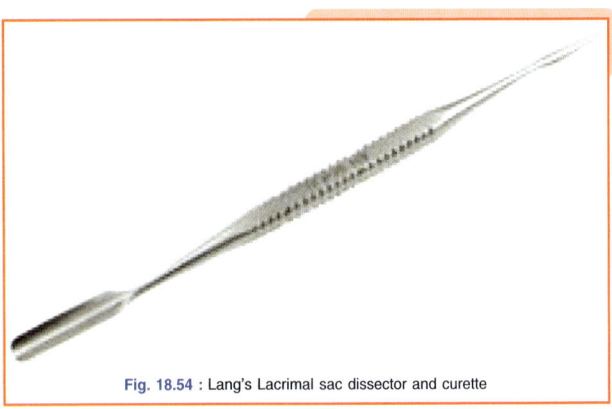

Fig. 18.54 : Lang's Lacrimal sac dissector and curette

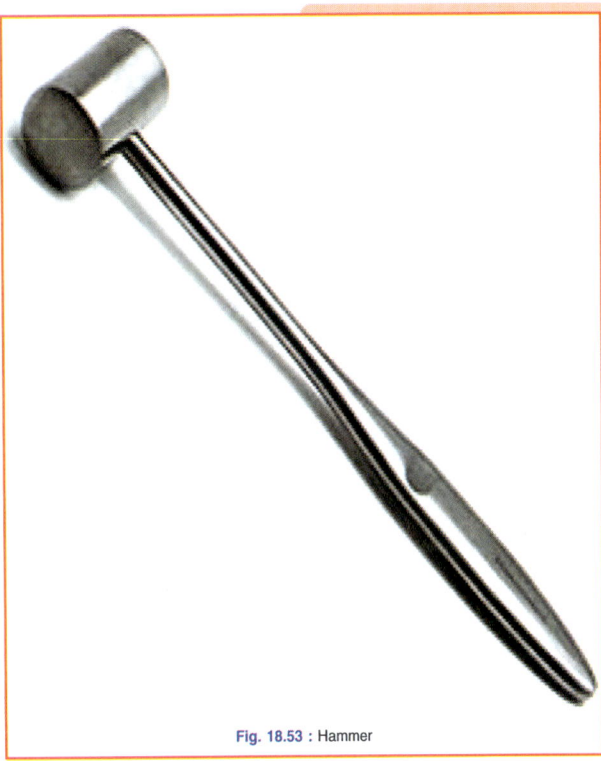

Fig. 18.53 : Hammer

54) Lang's Lacrimal sac dissector and curette : (Fig. 18.54)

➢   Blunt tipped instrument which is cylindrical.

➢   On one end there is blunt tip dissector and other end is curetted.

Uses :

i)   To dissect and separate the lacrimal sac from surrounding structures in DCT and DCR.

55) Bone gouge : (Fig. 18.55)

➢   Has a stout metal handle, one end of which is longitudinally scooped.

➢   Scoop has sharp edges.

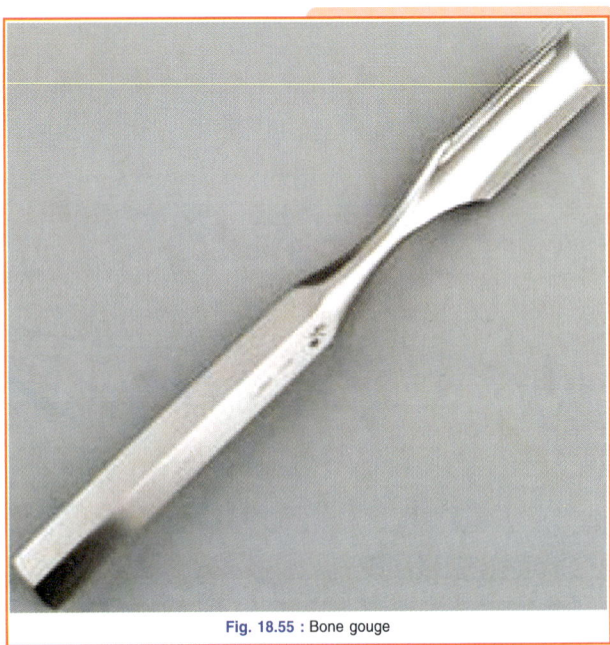

Fig. 18.55 : Bone gouge

Uses :

i)   To smoothen the irregularly cut margins of the bone by nibbling the small projecting bone.

ii) In DCR, Orbitotomy.

XI. INSTRUMENTS FOR ENUCLEATION :

56) Optic Nerve Guide (Enucleation spoon) : (Fig. 18.56)

➢   Has a spoon like end with a central cleavage.

Uses :

i)   Far enucleation to cut the optic nerve. Cleavage is used to engage the optic nerve and the surrounding spoon protects the globe.

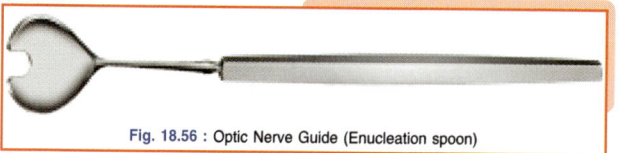

Fig. 18.56 : Optic Nerve Guide (Enucleation spoon)

XII. INSTRUMENTS FOR EVISCERATION :

57) Evisceration spatula : (Fig. 18.57)

➤ Has a small stout rectangular blade with convex surface.

➤ Blunt edge is attached to the handle.

Uses :

i) To separate uveal tissue from sclera in evisceration.

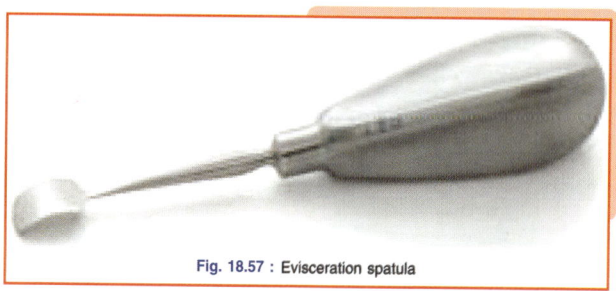

Fig. 18.57 : Evisceration spatula

58) Evisceration Curette : (Fig. 18.58)

➤ Has a rounded cup tip (bigger than chalazion curette) with blunt margins attached to a stout handle.

Uses :

i) To curette out intraocular contents during evisceration.

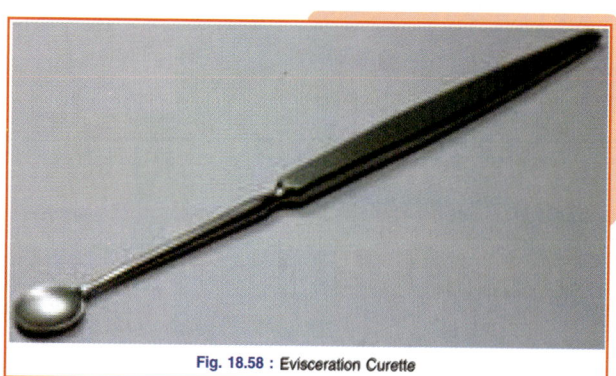

Fig. 18.58 : Evisceration Curette

XIII. INSTRUMENTS FOR LID SURGERY :

59) Lid Spatula : (Fig. 18.59)

➤ Flat solid instrument about 10 cm long.

➤ Both ends are round and convex.

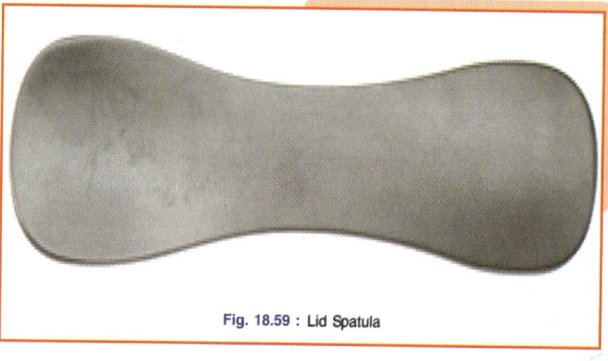

Fig. 18.59 : Lid Spatula

Uses :

i) To protect the globe and support the lid during ptosis, entropion, ectropion, other lid surgeries.

60) Meyerhoefer's Chalazion Scoop : (Fig. 18.60)

➤ Small scoop with sharp edge, attached to a handle.

Uses :

i) To scoop out the contents of chalazion during incision and curettage.

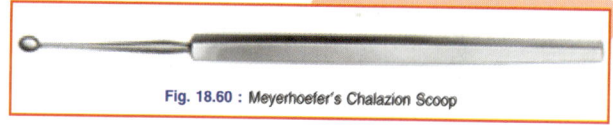

Fig. 18.60 : Meyerhoefer's Chalazion Scoop

XIV. ADDITIONAL INSTRUMENTS :

61) Thermal Ball point Cautery : (Fig. 18.61)

➤ Has a copper ball and a tip with a long handle.

➤ Instrument is heated with the copper ball held in the flame of spirit lamp and the heat which is retained by the copper ball is transmitted to the tip that is used to achieve hemostasis by thermal coagulation.

Uses :

i) To cauterize bleeding vessels in surgeries such as cataract, pterygium excision, trabeculectomy.

ii) To cauterize the margin of a progressive corneal ulcer.

iii) To cauterize small iris prolapse.

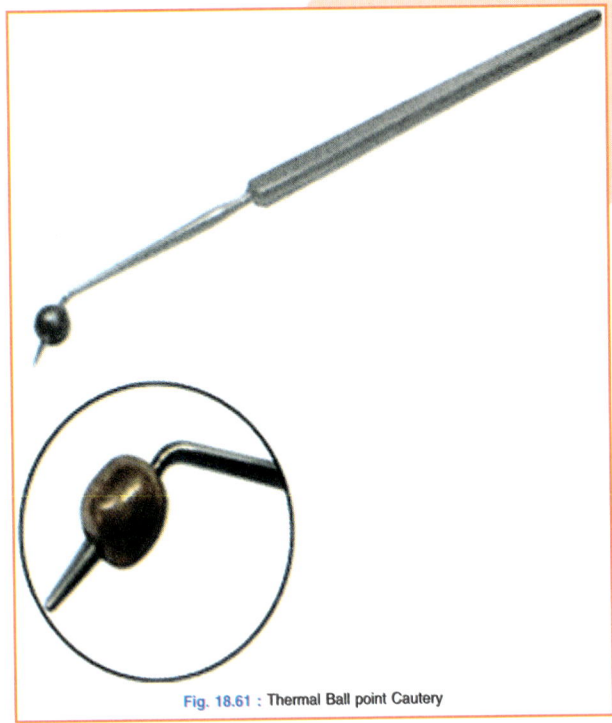

Fig. 18.61 : Thermal Ball point Cautery

Chapter 19

Ophthalmic Lens

BASICS :

A transparent refractive medium with two surfaces, which form a part of a sphere or a cylinder is called lens.

I) TYPES OF LENS :

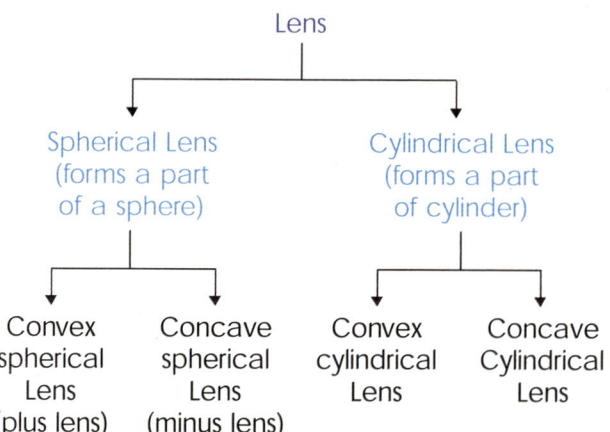

II) IDENTIFICATION OF LENS :

Lens
→ with handle → Spherical Lens
→ without handle → Cylindrical Lens and with a line marked on the frame holding the lens

➤ In cylindrical lenses, handle is absent to facilitate smooth rotatory movement to check the axis of cylinder and line marked on it is to identify the axis of cylinder.

Note : Lens shouldn't be identified by the above method, but should be identified by noticing and seeing what is happening to the object when the object is seen through the lens.

1) Magnification of object → Convex Lens
2) Minification of object → Concave Lens
3) Object moves in both axis → Spherical Lens
4) Object moves in only one axis → Cylindrical Lens
5) Object moves in opposite direction as the lens → Convex Lens
6) Object moves in same direction as the Lens → Concave Lens
7) Image distortion on rotation of lens → Cylindrical Lens

Spherical Lens	Cylindrical Lens
1) Object moves in both the axis	1) Object moves only in one axis
2) No Image distortion on rotating the lens	2) Image distortion on rotating the lens

III. INDIVIDUAL LENSES :

1) Convex Spherical Lens :

Characteristics :

a) Magnification of object when viewed through it.

b) Object moves in opposite direction as the lens.

c) Movement of object in both the axis.

d) No Image distortion on rotation of lens.

e) Lens is thicker in the centre, thin at the periphery.

Uses :

a) Far correcting hypermetropia, presbyopia, aphakia.

b) 20 D lens in Indirect Ophthalmoscopy.

c) + 78 D, + 90 D for slit lamp Biomicroscopy.

d) In loupe and lens examination.

2) Concave Spherical Lens :

Characteristics :

a) Minification of object when viewed through it.

b) Object moves in same direction as the lens.

c) Movement of object in both the axis.

d) No Image distortion on rotation of lens.

e) Lens is thin in the centre, thick at the periphery.

Uses :

a) For correction of Myopia.

b) Hruby lens - 58.6 D for slit lamp Biomicroscopy.

3) Convex cylindrical Lens :

Characteristics :

a) Magnification of object when viewed through it.

b) object moves in opposite direction as the lens.

c) Movement of object in only one axis.

d) Image distortion on rotation of lens.

e) Lens is thicker in the centre and thin at the periphery.

Uses :

a) For correction of hypermetropic Astigmatism.

b) In Jackson cross cylinder for verification of subjective Refraction.

4) Concave Cylindrical Lens :

Characteristics :

a) Minification of object when viewed through it.

b) Object moves in same direction as the lens.

c) Movement of object in only one axis.

d) Image distortion on rotation of lens.

e) Lens is thin in the centre and thick at the periphery.

Uses :

a) For correction of Myopic Astigmatism.

b) In Jackson cross cylinder for verification of subjective refraction.

5) Pinhole : **(Fig. 19.1)**

➤ It is a black disc with a small central hole, attached to a small handle.

➤ Size of pinhole is 1 mm.

Principle :

➤ Pinhole eliminates all the peripheral rays and allows only central parallel beam of rays to enter the eye, and visual improvement is seen in cases of Refractive errors.

➤ If the diminution of vision is not due to refractive error (as in retinal diseases or cataract), visual improvement is not seen.

Uses :

a) To differentiate diminution of vision is due to refractive error or due to organic

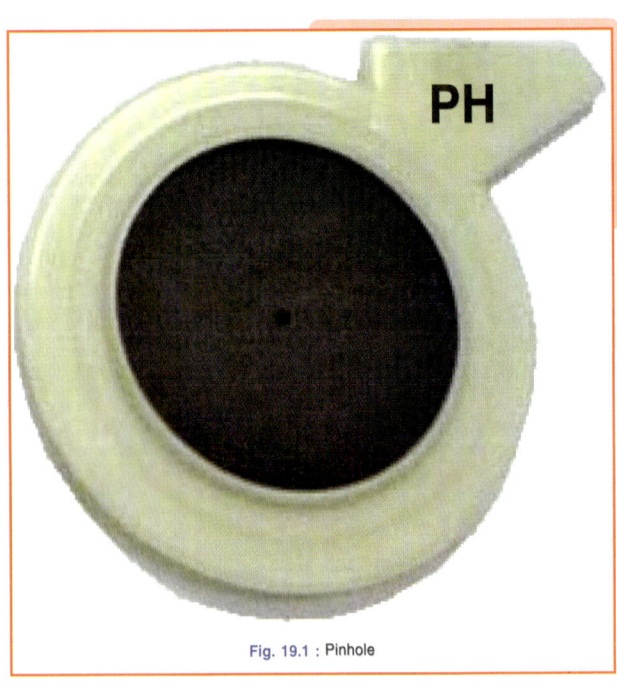

Fig. 19.1 : Pinhole

diseases of media, macular, neurophthalmologic disease.

b) During prescription of glasses in refractive error.

c) During follow up after cataract surgery or keratoplasty, potential visual acuity can be judged.

6) Stenopaeic slit : (Fig. 19.2)

➤ Black disc with a large slit like opening at the center. It has small handle, size of slit is 1 mm.

Principle :

➤ It allows clearest vision when it is rotated into the axis of Astigmatism. If the vision improves with stenopaeic slit when it is rotated, it indicates under correction.

Uses :

a) Detection of the axis for prescribing cylindrical lens for astigmatic correction.

b) Fincham's test to differentiate between halos of glaucoma and cataract.

c) To determine best meridian for optical Iridectomy.

d) As a part of Maddox wing.

7) Maddox Rod : (Fig. 19.3)

➤ Has series of parallel high power, plus cylinders (rods) of red glass placed side by side in a supporting disc.

➤ It converts a point light into a red streak light at right angle to the axis of rods.

Uses :

a) To test Macular function, in presence of opaque media :

Patient looks through Maddox rod at bright light

↓

Patient sees continuous unbroken and undistorted redline.

↓

Macula is normal (If line is broken, there is pathology of macula)

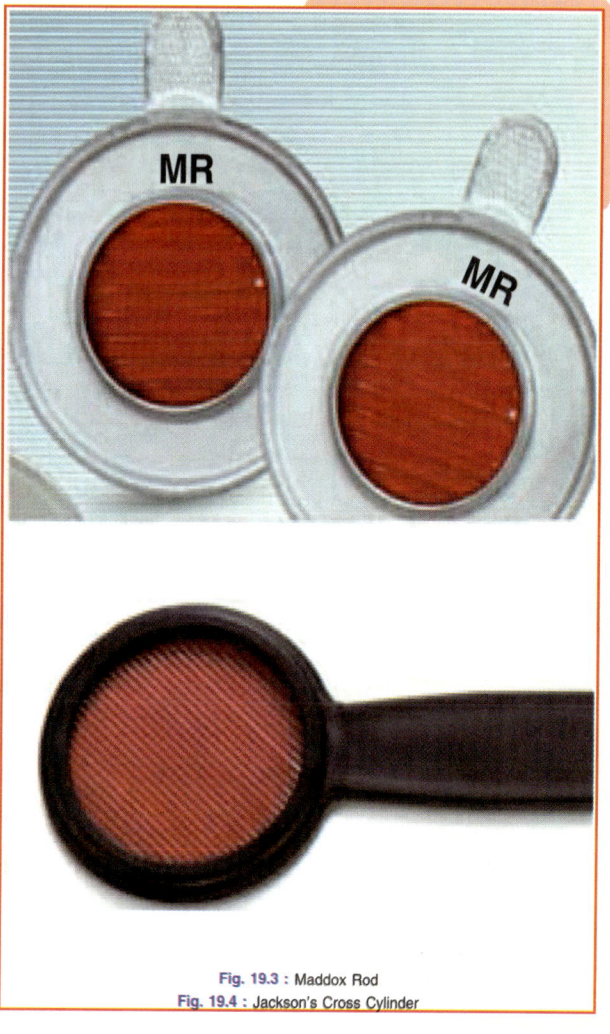

Fig. 19.3 : Maddox Rod
Fig. 19.4 : Jackson's Cross Cylinder

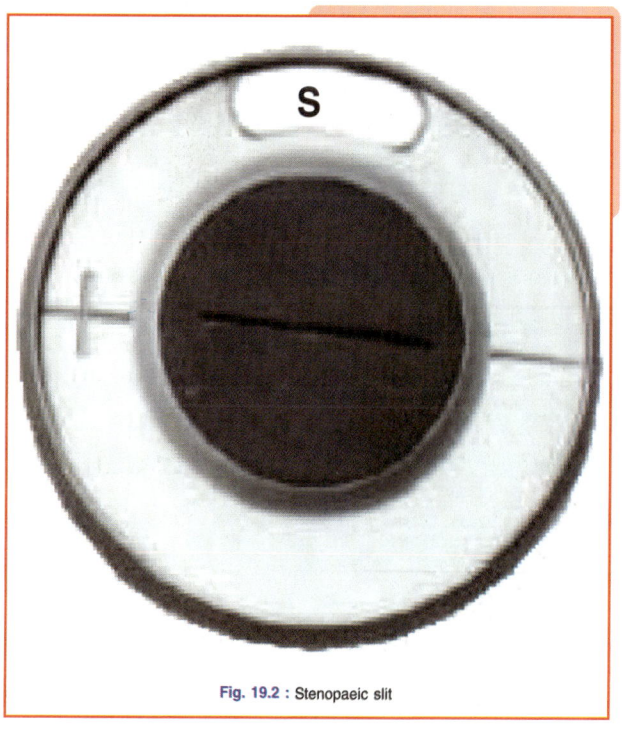

Fig. 19.2 : Stenopaeic slit

b) To test the latent squint for distance :

Maddox rod is held infront of one eye

↓

Image of point source of light becomes dissimilar between the two eyes as fusion is dissociated (Dissimilar image test). Performed at 6 metres and at 33 cm from bright spot light in dark room.

↓

Patient sees red line in one eye and a point source of light in other eye.

c) For orthoptic exercise in Cyclophoria : (Double Maddox Rod test)

↓

Two Maddox Rod placed as one each infront of each eye with the axis horizontally so that patient sees vertical lines.

↓

Patient without cyclophoria sees the lines parallel to each other.

8) Jackson's Cross Cylinder : (Fig. 19.4)

➤ Sphero-cylindrical combination of lens in which spherical component is half the power but of opposite sign of cylindrical component.

➤ Most convenient is combination of a –0.25 D spherical with + 0.5 D cylinder.

Uses :

a) To check the power and axis of the cylinder in refractive correction.

9) Prism : (Fig. 19.5)

➤ Wedge shaped refracting material (glass/plastic), with thin edge at one side and thick edge on opposite side.

➤ Triangular in cross section having an apex and a base.

Uses :

I) *Diagnostic :*

  a) Assessment of squint & Heterophoria.

  b) To detect malingering.

II) *Therapeutic :*

  a) To relieve diplopia.

  b) Convergence insufficiency - synoptophore.

III) *Instrumental use in :*

  a) Goldmann applanation tonometer

  b) Indirect Ophthalmoscope

  c) Slit lamp Biomicroscope

  d) Keratometer

  e) Synoptophore

  f) Koeppe's goniolens

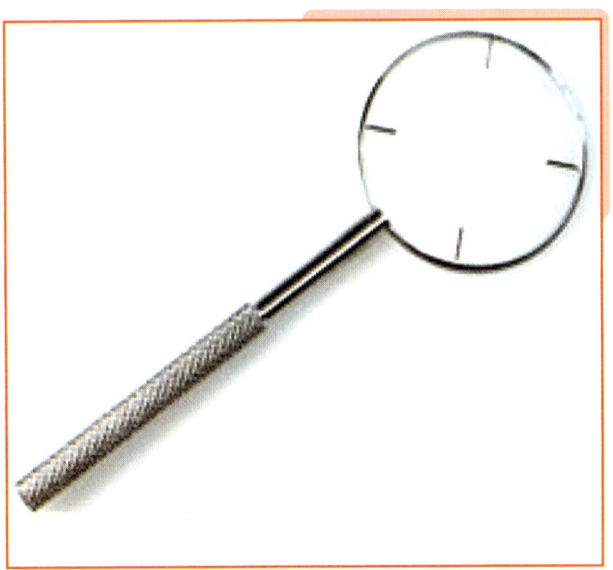

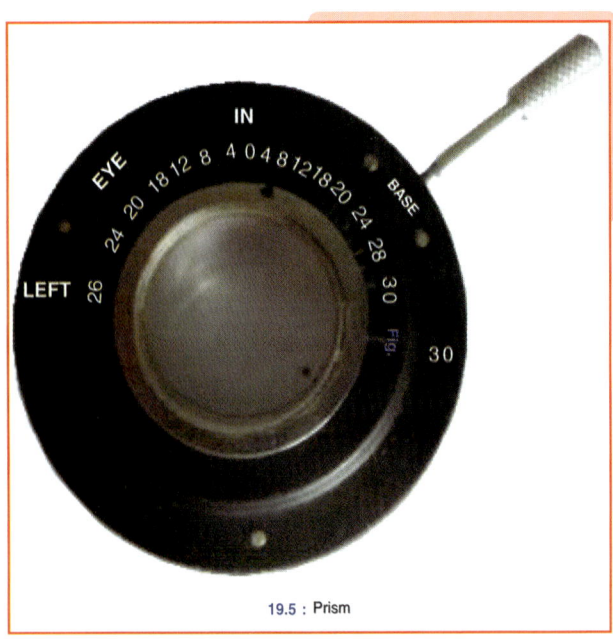

19.5 : Prism

IV) *Miscellaneous :*

    a) Recumbent spectacles

    b) Hemianopic spectacles

    c) Low visual aid (LVA)

10) Placido's Disc : (Fig. 19.6)

> Medium size circular disc with a central hole and is attached to a handle.

> On one surface of the disc there are alternate black and white circle like Bull's eye.

Uses :

a) To assess corneal anterior surface and anterior corneal curvature

    ➤ Loss in sharpness of image denotes corneal abrasion, dry eye.

    ➤ Elliptical image is seen in regular astigmatism.

    ➤ Irregular image is seen in keratoconus.

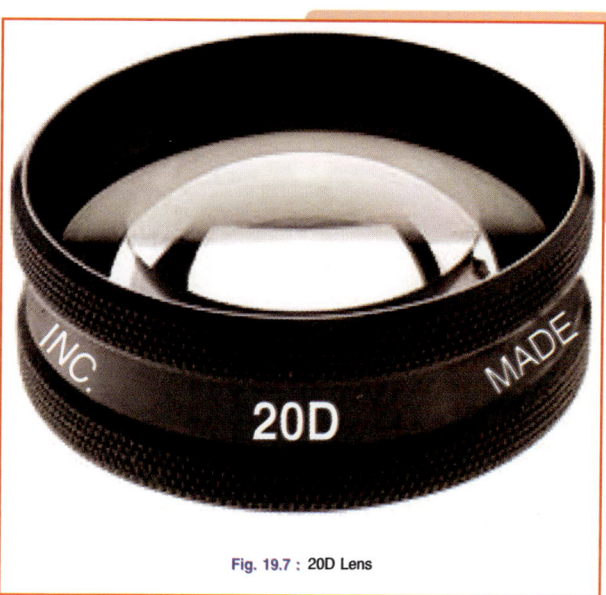

Fig. 19.7 : 20D Lens

12) + 78 D Lens : (Fig. 19.8)

Uses :

a) for slit lamp biomicroscopic examination of retina (other lenses for slit lamp biomicroscopy are + 90 D, – 58.6 D).

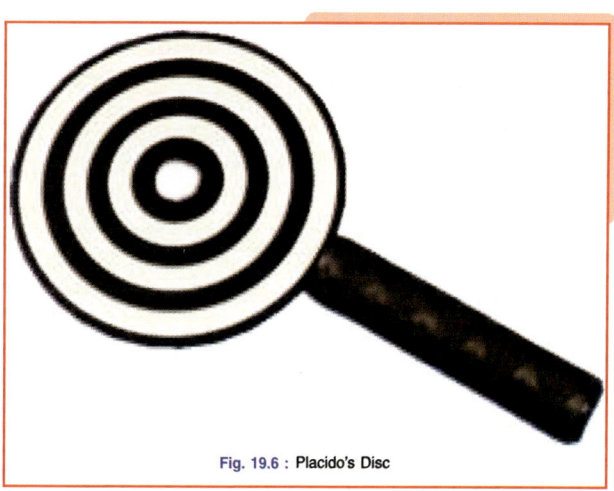

Fig. 19.6 : Placido's Disc

11) 20 D Lens : (Fig. 19.7)

Uses :

a) for Indirect ophthalmoscopy (for fundus examination).

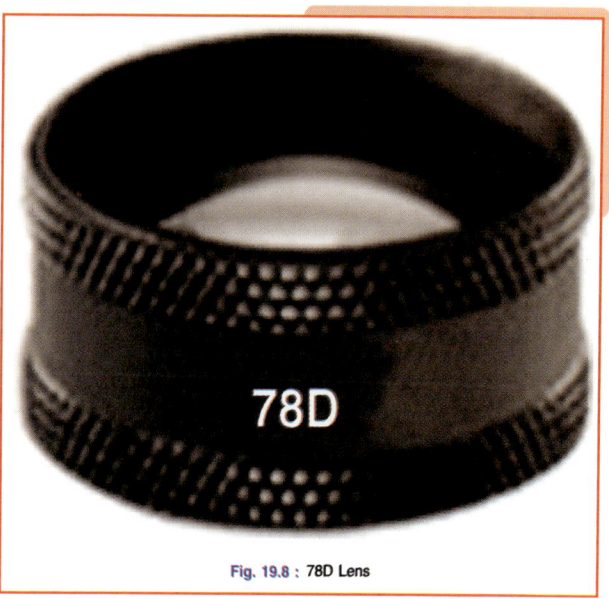

Fig. 19.8 : 78D Lens